Cytopathology

Editor

VICKIE Y. JO

SURGICAL PATHOLOGY CLINICS

www.surgpath.theclinics.com

Consulting Editor
JASON L. HORNICK

September 2018 • Volume 11 • Number 3

ELSEVIER

1600 John F. Kennedy Boulevard • Suite 1800 • Philadelphia, Pennsylvania, 19103-2899

http://www.theclinics.com

SURGICAL PATHOLOGY CLINICS Volume 11, Number 3
September 2018 ISSN 1875-9181, ISBN-13: 978-0-323-61414-6

Editor: Stacy Eastman
Developmental Editor: Donald Mumford

Surgical Pathology Clinics (ISSN 1875-9181) is published quarterly by Elsevier Inc., 360 Park Avenue South, New York, NY 10010. Months of issue are March, June, September, and December. Business and Editorial Office: Elsevier Inc., 1600 John F. Kennedy Blvd., Ste. 1800, Philadelphia, PA 19103-2899. Accounting and Circulation Offices: Elsevier Inc., 3251 Riverport Lane, Maryland Heights, MO 63043. Periodicals postage paid at New York, NY and at additional mailing offices. Subscription prices are $206.00 per year (US individuals), $279.00 per year (US institutions), $100.00 per year (US students/residents), $258.00 per year (Canadian individuals), $318.00 per year (Canadian Institutions), $258.00 per year (foreign individuals), $318.00 per year (foreign institutions), and $120.00 per year (international & Canadian students/residents). Foreign air speed delivery is included in all *Clinics'* subscription prices. All prices are subject to change without notice. **POSTMASTER:** Send address changes to *Surgical Pathology Clinics*, Elsevier, 3251 Riverport Lane, Maryland Heights, MO 63043. **Customer Service: 1-800-654-2452 (US). From outside the United States, call 1-314-447-8871. Fax: 1-314-447-8029. E-mail: JournalsCustomerServiceusa@elsevier.com (for print support) and JournalsOnlineSupport-usa@elsevier.com (for online support).**

Reprints. For copies of 100 or more, of articles in this publication, please contact the Commercial Reprints Department, Elsevier Inc., 360 Park Avenue South, New York, NY 10010-1710. Tel. 212-633-3874; Fax: 212-633-3820; E-mail: reprints@elsevier.com.

Surgical Pathology Clinics of North America is covered in *MEDLINE/PubMed (Index Medicus).*

Contributors

CONSULTING EDITOR

JASON L. HORNICK, MD, PhD
Director of Surgical Pathology and
Immunohistochemistry, Brigham and
Women's Hospital, Professor of Pathology,
Harvard Medical School, Boston,
Massachusetts

EDITOR

VICKIE Y. JO, MD
Assistant Professor of Pathology, Department
of Pathology, Brigham and Women's Hospital,
Harvard Medical School, Boston,
Massachusetts

AUTHORS

JUSTIN A. BISHOP, MD
Director of Surgical Pathology, Clements
University Hospital, Director of Head
and Neck Pathology, Associate Professor
of Pathology, Department of Pathology,
The University of Texas Southwestern
Medical Center, Dallas, Texas

DEBORAH J. CHUTE, MD
Associate Professor of Pathology and Staff
Pathologist, Department of Pathology,
Cleveland Clinic, Cleveland, Ohio

ERIKA E. DOXTADER, MD
Associate Staff, Department of Pathology,
Cleveland Clinic, Cleveland, Ohio

WILLIAM C. FAQUIN, MD, PhD
Director of Head and Neck Pathology,
Massachusetts Eye and Ear Infirmary,
Professor of Pathology, Department of
Pathology, Massachusetts General Hospital,
Harvard Medical School, Boston,
Massachusetts

LUIZ PAULO GUIDO, MD
Research Fellow, Department of
Pathology and Laboratory Medicine, University
of Miami Miller School of Medicine, Miami,
Florida

KRISZTINA Z. HANLEY, MD
Associate Professor, Department of
Pathology and Laboratory Medicine,
Emory University School of Medicine,
Atlanta, Georgia

RAZA S. HODA, MD
Resident, Department of Pathology,
Massachusetts General Hospital,
Harvard Medical School, Boston,
Massachusetts

VICKIE Y. JO, MD
Assistant Professor of Pathology, Department
of Pathology, Brigham and Women's Hospital,
Harvard Medical School, Boston,
Massachusetts

MERCE JORDA, MD, PhD, MBA
Professor and Chair of Pathology, Department of Pathology and Laboratory Medicine, University of Miami Miller School of Medicine, Miami, Florida

JEFFREY F. KRANE, MD, PhD
Chief, Head and Neck Pathology Service, Associate Director, Cytology Division, Associate Professor, Department of Pathology, Brigham and Women's Hospital, Harvard Medical School, Boston, Massachusetts

CHRISTIN M. LEPUS, MD, PhD
Resident, Department of Pathology, Brigham and Women's Hospital, Harvard Medical School, Boston, Massachusetts

ALARICE C. LOWE, MD
Assistant Professor of Pathology, Director of the Circulating Tumor Cell Lab, Department of Pathology, Brigham and Women's Hospital, Harvard Medical School, Boston, Massachusetts

EMILIO MADRIGAL, DO
Fellow, Department of Pathology, Massachusetts General Hospital, Harvard Medical School, Boston, Massachusetts

MICHIYA NISHINO, MD, PhD
Director, Head and Neck Pathology, Assistant Professor, Department of Pathology, Beth Israel Deaconess Medical Center, Harvard Medical School, Boston, Massachusetts

MARTHA B. PITMAN, MD
Professor of Pathology, Director of Cytopathology, Department of Pathology, Massachusetts General Hospital, Harvard Medical School, Boston, Massachusetts

XIAOHUA QIAN, MD, PhD
Director of Fine Needle Aspiration Service, Assistant Professor of Pathology, Department of Pathology, Brigham and Women's Hospital, Harvard Medical School, Boston, Massachusetts

JORDAN P. REYNOLDS, MD
Associate Professor of Pathology, Laboratory Medicine Institute, Cleveland Clinic Foundation, Cleveland Clinic, Cleveland, Ohio

CATHERINE J. ROE, MD
Resident, Department of Pathology and Laboratory Medicine, Emory University School of Medicine, Atlanta, Georgia

SINCHITA ROY-CHOWDHURI, MD, PhD
Associate Professor, Department of Pathology, Division of Pathology and Laboratory Medicine, The University of Texas MD Anderson Cancer Center, Houston, Texas

EDWARD B. STELOW, MD
Professor, Department of Pathology, UVA Hospital, University of Virginia, Charlottesville, Virginia

PAUL A. VANDERLAAN, MD, PhD
Director of Cytopathology, Director of Thoracic Pathology, Assistant Professor of Pathology, Department of Pathology, Beth Israel Deaconess Medical Center, Harvard Medical School, Boston, Massachusetts

JAYLOU VELEZ-TORRES, MD
Professor of Pathology, Department of Pathology and Laboratory Medicine, University of Miami Miller School of Medicine, Miami, Florida

MARINA VIVERO, MD
Associate Pathologist, Instructor of Pathology, Department of Pathology, Brigham and Women's Hospital, Harvard Medical School, Boston, Massachusetts

JUAN XING, MD
Assistant Professor, University of Pittsburgh Medical Center, UPMC Shadyside Hospital, Pittsburgh, Pennsylvania

Contents

Genomic, clinical, and pathologic studies have prompted a more risk-stratified approach to the management of patients with thyroid nodules. The recent nomenclature change concerning noninvasive follicular thyroid neoplasm with papillary-like nuclear features reflects the clinical trend toward conservative treatment choices for carefully selected low-risk thyroid neoplasms. These developments have occurred in parallel with a growing array of molecular tests intended to improve clinical triage for patients with indeterminate fine-needle aspiration diagnoses. This article discusses the implications of the nomenclature revision on the interpretation of thyroid fine-needle aspiration and updates available on ancillary molecular tests for thyroid fine needle aspirations.

Salivary gland fine-needle aspiration biopsies remain common specimens seen by most cytology services. The diagnostic diversity and overlap between many of the lesions seen with these biopsies impart many challenges for the cytopathologist, rendering most specific diagnoses impossible with cytology alone. Here, the use of the Milan System for the classification of salivary gland fine-needle aspiration biopsy is discussed, together with the potential use of ancillary testing in arriving at definitive diagnoses.

Oropharyngeal squamous cell carcinoma caused by transcriptionally active human papillomavirus (HPV) is now well established as a unique form of head and neck cancer. Given the high frequency of metastasis to cervical lymph nodes by HPV-positive oropharyngeal squamous cell carcinomas, fine-needle aspiration (FNA) represents a widely accepted method for the sampling and diagnosis of these cancers. The recently published College of American Pathologists Guideline (2017) provides recommendations for the effective performance and interpretation of high-risk (HR) HPV testing in head and neck squamous cell carcinoma (HNSCC), including testing on FNA samples of metastatic HNSCC to cervical lymph nodes. There is a wide range of options available for HR-HPV testing in cytologic specimens.

Lung cancer diagnosis and ancillary testing are increasingly relying on cytology and small biopsy specimens obtained via minimally invasive means. Paired with traditional immunohistochemical characterization of tumors, biomarker testing and comprehensive genomic profiling are becoming essential steps in the workup of lung cancer to identify targetable alterations and guide optimal therapy selection. Recent advances in immune checkpoint inhibitor therapy have led to an increasingly complex and unresolved landscape for tumor PD-L1 testing. The prevalence and importance of lung cancer cytology specimens are growing, with more required by the cytopathologist in directing the care of patients with lung cancer.

Christin M. Lepus and Marina Vivero

Effusion cytology plays multiple roles in the management of benign and malignant disease, from primary diagnosis to tissue allocation for ancillary diagnostic studies and biomarker testing of therapeutic targets. This article summarizes recent advances in pleural effusion cytology, with a focus on the practical application of immunohistochemical markers, cytogenetic techniques, flow cytometry, and molecular techniques for the diagnosis and management of primary and secondary neoplasms of the pleura.

Erika E. Doxtader and Deborah J. Chute

Carcinoma of unknown primary is defined as metastatic carcinoma without a clinically obvious primary tumor. Determining the tissue of origin in carcinoma of unknown primary is important for site-directed therapy. Immunohistochemistry is the most widely used tool for the workup of metastases, but molecular profiling assays are also available. This article provides an overview of immunohistochemical stains in the workup of metastatic carcinoma, with a focus on newer site-specific markers, and discusses the role of gene expression profiling assays for determining the tissue of origin. The utility of cytopathology specimens in the evaluation of carcinoma of unknown primary also is highlighted.

Raza S. Hoda and Martha B. Pitman

The diagnostic approach to pancreaticobiliary disease requires a multidisciplinary team in which the cytopathologist plays a crucial role. Fine-needle aspiration, obtained by endoscopic ultrasonography, is the diagnostic test of choice for pancreatic lesions. Preoperative clinical management depends on many factors, some of which rely on accurate cytologic assessment. Pancreaticobiliary cytology is wrought with diagnostic pitfalls. Clinical history, imaging studies, cytology samples, and ancillary tests, including immunohistochemistry, biochemical analysis, and genetic sequencing, are integral in forming a complete diagnosis and guiding optimal patient management. This article reviews the clinical aspects and diagnostic workup of common diagnostic entities within the field of pancreaticobiliary cytology.

Catherine J. Roe and Krisztina Z. Hanley

Ninety years ago, at the Battle Creek conference, Papanicolaou introduced cervical exfoliative cytology. Since then, the "Pap test" has come a long way. The discovery of a causal relationship between cervical carcinoma and HPV infection opened the door for molecular testing and immunomarkers for HPV. The Clinical Laboratory Improvement Amendments, 1988, established quality assurance and quality control programs to monitor performance of cytology laboratories. The Bethesda System for reporting cervical cytology laid the foundations for cervical cytology education, implementation of management guidelines, and further research on cervical carcinogenesis. HPV vaccine penetration in both genders remains 62% or less.

The utility of urine cytology has shifted from the identification of red blood cells, crystals, or parasites to its currently used role of detection of cancer cells exfoliated in urine samples. A variety of ancillary tests have been developed to complement the diagnostic ability of urine cytology. Furthermore, urine testing will continue to evolve as the pathogenesis of genitourinary tract diseases in depth is understood. This article focuses on the diagnostic advances in urine cytology from the cytomorphological perspective, past and current reporting schemes, and the application of ancillary testing in urine samples.

Tissue sampling of renal masses is traditionally performed using percutaneous sonographic or computed tomographic guidance core biopsy (CB) with or without touch preparation cytology and/or fine-needle aspiration cytology (FNAC). The combined use of CB and FNAC is expanding in clinical practice, especially in small renal masses, and plays a pivotal role in therapeutic decision-making. Grouping the renal neoplasms in differential diagnostic groups helps in choosing specific immunohistochemical markers and reaching an accurate diagnosis.

Soft tissue neoplasms are diagnostically challenging, although many advances in ancillary testing now enable accurate classification of fine-needle aspiration biopsies by detection of characteristic immunophenotypes (including protein correlates of molecular alterations) and molecular features. Although there are many useful diagnostic immunohistochemical markers and molecular assays, their diagnostic utility relies on correlation with clinical and morphologic features, judicious application, and appropriate interpretation because no single test is perfectly sensitive or specific. This article discusses applications of ancillary testing for commonly encountered soft tissue neoplasms in cytopathologic practice in the context of a pattern-based approach.

This article summarizes the current diagnostic challenges in fine-needle aspiration of primary bone tumors, with focus on the application of new molecular and immunohistochemical techniques in the diagnosis of giant cell–rich neoplasms, chondrosarcomas, and notochordal tumors.

Sinchita Roy-Chowdhuri

There has been a paradigm shift in the practice of cytopathology with the advent of highly sensitive molecular tests using small amounts of tissue that can provide diagnostic, prognostic, and predictive information for clinical management. The cytopathologist plays a key role in providing a timely and accurate diagnosis as well as ensuring appropriate processing and handling of the specimen and judicious triaging of the tissue for molecular testing that guide therapeutic decisions. As the era of "precision medicine" continues to evolve and expand, cytopathology remains a dynamic field with advances in the practice of molecular cytopathology providing new paradigms in clinical care.

Alarice C. Lowe

Circulating tumor cells (CTCs) are rare tumor cells found in the blood of patients with cancer that can be reliably detected by CTC technologies to provide prognostic, predictive, and diagnostic information. CTC sampling better reflects intratumoral and intertumoral heterogeneity than targeted biopsy. CTC samples are minimally invasive and amenable to repeated sampling, allowing real-time evaluation of tumor in response to therapy-related pressures and possibly early detection. Cytology is the most natural arena for integration of CTC testing. CTC technology may also be deployed to enhance and facilitate the practice of cytology and surgical pathology.

SURGICAL PATHOLOGY CLINICS

RELATED INTEREST

Otolaryngologic Clinics, August 2014 (Vol. 47, No. 4)
Thyroid Cancer: Current Diagnosis, Management, and Prognostication
Robert L. Witt, *Editor*

THE CLINICS ARE AVAILABLE ONLINE!
Access your subscription at:
www.theclinics.com

Preface
Cytopathology: Diagnostic Updates and Advances in Ancillary Testing

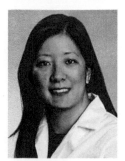

Vickie Y. Jo, MD
Editor

This issue of *Surgical Pathology Clinics* is devoted to cytopathology, with an emphasis on recent developments in common and challenging areas of practice. In the era of subspecialization and ancillary testing, cytopathologists remain true generalists and morphologists. However, cytologic practice now requires understanding and adapting the parallel advances in tumor classification, ancillary testing, and clinical management occurring across numerous subspecialties. Nonetheless, this is an exciting time for the field, as our ability as cytopathologists to "do more with less" with small tissue samples at the front lines of patient care is expanding greatly.

This issue provides systematic overviews and updated synopses of diagnostic criteria, ancillary testing, established and recently implemented standardized reporting schemes, and common challenges in selected areas of cytology. Covered topics include frequently encountered yet evolving areas of thyroid, gynecologic Pap smears, urine specimens, effusions, and lung cytology; challenging organ systems such as salivary gland, pancreaticobiliary, and kidney; rare and notoriously difficult bone and soft tissue tumors; and recent insights and issues with HPV-associated carcinomas of the head and neck and carcinomas of unknown primary. There are also two articles dedicated to molecular testing techniques and circulating tumor cell technology, aimed to serve as practical guides for applying these innovations to cytology.

The numerous advances in cytology enhance our diagnostic capabilities to enable accurate diagnoses and risk stratification and to detect prognostic and predictive information, which ultimately improve the care of patients with cancer. It is hoped that this collection of articles will benefit a wide audience, including cytopathologists, general pathologists, and pathologists-in-training, and will provide readers with a current and comprehensive overview of the ongoing developments in cytology and guide the integration of relevant advances (such as immunohistochemical and molecular testing) in routine practice.

Vickie Y. Jo, MD
Department of Pathology
Brigham and Women's Hospital and
Harvard Medical School
75 Francis Street
Boston, MA 02115, USA

E-mail address:
vjo@partners.org

Surgical Pathology 11 (2018) xi
https://doi.org/10.1016/j.path.2018.06.005
1875-9181/18/

Updates in Thyroid Cytology

Michiya Nishino, MD, PhD[a],*, Jeffrey F. Krane, MD, PhD[b]

KEYWORDS

- Thyroid nodule • Thyroid cancer
- Noninvasive follicular thyroid neoplasm with papillary-like nuclear features • NIFTP
- Indeterminate cytology • Molecular testing • Fine needle aspiration

Key points

- Noninvasive follicular thyroid neoplasm with papillary-like nuclear features (NIFTP) are indolent neoplasms for which lobectomy is diagnostically necessary and therapeutically sufficient.

- Awareness of cytologic features suggestive of NIFTP on preoperative fine needle aspiration may help triage patients to lobectomy rather than near-total thyroidectomy.

- Commercially available molecular tests aim to improve the preoperative risk stratification of thyroid nodules with indeterminate fine needle aspiration cytology.

- The 4 molecular tests described in this review all aim to have a high negative predictive value for "ruling out" cancer among thyroid nodules with indeterminate cytology.

ABSTRACT

Genomic, clinical, and pathologic studies have prompted a more risk-stratified approach to the management of patients with thyroid nodules. The recent nomenclature change concerning noninvasive follicular thyroid neoplasm with papillary-like nuclear features reflects the clinical trend toward conservative treatment choices for carefully selected low-risk thyroid neoplasms. These developments have occurred in parallel with a growing array of molecular tests intended to improve clinical triage for patients with indeterminate fine needle aspiration diagnoses. This review discusses the implications of the nomenclature revision on the interpretation of thyroid fine needle aspiration and updates available ancillary molecular tests for thyroid fine needle aspirations.

OVERVIEW

Fine needle aspiration (FNA) plays an important role in the evaluation of thyroid nodules that meet clinical, laboratory, and radiographic criteria for biopsy evaluation. The Bethesda System for Reporting Thyroid Cytopathology (TBSRTC) provides a standardized framework for the classification of thyroid FNA specimens based on cytomorphologic criteria. Each of the 6 interpretive categories of TBSRTC is associated with an approximate risk of malignancy, which clinicians may use to guide management of patients with a thyroid nodule.

Disclosure Statement: The authors have no relevant funding source or commercial/financial conflicts of interest.
[a] Department of Pathology, Harvard Medical School and Beth Israel Deaconess Medical Center, 330 Brookline Avenue, Boston, MA 02215, USA; [b] Department of Pathology, Harvard Medical School and Brigham and Women's Hospital, 75 Francis Street, Amory 3, Boston, MA 02115, USA
* Corresponding author.
E-mail address: mnishin1@bidmc.harvard.edu

Surgical Pathology 11 (2018) 467–487
https://doi.org/10.1016/j.path.2018.05.002
1875-9181/18/© 2018 Elsevier Inc. All rights reserved.

surgpath.theclinics.com

The recently published seond edition of TBSRTC has updated the implied cancer risk for each interpretive category, partially in response to the recent reclassification of noninvasive, encapsulated follicular variant of papillary thyroid carcinoma (FV-PTC) as an indolent neoplasm known as noninvasive follicular thyroid neoplasm with papillary-like nuclear features (NIFTP). These changes have occurred in parallel with an increasing shift toward a more refined approach to the treatment of thyroid nodules. The development of ancillary molecular diagnostic tests for thyroid FNA specimens has encouraged this trend. Although specific, evidence-based guidelines for the optimal application and interpretation of molecular tests in thyroid FNAs have yet to be established, these tests have begun to influence clinical practice. In that context, this review covers 2 main topics: (a) the NIFTP nomenclature change and its impact on cytopathology practice and (b) an appraisal of the ancillary molecular tests that are commercially available for thyroid FNA specimens: Afirma (Veracyte, Inc., South San Francisco, CA), RosettaGX Reveal (Rosetta Genomics, Inc., Philadelphia, PA), ThyGenX/ThyraMIR (Interface Diagnostics, Inc., Parsippany, NJ), and ThyroSeq (University of Pittsburgh Medical Center, Pittsburgh, PA, and CBLPath, Inc., Rye Brook, NY).

PART 1: NONINVASIVE FOLLICULAR THYROID NEOPLASM WITH PAPILLARY-LIKE NUCLEAR FEATURES AND ITS IMPACT ON THYROID CYTOLOGY

ORIGINS OF NONINVASIVE FOLLICULAR THYROID NEOPLASM WITH PAPILLARY-LIKE NUCLEAR FEATURES: RECLASSIFICATION OF A SUBSET OF FOLLICULAR VARIANT OF PAPILLARY THYROID CARCINOMA

PTC has encompassed thyroid tumors with characteristic nuclear morphology and a wide variety of cytologic and architectural patterns. The designation of a number of PTC variants reflects this morphologic heterogeneity. In particular, thyroid tumors with the nuclear atypia of PTC and a follicular growth pattern have historically been classified as FV-PTC, which has been further subclassified based on histopathologic assessment of their circumscription and tumor invasion, molecular alterations, and clinical behavior. FV-PTCs that demonstrate diffuse growth into the surrounding thyroid parenchyma (infiltrative FV-PTC; **Fig. 1**A) have a tendency to harbor *BRAF*-like genetic alterations and have increased risk for local recurrence and cervical lymph node metastasis, similar to classical PTC (cPTC).[1–4]

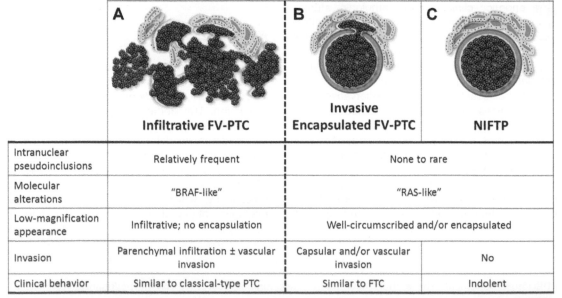

	Infiltrative FV-PTC	Invasive Encapsulated FV-PTC	NIFTP
Intranuclear pseudoinclusions	Relatively frequent	None to rare	
Molecular alterations	"BRAF-like"	"RAS-like"	
Low-magnification appearance	Infiltrative; no encapsulation	Well-circumscribed and/or encapsulated	
Invasion	Parenchymal infiltration ± vascular invasion	Capsular and/or vascular invasion	No
Clinical behavior	Similar to classical-type PTC	Similar to FTC	Indolent

Fig. 1. Comparison of the pathology, molecular alterations, and clinical behavior of thyroid neoplasms with the nuclear atypia of papillary carcinoma and an exclusively follicular growth pattern. Historically, each of these 3 categories of tumors had been subsumed under the umbrella term follicular variant of papillary thyroid carcinoma (FV-PTC). Studies over the past decade have underscored pathologically, molecularly, and clinically distinct subcategories among these tumors: (*A*) Infiltrative FV-PTC, (*B*) invasive encapsulated FV-PTC, and (*C*) Noninvasive Follicular Thyroid Neoplasm with Papillary-like Nuclear Features (NIFTP). See text for details. FTC, follicular thyroid carcinoma; PTC, papillary thyroid carcinoma.

In contrast, FV-PTCs that are well-circumscribed and/or encapsulated show clinical behavior that parallels follicular adenoma/carcinoma.[5] In the presence of capsular or vascular invasion, well-circumscribed/encapsulated FV-PTCs demonstrate a propensity for hematogenous spread and distant metastasis, more similar to follicular carcinomas than cPTC (invasive encapsulated FV-PTC; **Fig. 1B**).[6] In contrast, when well-circumscribed/encapsulated FV-PTCs show evidence of neither capsular nor vascular invasion, their subsequent clinical course is indolent, mirroring that of follicular adenomas.[4,6–13] Based on their exceptionally low malignant potential, this noninvasive subset of well-circumscribed/encapsulated FV-PTC was recently reclassified as NIFTP (**Fig. 1C**).[11]

Molecular analysis further reinforces the notion that encapsulated FV-PTC and NIFTP are more closely related to follicular adenomas and carcinomas than to cPTC. Although *BRAF*-like genetic alterations are found in infiltrative FV-PTC and cPTC, *RAS*-like genetic alterations are characteristic of both invasive encapsulated FV-PTC and NIFTP.[1,3,5,9,14–16] Molecular studies of NIFTPs in particular have identified a variety of genetic driver alterations, including mutations in *RAS*, *BRAF* K601E, and *EIF1AX*, as well as gene fusions involving *THADA* or *PAX8-PPARG*.[11,17] Notably, NIFTP and invasive encapsulated FV-PTC have overlapping molecular profiles and the only distinction between these tumors to date is the histologic detection of capsular/vascular invasion in the latter.

NIFTP may be considered a premalignant neoplasm, for which conservative surgical treatment (thyroid lobectomy) is generally considered adequate treatment, without the need for completion thyroidectomy and radioactive iodine treatment.[6,11] The histopathologic features of NIFTP are summarized in **Table 1**.[11,18] Pathologists should strictly adhere to these inclusionary and exclusionary criteria to help maintain the reproducibility and the very low malignant potential of the NIFTP diagnosis. Histologic examination of the entire interface between the tumor and adjacent thyroid parenchyma is essential to exclude capsular/vascular invasion or infiltrative growth.

DOES NONINVASIVE FOLLICULAR THYROID NEOPLASM WITH PAPILLARY-LIKE NUCLEAR FEATURES HAVE DISTINCTIVE CYTOLOGIC FEATURES?

Several retrospective studies have examined the cytologic features of NIFTP (or equivalent tumors

Table 1
Histologic inclusion and exclusion criteria for NIFTP

Inclusion Criteria for NIFTP	Exclusion Criteria for NIFTP
Encapsulation or clear demarcation	Capsular or vascular invasion
Predominantly follicular growth pattern	True papillary architecture
Nuclear score of 2 or 3[a]	>30% solid, insular, or trabecular architecture
	Psammoma bodies
	Features of tall cell or columnar cell variant of PTC
	Tumor necrosis
	>3 mitoses per 10 high-power (400×) fields

Abbreviations: NIFTP, noninvasive follicular thyroid neoplasm with papillary-like nuclear features; PTC, papillary thyroid carcinoma.

[a] Nuclear score refers to a 3-point scoring system for assessing the nuclear atypia, whereby 1 point is assigned for (a) nuclear size and shape (enlargement, elongation, overlapping), (b) nuclear membrane irregularities (irregular contours, grooves, pseudoinclusions), and (c) chromatin changes (pallor/clearing, margination of chromatin to membrane).

Adapted from Inclusion and exclusion criteria adapted from Nikiforov YE, Seethala RR, Tallini G, et al. Nomenclature Revision for Encapsulated Follicular Variant of Papillary Thyroid Carcinoma: A Paradigm Shift to Reduce Overtreatment of Indolent Tumors. JAMA Oncol 2016;2(8):1023–29; and Seethala RR, Baloch ZW, Barletta JA, et al. Noninvasive follicular thyroid neoplasm with papillary-like nuclear features: a review for pathologists. Mod Pathol 2018;31(1):39–55.

with the former appellation, noninvasive encapsulated FV-PTC). In keeping with its name, aspirates of NIFTPs may be distinguished from those of benign follicular nodules (eg, follicular adenomas and adenomatous/hyperplastic nodules) based on the presence of papillary-like nuclear features, including nuclear enlargement and crowding, nuclear contour irregularity, nuclear molding, and chromatin pallor.[19–21]

Early studies suggest that NIFTP can be distinguished cytologically from some malignant tumors but not from others. NIFTP and invasive encapsulated FV-PTC have overlapping cytoarchitectural and nuclear features, precluding reliable distinction between these tumors on FNA cytology.[2,3,20,22,23] In contrast, NIFTP and cPTC have distinctive architectural and nuclear features that may permit their separation on FNA cytology.[23,24] For NIFTP, the arrangement of cellular groups on FNA cytology specimens is predominantly microfollicular, whereas that of cPTC is typically papillary or sheet-like. NIFTPs also demonstrate lesser degrees of nuclear atypia relative to cPTC. In particular, intranuclear pseudoinclusions—an extreme manifestation of the nuclear contour irregularity characteristic of cPTC—are infrequent or absent in NIFTP with only rare exceptions.[25] Likewise, cytologic distinction between NIFTP and infiltrative FV-PTC may be possible based on nuclear features. Aspirates of NIFTP are less frequently classified as suspicious for malignancy or malignant compared with infiltrative FV-PTC, which may reflect the more modest nuclear atypia characteristic of the former.[3,26]

Taken together, the cytologic differential diagnosis of follicular-patterned lesions could be organized as a simplified matrix with nuclear atypia and architectural atypia as its axes (**Fig. 2**). In this matrix, the cytology of NIFTP occupies the intersection between moderate levels of nuclear atypia and the architectural features of a follicular neoplasm. Aspirates of NIFTPs can be distinguished from most benign follicular nodules (hyperplastic/adenomatous nodules and follicular adenomas) based on greater degrees of nuclear atypia in NIFTPs. Aspirates of NIFTPs may in turn be distinguished from cPTC (and related tumors, including the tall cell variant of PTC) based on both nuclear and architectural features, with

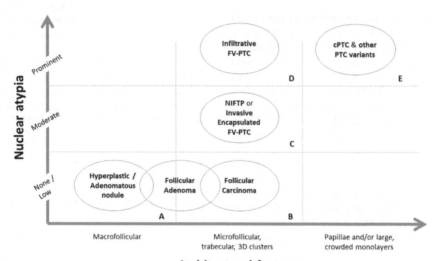

Architectural features

Fig. 2. Idealized conceptual model of follicular-patterned lesions and differentiated thyroid carcinoma based on nuclear atypia and architectural features. The cytologic features of many thyroid aspirates can be conceptually compartmentalized based on nuclear atypia and architectural features. Nuclear atypia (y-axis) refers to the nuclear features that are characteristic of papillary thyroid carcinoma (nuclear enlargement, nuclear contour irregularity, and/or chromatin pallor). In this chart, nuclear atypia is qualitatively stratified as none/low, moderate (ie, aspirates demonstrating ≥2 of these features), or prominent (ie, aspirates showing all 3 of these features, with numerous intranuclear inclusions). Thyroid aspirates can also be arranged by architectural features (x-axis), which can vary from macrofollicular (cells arranged in flat sheets with evenly spaced nuclei), microfollicular (architectural features of a follicular-patterned neoplasm), to papillary (including large, crowded monolayers). Aspirates demonstrating macrofollicular architecture and no/minimal nuclear atypia (A) are characteristic of benign follicular nodules (hyperplastic/adenomatous nodules as well as follicular adenomas). In contrast, tumors with microfollicular architecture have a broad differential diagnosis that includes benign, premalignant, and malignant lesions. Follicular carcinoma and follicular adenoma can show overlapping cytologic features (microfollicular architecture and no/low nuclear atypia; B) and are distinguished by the histologic detection of invasive growth in the former. Similarly, the cytologic features of invasive encapsulated follicular variant of papillary thyroid carcinoma (FV-PTC) and its presumed precursor, noninvasive follicular thyroid neoplasm with papillary-like nuclear features (NIFTP), are similar, with both lesions demonstrating microfollicular architecture and moderate degrees of nuclear atypia (C). The distinction between these entities relies on the histologic detection of invasion in encapsulated FV-PTC. In this model, thyroid aspirates with prominent nuclear atypia (particularly with numerous intranuclear pseudoinclusions) represent infiltrative FV-PTC (D), classical papillary thyroid carcinoma (cPTC), or other PTC variants (E). In actual practice, many of these entities can show considerable cytologic overlap with each other. Likewise, the boundaries between categories in real life are not as sharply demarcated as indicated in this figure. Nevertheless, this idealized vision of how these entities present cytologically may provide a structure for generating a differential diagnosis based on cytologic findings. 3D, 3-dimensional.

NIFTPs demonstrating more subtle nuclear atypia (including rare or absent intranuclear pseudoinclusions) and microfollicular (rather than papillary or sheetlike) architecture. Early studies indicate that NIFTPs can also be distinguished cytologically from infiltrative FV-PTC based on nuclear (but not architectural) features, in keeping with biologic similarity between infiltrative FV-PTC and cPTC.

Importantly, NIFTP shares its spot in this idealized matrix with malignant tumors (see **Fig. 2**). Analogous to follicular adenoma/carcinoma, the distinction between NIFTP and invasive encapsulated FV-PTC is based on histologic demonstration of capsular and/or angioinvasion, attributes that cannot be evaluated cytologically.

The NIFTP nomenclature change was prompted in part to curb the overtreatment of low-risk thyroid neoplasms.[11] For thyroid FNA specimens that are suggestive of NIFTP, classification in one of the indeterminate categories of TBSRTC—atypia (or follicular lesion) of undetermined significance (AUS/FLUS, Bethesda-III), follicular neoplasm (or suspicious for follicular neoplasm; FN/SFN [Bethesda-IV]), or suspicious for malignancy (Bethesda-V)—may encourage lobectomy instead of total thyroidectomy. For aspirates in the suspicious for malignancy category in particular, an explanatory note that includes NIFTP in the differential diagnosis may be helpful to prompt consideration for lobectomy as the initial surgical approach.[25,27] To minimize the diagnosis of NIFTPs as malignant and avoid overtreatment, some authors recommend limiting malignant cytologic diagnoses to those aspirates with features favoring cPTC, such as overt nuclear atypia (including the detection of intranuclear pseudoinclusions), psammomatous calcifications, and/or cytologic evidence of true papillary architecture.[23,27] This approach has been adopted in the recent update to TBSRTC.[28]

WHAT ARE THE IMPLICATIONS OF THE NONINVASIVE FOLLICULAR THYROID NEOPLASM WITH PAPILLARY-LIKE NUCLEAR FEATURES RECLASSIFICATION FOR THE BETHESDA SYSTEM FOR REPORTING THYROID CYTOPATHOLOGY?

One of the early questions surrounding the reclassification of noninvasive encapsulated FV-PTC as NIFTP was its impact on the cancer risks associated with each TBSRTC category. Retrospective studies have demonstrated that aspirates of NIFTPs are predominantly classified in the indeterminate categories of TBSRTC. Consequently, if NIFTPs are considered benign tumors for the purposes of cancer risk calculations, the most pronounced decreases in cancer risk would occur in the AUS/FLUS, FN/SFN, and suspicious for malignancy categories of TBSRTC.[20,24,29–35]

Yet, there are arguments against equating NIFTP's new nonmalignant status with benignity. Although NIFTP is considered an indolent neoplasm with very low malignant potential, surgery (ie, lobectomy) is considered the standard of care and is necessary to establish the diagnosis of NIFTP definitively. Given this, it may not make sense to conflate NIFTPs with histologically benign nodules, for which nonsurgical follow-up is generally accepted.

In recognition of these conflicting perspectives, the second edition of TBSRTC offers 2 updated versions of the cancer risks associated with each interpretive category: one that considers NIFTP as benign and another that considers NIFTP as malignant (**Table 2**).[28] Ultimately, the binary benign versus malignant histopathologic classification scheme—although straightforward for statistical analysis—may prove to be inadequate to capture the progressive nature of thyroid neoplasia.

PART 2: ANCILLARY MOLECULAR TESTING IN THE EVALUATION OF THYROID NODULES

BACKGROUND: FINE NEEDLE ASPIRATION AS A RISK STRATIFICATION TOOL FOR THYROID NODULES

The 6 interpretive categories of TBSRTC help to translate cytomorphologic findings from an FNA biopsy into a practical approximation of thyroid cancer risk (see **Table 2**). At the extreme ends of this tiered reporting system, the appropriate management is fairly straightforward (although management may be modified in individual cases by clinical and sonographic risk factors). Thyroid nodules classified as cytologically benign by FNA (Bethesda-II) have a low malignancy risk (0%–3%) and are generally safe to follow by clinical observation (**Fig. 3**). Alternatively, nodules classified as cytologically malignant (Bethesda-VI) are associated with a 94% to 96% cancer risk and are generally referred for surgical resection (see **Fig. 3**).

Historically, near-total thyroidectomy was recommended for most FNA-proven PTCs larger than 1 cm.[36] However, concepts regarding the extent of surgery that patients with cytologically malignant thyroid nodules should undergo (ie, lobectomy vs near-total thyroidectomy) have evolved in recent years. Some cytologically

Table 2
Updated risks of malignancy in the second edition of The Bethesda System for Reporting Thyroid Cytopathology

Category	Risk of Malignancy (%)		Usual Management
	If NIFTP Considered Nonmalignant	If NIFTP Considered Malignant	
Nondiagnostic	5–10	5–10	Repeat FNA with ultrasound imaging
Benign	0–3	0–3	Clinical and follow-up with ultrasound imaging
Atypia/follicular lesion of undetermined significance	6–18	10–30	Repeat FNA, molecular testing, or lobectomy
Follicular neoplasm/suspicious for follicular neoplasm	10–40	25–40	Molecular testing, lobectomy
Suspicious for malignancy	45–60	50–75	Near-total thyroidectomy or lobectomy
Malignant	94–96	97–99	Near-total thyroidectomy or lobectomy

The 6 interpretive categories of The Bethesda System for Reporting Thyroid Cytopathology are listed in the first column, and the approximate cancer risks associated with each category are noted in subsequent columns, based on whether noninvasive follicular thyroid neoplasm with papillary-like nuclear features (NIFTP) are considered nonmalignant (second column) or malignant (third column).

Abbreviations: FNA, fine needle aspiration; NIFTP, noninvasive follicular thyroid neoplasm with papillary-like nuclear features.

Adapted from Baloch ZW, Cooper DS, Gharib HS, et al. Overview of diagnostic terminology and reporting. In: Ali SZ, Cibas ED, editors. The Bethesda system for reporting thyroid cytopathology. Springer, Cham, Switzerland 2018; 3–4; with permission. Copyright 2018.

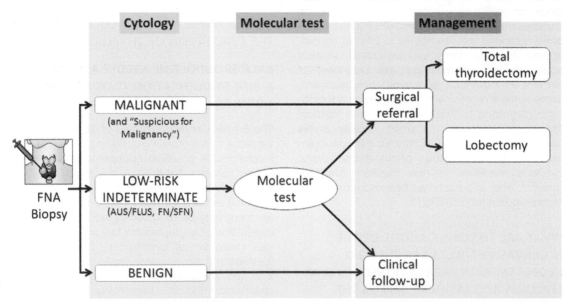

Fig. 3. Simplified algorithm for how cytologic and molecular testing results can guide management of thyroid nodules. Most of the molecular tests described in this review are primarily indicated for aspirates classified in the "low-risk" indeterminate categories of the Bethesda System for Reporting Thyroid Cytopathology (atypia of undetermined significance/follicular lesion of undetermined significance [AUS/FLUS], follicular neoplasm/suspicious for follicular neoplasm [FN/SFN]). The results of molecular testing in this setting help to direct patients toward either surgical referral or clinical follow-up. The extent of surgical resection may be determined by multiple factors, including clinical/radiographic assessment of tumor size, extrathyroidal spread, nodal metastasis, and distant metastasis; ultrasonographic and cytologic findings in the contralateral lobe; patient/clinician preference; and cytomorphologic or molecular features that may distinguish indolent/precancerous neoplasms from more aggressive disease. Regarding the latter, molecular tests that can detect genetic alterations characteristic of classical papillary thyroid carcinoma (eg, *BRAF* V600E mutations, *RET-PTC1/3* fusions) could also be considered for aspirates in the higher risk indeterminate category (suspicious for malignancy) to help guide the extent of initial surgical resection. FNA, fine needle aspiration.

malignant tumors represent low- to intermediate-risk cancers (eg, encapsulated FV-PTC, minimally invasive FTC) or potentially premalignant neoplasms (eg, NIFTP) for which lobectomy may be sufficient treatment.[11,37–39] In recognition of this observation, the American Thyroid Association's latest management guidelines include the option of lobectomy as the initial surgical approach for cytologically malignant tumors that are unifocal, smaller than 4 cm, and do not show clinical/radiologic evidence of extrathyroidal extension or metastasis (see **Fig. 3**).[40] Near-total thyroidectomy may thus be reserved for cytologically malignant tumors that do not fulfill the selection criteria for lobectomy, as well as for tumors that otherwise merit more extensive surgery based on patient/physician preference and/or cytologic or molecular features associated with aggressive clinical behavior. Most thyroid nodules classified as suspicious for malignancy on FNA biopsy follow similar recommendations for surgical resection as cytologically malignant nodules, owing to a risk of cancer estimated to be 45% to 60%.[28] As indicated, the extent of surgery for nodules in this setting may be influenced by clinical (including patient/physician preference), sonographic, and possibly molecular features of the nodule.[40] Cytologic concern for NIFTP may also influence the extent of surgery for a suspicious for malignancy diagnosis.[25]

In contrast, the most suitable management is not as clear-cut for the 15% to 30% of thyroid nodules that fall into the remaining 2 cytologically indeterminate categories of TBSRTC: AUS/FLUS and FN/SFN.[41] These cytologic categories are associated with modest but not negligible cancer risks (6%–18% for AUS/FLUS and 10%–40% for FN/SFN).[28] For nodules in the AUS/FLUS category, management options have historically ranged from surveillance with repeat FNA to diagnostic lobectomy, particularly for nodules with concerning clinical/ultrasound findings and/or persistently indeterminate cytology on repeat FNA. Likewise, nodules in the FN/SFN category have traditionally been referred for diagnostic lobectomy. Nevertheless, the majority of resected nodules in the AUS/FLUS and FN/SFN categories are found to be histologically benign. For these nodules, surgical resection may have been warranted for establishing a benign diagnosis, but unnecessary from a therapeutic standpoint.

MOLECULAR TESTING FOR CYTOLOGICALLY INDETERMINATE THYROID NODULES

Ancillary molecular testing on FNA material provides opportunities to refine the risk stratification of cytologically indeterminate nodules (see **Fig. 3**). The goals of molecular testing in this setting are 2-fold: (a) to help distinguish biologically benign nodules that are safe to follow clinically from those that merit surgical resection, and for nodules in the latter category, (b) to help guide the extent of the initial surgical approach (lobectomy vs near-total thyroidectomy). It is important to emphasize that molecular characteristics alone are inadequate to guide clinical management decisions; the results of molecular testing should always be considered in the context of a nodule's cytomorphology, clinical history, and ultrasound features.[40]

Currently, 4 ancillary molecular tests are commercially available for thyroid FNA specimens with indeterminate cytology. These tests can be broadly grouped by their methodology: (a) expression profiling for selected messenger RNAs (mRNA) or microRNAs (miRNAs), (b) genotyping for oncogenic driver mutations and gene fusions, or (c) a combination thereof. We review the design, performance, and usefulness of each of these tests. In appraising the published literature regarding the performance of molecular tests on cytologically indeterminate thyroid FNA specimens, several points of caution should be kept in mind.

- A test's positive predictive value (PPV) reflects the risk of cancer associated with a positive test result, whereas the negative predictive value (NPV) indicates the likelihood of benignity associated with a negative test result. Test performance is extrapolated from these predictive values, which in turn varies with the pretest probability of cancer in the tested population.[42,43] Pretest cancer risk may be estimated from the prevalence of cancer associated with the AUS/FLUS and FN/SFN Bethesda categories for each institution; integration of clinical, ultrasound, and cytologic features into pretest cancer risk calculations may provide a more clinically meaningful understanding of molecular testing results.
- The histopathologic diagnosis of resected nodules serves as the gold standard by which these molecular tests are evaluated. Yet, histopathology is an imperfect gold standard for thyroid tumors, with well-documented examples of discordance among pathologists in the classification of resected thyroid tumors as benign or malignant.[44–47]
- Furthermore, statistical analyses for validation studies generally consider the reference histopathologic diagnosis to be binary variables (benign or malignant). This practice does not

reflect evolving concepts of thyroid neoplasia as a continuous rather than dichotomous process.[11,40]

- Likewise, the validation studies for these molecular tests reduce test results into dichotomous outcomes (negative or positive) for the purposes of statistical analysis. Although this approach may be suitable for analyzing the performance of Afirma gene expression classifier (GEC) and RosettaGX Reveal (both of which report binary outcomes in practice), it does not capture the gradation of risk estimates offered by genotyping-based tests such as ThyroSeq and ThyGenX/ThyraMIR.

EXPRESSION PROFILING APPROACHES TO RISK STRATIFY CYTOLOGICALLY INDETERMINATE THYROID NODULES

Studies have identified various genes[48–51] and miRNAs[52–57] that are differentially expressed by benign versus malignant thyroid tumors. The Afirma GEC and RosettaGX Reveal tests analyze gene or miRNA expression patterns, respectively, in aspirates from cytologically indeterminate thyroid nodules. Both of these tests have been optimized to have high sensitivity and NPV for cancer; therefore, their usefulness is in recognizing those nodules with a very low risk of malignancy that are safe to monitor by clinical observation rather than surgical resection.

AFIRMA GENE EXPRESSION CLASSIFIER

The Afirma GEC uses a DNA microarray-based platform to analyze the gene (mRNA) expression profiles of cytologically indeterminate thyroid nodules. The test requires 2 dedicated FNA passes to be collected from each nodule into a vial of nucleic acid preservative, in addition to separate FNA passes collected for standard cytomorphologic evaluation. For aspirates classified as cytologically indeterminate (AUS/FLUS or SFN/FN), the concurrent sample collected for molecular testing is processed reflexively as follows (Fig. 4).

- The sample is first screened for the expression profiles of 25 genes associated with less common entities in the thyroid, including metastatic tumors (breast, renal, and melanoma), parathyroid tissue, and medullary thyroid carcinoma (MTC). A sample that triggers one of these screening cassettes is reported as having a suspicious Afirma result and does not undergo further analysis by the main GEC. A sample that harbors the expression profile of MTC in particular is reported as positive for the Afirma MTC test (discussed elsewhere in this article).
- For samples that are negative for the screening cassettes, the expression profile of 142 genes is analyzed by the main GEC, which categorizes each nodule as having either a benign or suspicious gene expression profile.

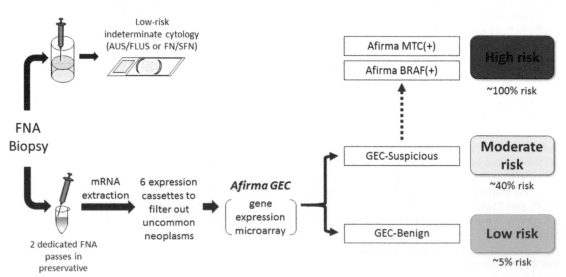

Fig. 4. Afirma GEC and malignancy classifiers. See text for details. AUS/FLUS, atypia of undetermined significance/follicular lesion of undetermined significance; FNA, fine needle aspiration; FN/SFN, follicular neoplasm/suspicious for follicular neoplasm; GEC, gene expression classifier; mRNA, messenger RNA; MTC, medullary thyroid carcinoma. (*Adapted from* Nishino M, Nikoforova M. Update on molecular testing for cytologically indeterminate thyroid nodules. Arch Pathol Lab Med. https://doi.org/10.5858/arpa.2017-0174-RA; with permission from Archives of Pathology & Laboratory Medicine. Copyright 2018 College of American Pathologists.)

In a prospective, multiinstitutional clinical validation study of 210 cytologically low-risk indeterminate nodules (129 AUS/FLUS and 81 FN/SFN), the Afirma GEC was found to have 90% sensitivity and approximately 50% specificity for cancer.[58] Based on these figures, the test has an NPV of 94% to 95% and a PPV of 37% to 38% among cytologically low-risk indeterminate nodules with a 24% to 25% prevalence of cancer. For clinical settings where the baseline cancer risk among cytologically indeterminate nodules is similar to that of the validation study, the Afirma results may be interpreted as follows (see **Fig. 4**).

- Cytologically indeterminate nodules with benign Afirma results are associated with a low risk of cancer (5%–6%, corresponding with 1 – NPV), similar to cytologically benign nodules. These nodules may be safe to follow by clinical observation.
- Cytologically indeterminate nodules with suspicious Afirma results are associated with an approximately 40% risk of cancer (corresponding with the PPV). At this intermediate risk level, a diagnostic lobectomy is generally advised.
- Among nodules with suspicious Afirma results, the Afirma malignancy classifiers can be used to identify a subset of cases with a near 100% risk of cancer (discussed elsewhere in this article).

Afirma Malignancy Classifiers

Veracyte offers opportunities for further risk stratification among nodules with suspicious Afirma GEC results with 2 additional tests: Afirma MTC and Afirma BRAF tests.

- The Afirma MTC test examines samples for the expression levels of 5 genes (*CALCA*, *CEACAM5*, *SCG3*, *SCN9A*, and *SYT4*), which identify MTC with high sensitivity and specificity.[59,60] Although MTC is uncommon among nodules classified as AUS/FLUS or FN/SFN, the preoperative detection of MTC can prompt genetic testing for germline *RET* mutations, laboratory and/or radiographic evaluation for pheochromocytoma (with adrenergic blockade and surgical resection thereof, before thyroid surgery), and surgical planning for total thyroidectomy with central lymph node dissection.[61]
- The Afirma BRAF test assays for the gene expression profile associated with a *BRAF* V600E mutation; the test is offered reflexively for samples with suspicious Afirma GEC

results. Owing to the high specificity of the *BRAF* V600E mutation for PTC, a positive test is associated with a near 100% risk of malignancy and may influence decisions regarding the extent of initial surgery. Nonetheless, because the prevalence of papillary carcinomas with *BRAF* V600E mutations is low among AUS/FLUS and FN/SFN nodules in Western populations, the cost effectiveness of routinely ordering the Afirma BRAF test for all nodules with suspicious Afirma GEC results has yet to be determined.[62,63]

Key Features
AFIRMA GENE EXPRESSION CLASSIFIER

1. Afirma GEC (Veracyte, Inc.) assesses the expression profiles of a large panel of genes with microarrays and uses a proprietary algorithm to classify samples as having a benign or suspicious gene expression profile.

2. Among thyroid FNAs classified as AUS/FLUS or FN/SFN, benign GEC results correspond with a low risk of cancer, comparable with a cytologically benign aspirate. Alternatively, suspicious GEC results correspond with a moderate risk of cancer, for which diagnostic surgery (lobectomy) is generally indicated.

3. Afirma Malignancy Classifiers assay for the expression of genes associated with MTC and PTCs harboring the *BRAF* V600E mutation. Positive Afirma MTC or Afirma BRAF results are associated with a high risk of cancer.

4. The cellular composition of the FNA sample used for Afirma testing is determined in part by screening for the expression profiles of MTC, metastatic tumors, and parathyroid tissue.

5. An updated version of the test known as the Afirma Gene Sequencing Classifier was recently released. The updates include (a) testing for *RET-PTC1/3* gene fusion and (b) optimization of algorithms for improved specificity for cancer, particularly among aspirates rich in Hürthle cells.

Real-World Clinical Experiences with Afirma Gene Expression Classifier

Many groups have published their institutional experiences with the Afirma GEC in real-world clinical practice.[64–78] Collectively, the proportion of cytologically indeterminate cases classified as benign by Afirma in these studies is approximately

40%, similar to what was reported in the Afirma clinical validation study.[58] These studies support the notion that Afirma is helpful for stratifying nearly one-half of cytologically indeterminate nodules into a low-risk category that may be safe to monitor by clinical observation. At the same time, because most cytologically indeterminate nodules with benign (or negative) molecular testing results are not resected in real-world clinical practice, the true-negative and false-negative rates of these tests using a histopathologic gold standard remain unknown outside of the clinical validation study.[58] This realization has prompted some authors to call for clinical and/or sonographic features to serve as surrogate endpoints for benign histopathology.[79] As a case in point, Angell and colleagues[66] used sonographic assessments of nodule growth to conclude that thyroid nodules with indeterminate cytology and benign Afirma results may be clinically observed similarly to cytologically benign nodules. Concerns have also been raised that the Afirma GEC shows relatively diminished specificity for Hürthle cell lesions.[70,73,74,76]

Recent Updates to the Afirma Test

Veracyte released the Afirma Genomic Sequencing Classifier in 2017. This updated version of the Afirma test incorporates RNA sequencing methodology (notably for *RET-PTC* fusions) and new machine-learning processes to the gene expression profiling and malignancy classifiers described elsewhere in this article. Thus, in its current form, Afirma combines its binary (benign vs suspicious) gene expression profiling with testing for MTC, *BRAF* V600E mutation, and *RET-PTC1/3* gene fusions. Published data regarding performance of the updated test are not available at the time of this writing, but the test provider describes improved specificity overall and with Hürthle cell-rich aspirates using the

same case cohort from the prior multiinstitutional validation study.

RosettaGX REVEAL microRNA CLASSIFIER

RosettaGX Reveal risk stratifies cytologically indeterminate thyroid nodules based on miRNA expression profiles. The nucleic acid for miRNA expression profiling is extracted from the cellular material on routinely prepared and stained cytology specimens (**Fig. 5**). The advantages of using existing cytology slides as substrates for molecular testing are 2-fold. First, this approach should decrease the number of FNA passes needed from each nodule, because the slides used for cytomorphologic examination can be repurposed for molecular testing. Second, miRNA profiling is performed on the same cells that are examined microscopically. This approach theoretically decreases the risk of sampling discrepancy compared with testing approaches that require separate, dedicated FNA passes for molecular analysis. The primary disadvantage of using routine cytology slides as a substrate for molecular testing may be the sacrifice of a diagnostic cytology slide. Rosetta Genomics offers a slide scanning service to maintain a digital record of the cytology specimen before processing the slide for nucleic acid extraction.

RosettaGX Reveal evaluates the expression levels of 24 miRNAs by quantitative reverse transcriptase polymerase chain reaction to classify each sample as having either a benign or a suspicious miRNA profile. The test was clinically validated in a retrospective multicenter study of 189 cases from the AUS/FLUS, SFN/FN, and suspicious for malignancy categories, with a combined 32% cancer prevalence. Among this validation set, RosettaGX Reveal demonstrated 85% sensitivity, 72% specificity, 91% NPV, and 59% PPV.[80]

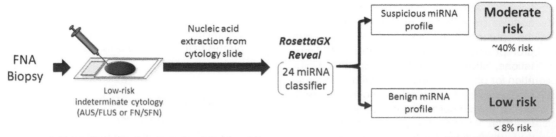

Fig. 5. RosettaGX reveal. See text for details. AUS/FLUS, atypia of undetermined significance/follicular lesion of undetermined significance; FN/SFN, follicular neoplasm/suspicious for follicular neoplasm; FNA, fine needle aspiration; miRNA, microRNA. (*Adapted from* Nishino M, Nikoforova M. Update on molecular testing for cytologically indeterminate thyroid nodules. Arch Pathol Lab Med. https://doi.org/10.5858/arpa.2017-0174-RA; with permission from Archives of Pathology & Laboratory Medicine. Copyright 2018 College of American Pathologists.)

The authors of the validation study also analyzed a subset of cases for which all 3 pathologists reviewing the resection specimen (ie, the original pathologist who signed out the case and 2 study pathologists) concurred on the reference histopathologic diagnosis. Among this agreement set of 150 cases (27% prevalence of cancer), RosettaGX Reveal was found to have 98% sensitivity, 78% specificity, 99% NPV, and 62% PPV. The superior sensitivity and NPV in this subset analysis is likely due in part to the omission of 14 encapsulated FVPTCs from the agreement set, 5 of which were classified as having a benign miRNA profile by RosettaGX Reveal.

Validation studies for the other commercially available molecular tests reviewed in this article have generally excluded nodules interpreted as suspicious for malignancy. Variations in the makeup of the validation cohort such as this underscore the challenges of comparing the performance of these molecular tests across different studies. With that caveat in mind, we provide sensitivity, specificity, and predictive value calculations based on only the AUS/FLUS and FN/SFN cases in the RosettaGX Reveal clinical validation study.

- Among all the AUS/FLUS and FN/SFN cases in their study (n = 150; 21% prevalence of cancer), Rosetta's miRNA classifier had a sensitivity and specificity of 74%, NPV of 92%, and PPV of 43%.
- For the AUS/FLUS and SFN/FN cases in their agreement set (n = 116; 12% prevalence of cancer), the miRNA classifier had 100% sensitivity, 80% specificity, 100% NPV, and 41% PPV.

Therefore, like the Afirma GEC, Rosetta's miRNA classifier demonstrates a high NPV and modest PPV. Cytologically indeterminate nodules with a benign miRNA profile have a low risk of malignancy (0%–8%, depending on which subset analysis from the validation cohort is used) and may be triaged for clinical observation. In contrast, nodules that are suspicious for malignancy by miRNA profiling have an intermediate cancer risk (41%–62%, depending on subset analysis) and should be referred for surgical resection (see **Fig. 5**).

Of note, RosettaGX Reveal is advertised to distinguish MTCs based on the inclusion of hsa-miR-375 (an miRNA that is often expressed at high levels in MTC) among its 24-miRNA panel. However, broader confirmation of this claim is needed based on the low number of MTC cases in their validation study.[80]

Key Features
RosettaGX Reveal

1. RosettaGX Reveal (Rosetta Genomics, Inc.) assesses the expression profiles of 24 miRNAs with reverse transcriptase polymerase chain reaction and uses a proprietary algorithm to classify samples as having a "benign" or "suspicious for malignancy by miRNA profiling" result.

2. Among AUS/FLUS and FN/SFN aspirates, benign miRNA results correspond with a low risk of cancer, comparable with cytologically benign aspirates. Samples with suspicious miRNA profiles have a moderate risk of cancer for which surgery is generally indicated.

3. The test is designed to detect MTC by including hsa-miR-375 in the miRNA panel.

4. Cells on routinely prepared and stained cytology slides serve as the starting material for nucleic acid extraction, obviating the need for separate FNA passes dedicated to collecting cells for molecular testing.

5. The cellular composition of the material used for molecular testing can be verified by visual microscopic examination (because cytology slides serve as the source material for molecular testing), as well as by assaying for epithelial markers.

GENOTYPING-BASED APPROACHES TO RISK STRATIFY CYTOLOGICALLY INDETERMINATE THYROID NODULES

An alternative approach to gene- or miRNA-based expression profiling is to test FNA material for a panel of mutations or gene fusions that are associated with thyroid cancer. Early generations of a genotyping panel for risk stratifying cytologically indeterminate thyroid FNAs focused on detecting hotspot mutations in *BRAF, HRAS, NRAS, KRAS,* as well as chromosomal rearrangements resulting in *PAX8-PPARG, RET-PTC1,* or *RET-PTC3* gene fusions. Several validation studies of this 7-marker panel reported high PPVs among cytologically indeterminate nodules.[81–86] Based on such studies, this 7-marker panel was suggested as a useful test for ruling in cancer, whereby AUS/FLUS and FN/SFN nodules with a positive molecular result could be referred for definitive surgical management (total thyroidectomy) rather than having to undergo a

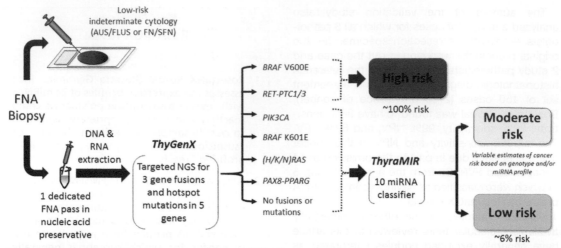

Fig. 6. ThyGenX/ThyraMIR. See text for details. AUS/FLUS, atypia of undetermined significance/follicular lesion of undetermined significance; FN/SFN, follicular neoplasm/suspicious for follicular neoplasm; FNA, fine needle aspiration; miRNA, microRNA; NGS, next-generation sequencing. (*Adapted from* Nishino M, Nikoforova M. Update on molecular testing for cytologically indeterminate thyroid nodules. Arch Pathol Lab Med. https://doi.org/10.5858/arpa.2017-0174-RA; with permission from Archives of Pathology & Laboratory Medicine. Copyright 2018 College of American Pathologists.)

2-staged diagnostic and therapeutic procedure (diagnostic lobectomy followed by completion thyroidectomy).

Nonetheless, the high PPV reported by these studies has not necessarily translated into a high posttest cancer risk for mutation/fusion-positive nodules. Although the presence of any gene mutation or fusion is often considered a positive result in validation studies to simplify statistical analysis, genotyping-based tests do not report binary outcomes (ie, positive vs negative) in practice. Rather, the genetic alterations in this and other genotyping panels are associated with a spectrum of cancer risk. For instance, the *BRAF* V600E mutation and *RET-PTC1/3* gene fusions are associated with near 100% cancer risks.[81–86] In contrast, *RAS* mutations and *PAX8-PPARG* gene fusions have been identified in a continuum of benign, premalignant, and malignant follicular-patterned lesions (ie, follicular adenoma, follicular carcinoma, NIFTP, or encapsulated FV-PTC).[11,83,87–96] Thus, these latter genetic changes may be best considered a marker of neoplasia rather than malignancy per se.

An additional limitation of the 7-marker panel has been its relatively low sensitivity and low NPV. Even in the absence of a genetic alteration from this panel, the residual cancer risk was considered too high to recommend a watchful waiting approach.[83–86,97] In other words, a negative 7-marker panel could not rule out malignancy.

Two companies have taken different approaches to overcome the shortcomings in the NPV of this limited genotyping panel. ThyGenX/ThyraMIR combines genotyping (ThyGenX) with a miRNA-based expression classifier (ThyraMIR) to achieve high sensitivity and NPV for malignancy. In contrast, ThyroSeq uses a vastly expanded panel of mutations and gene fusions to improve the sensitivity and NPV of the genotyping panel.

ThyGenX/ThyraMIR: INCREASING TEST SENSITIVITY BY COMBINING GENOTYPING WITH microRNA EXPRESSION-BASED TESTING

ThyGenX uses targeted next-generation sequencing to detect mutations in 5 genes (*BRAF, HRAS, KRAS, NRAS, PIK3CA*) and 3 chromosomal rearrangements (*RET-PTC1, RET-PTC3, PAX8-PPARG*; **Fig. 6**). Although nodules with *BRAF* V600E mutations and *RET-PTC1/3* rearrangements have a near 100% cancer risk, the panel is limited by both the low specificity of the remaining markers for cancer as well as the nonnegligible residual cancer risk that remains in the absence of mutation/fusion detection. To overcome these challenges, Interpace Diagnostics offers an miRNA-based expression profiler known as ThyraMIR in conjunction with the ThyGenX genotyping panel. ThyraMIR uses quantitative reverse transcriptase polymerase chain reaction to analyze the expression levels of 10 miRNAs and classifies each sample as having either a low-risk or high-risk miRNA profile.

ThyraMIR is intended as a reflex test for samples that are either (a) positive for mutations or gene fusions other than *BRAF* V600E and *RET-PTC1/3* or (b) negative for all the genetic alterations in the panel (see **Fig. 6**). In a prospective multicenter validation study of 109 AUS/FLUS and FN/SFN cases with 32% cancer prevalence, the NPV of the combined testing approach was 94%. In other words, cytologically indeterminate nodules with no mutations/fusions detected by ThyGenX and a low-risk miRNA profile by ThyraMIR have an approximately 6% cancer risk. Such nodules may be appropriate for clinical observation. For other combinations of ThyGenX results (no mutation, *H/K/NRAS* mutations, *PIK3CA* mutation, *BRAF* K601E mutation) and ThyraMIR results (low-risk vs high-risk miRNA profile), Interpace Diagnostics offers variable estimates of cancer risk based on their laboratory data. Lobectomy or near-total thyroidectomy may be considered for these nodules commensurate to the estimated risk and clinical scenario.

Key Features
ThyGenX and ThyraMIR

1. ThyGenX (Interpace Diagnostics, Inc.) uses next-generation sequencing to assay samples for hotspot mutations and fusions in 8 genes (*HRAS, KRAS, NRAS, BRAF, PIK3CA, RET-PTC1i, RET-PTC3,* and *PAX8-PPARG*).

2. ThyraMIR (Interpace Diagnostics, Inc.) assays samples for the expression profiles of 10 miRNAs and uses a proprietary algorithm to classify samples as having a low-risk or high-risk miRNA profile.

3. Samples that are positive for *BRAF* V600E mutation or *RET-PTC1/3* gene fusions by the ThyGenX test are associated with a high cancer risk and generally require surgical referral. ThyraMIR testing is not indicated for these cases.

4. Samples that are (a) positive for the remaining genetic alterations in the ThyGenX panel or (b) negative for all the genetic alterations in the panel are further risk stratified using ThyraMIR. For these cases, variable estimates of cancer risk are provided based on combined ThyGenX/ThyraMIR results.

5. Cases that are negative for both ThyGenX and ThyraMIR testing have a low risk of cancer and may be safe to follow clinically.

ThyroSeq: INCREASING TEST SENSITIVITY BY EXPANDING THE GENOTYPING PANEL

An alternative strategy to improve the performance of the 7-marker genotyping panel has been to augment the number of mutations and fusions in the test panel based on data from large-scale tumor sequencing efforts.[14] ThyroSeq v2 uses targeted next-generation sequencing to assay for 42 gene fusions as well as point mutations and insertions/deletions in 14 genes among cytologically indeterminate thyroid aspirates (**Fig. 7**). ThyroSeq v2 also analyzes samples for the expression of several mRNAs, including those associated with thyroid follicular cells (thyroglobulin [*TG*], *TTF1*, sodium-iodide symporter [*SLC5A5/NIS*], cytokeratin 7 [*KRT7*]), C-cells (calcitonin-related peptide alpha [*CALCA*]), and parathyroid cells (parathyroid hormone [*PTH*]).[98,99] This gene expression analysis helps to establish the cellular composition of the sample (including assessment of follicular cell adequacy), as well as flagging aspirates that are suspicious for medullary carcinoma or parathyroid tissue (based on expression of *CALCA* mRNA or *PTH* mRNA, respectively). Similar to the ThyGenX/ThyraMIR, the ThyroSeq v2 reports a spectrum of cancer risk based on genotype rather than a binary "positive" or "negative" test result.

The ThyroSeq v2 was clinically validated in a single-institution studies involving 239 cytologically indeterminate nodules (96 AUS/FLUS and 143 FN/SFN; combined prevalence of cancer of 26%), where the test was found to have high sensitivity (approximately 90%) and specificity (approximately 93%) for cancer, corresponding with an NPV of approximately 96% and a PPV of approximately 81% in the validation cohorts.[98,99] Postvalidation analyses of ThyroSeq v2 performance from different institutions have confirmed the high NPV of the test in real-world clinical practice.[100–102]

However, these independent institutional experiences with ThyroSeq also highlight a lower PPV (22%–63%) for cancer among cytologically indeterminate nodules than the 81% PPV reported by the validation study. The lower PPV among these postvalidation studies can be attributed to the relative preponderance of histologically benign or premalignant neoplasms harboring *RAS*, *RAS*-like, or *EIF1AX* mutations.[100–103] With the caveats discussed elsewhere in this article, for genotyping tests such as ThyroSeq or ThyGenX/ThyraMIR that offer granular estimates of cancer risk, the overall PPV advertised by the test does not necessarily convert to an approximation of posttest cancer risk.

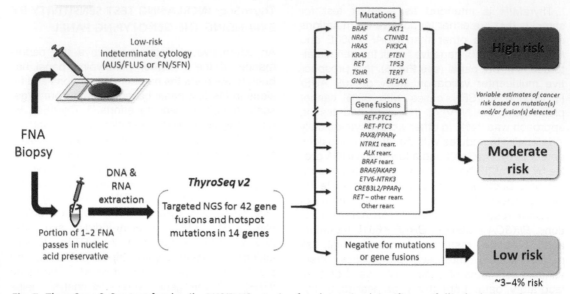

Fig. 7. ThyroSeq v2. See text for details. AUS/FLUS, atypia of undetermined significance/follicular lesion of undetermined significance; FN/SFN, follicular neoplasm/suspicious for follicular neoplasm; FNA, fine needle aspiration; NGS, next-generation sequencing. (*Adapted from* Nishino M, Nikoforova M. Update on molecular testing for cytologically indeterminate thyroid nodules. Arch Pathol Lab Med. https://doi.org/10.5858/arpa.2017-0174-RA; with permission from Archives of Pathology & Laboratory Medicine. Copyright 2018 College of American Pathologists.)

ThyroSeq's broad genotyping panel offers additional opportunities for risk stratification. Genomic profiling studies of clinically aggressive thyroid cancers, including poorly differentiated thyroid cancer and undifferentiated (anaplastic) thyroid cancer, have highlighted an association with *TERT* promoter mutations and *TP53* mutations.[104–109] Even among differentiated thyroid cancers, *TERT* promoter mutation has been associated with more aggressive clinical parameters.[108,110,111] Although broader confirmation of how ThyroSeq v2 results should impact management decisions is still pending, the existing data suggests that the test may help to stratify cytologically indeterminate nodules as follows (see **Fig. 7**).

- Nodules with genetic changes associated with near 100% cancer risks (eg, *BRAF* V600E mutation, *RET-PTC1/3* fusion), as well as nodules harboring markers of aggressive behavior such as *TERT* promoter mutations (either alone or concurrently with other genetic alterations): total thyroidectomy may be considered for such nodules in the appropriate clinical setting.
- Nodules with moderate cancer risks (eg, *RAS*, *RAS*-like, *EIF1AX* mutations): a diagnostic lobectomy may be suitable as the initial surgery.
- Nodules with low cancer risk (ie, negative for all mutations/fusions in the test panel, or positive for a marker associated with benignity): clinical observation may be appropriate.

Key Features
THYROSEQ V2

1. ThyroSeq v2 (University of Pittsburgh Medical Center and CBLPath, Inc.) uses next-generation sequencing to assay samples for genetic changes in 56 genes (hotspot mutations in 14 genes, 42 types of gene fusions).

2. Samples that are negative for ThyroSeq v2 have a low risk of cancer and are generally considered safe to follow clinically.

3. For samples that are positive for ThyroSeq v2, cancer risk estimates are made based on the type of genetic alteration(s) identified. Surgery (either lobectomy or near-total thyroidectomy) is typically indicated in this scenario.

4. The cellular composition of the FNA sample used for ThyroSeq testing is determined by testing for the expression of genes associated with thyroid follicular cells, C-cells/MTC, and parathyroid cells.

5. An updated version of the test known as ThyroSeq v3 was recently released, expanding the test panel to 112 genes. One aim of the updated test is to improve the risk stratification of Hürthle cell rich aspirates.

Recent Updates to ThyroSeq

An updated version of this test analyzing a total of 112 genes has been recently implemented commercially as ThyroSeq v3. In addition to augmenting the panel of genetic alterations from earlier versions of the test, ThyroSeq v3 also assays several genomic regions for copy number alterations that are associated with cancer. ThyroSeq v3 uses a proprietary point-based scoring scheme to weigh different genetic alterations based on their respective cancer risks. The total genetic alterations (or lack thereof) that are detected in a sample are represented as a weighted sum known as the genomic classifier score. Samples with a genomic classifier score below the threshold are reported as negative (ie, favoring benignity), whereas those that are at or beyond the cutoff are reported as positive.[112] Similar to previous versions of ThyroSeq, further cancer risk stratification among positive genomic classifier results should be possible based on the specific genetic alteration. Among 175 thyroid FNAs in the analytical validation study that were enriched for malignancy (52.6% prevalence of cancer), ThyroSeq v3 demonstrated 98.0% specificity and 90.9% sensitivity for cancer.[112] Of note, the resection specimens comprising the training set for ThyroSeq v3 were also enriched for Hürthle cell nodules, with the aim of improving risk stratification among nonneoplastic, benign neoplastic, and malignant Hürthle cell nodules. Clinical validation of ThyroSeq v3 in a prospective, blinded, multicenter study is in progress.

IS ONE MOLECULAR TEST BETTER THAN THE OTHERS?

The 4 commercially available molecular tests summarized herein take different approaches to improve the risk-stratification of cytologically indeterminate thyroid nodules. However, it is uncertain whether these tests are so dissimilar from the end-user's perspective.

- A high NPV is a key objective for each of these tests. Given that the majority of cytologically indeterminate nodules are benign, the ability to select those that are safe to monitor by nonsurgical means is a common and fundamental goal.
- Although the granular cancer risk estimate offered by genotyping-based tests differs from the relatively constrained risk stratification provided by expression classifier-based tests, the impact of these results on subsequent management recommendations seems

to converge for most cytologically indeterminate nodules. As a case in point, the detection of *RAS* and *RAS*-like mutations by genotyping-based tests may offer a more nuanced glimpse into the phenotype and molecular underpinnings of a nodule compared with a suspicious Afirma GEC result with negative Afirma Malignancy Classifiers. However, a similar risk-based management recommendation (diagnostic lobectomy) is generally made for both results, provided that more extensive surgery is not indicated based on clinical and/or ultrasound findings.

Furthermore, although test performance is reflected to some extent by the NPV and PPV reported in validation studies, differences in test design and dissimilarities in their respective validation cohorts limit our ability to compare the clinical usefulness of these tests across studies. In keeping with these observations, the American Thyroid Association's 2015 management guidelines refrain from recommending a particular molecular test for cytologically indeterminate thyroid nodules.[40]

HAS THE NONINVASIVE FOLLICULAR THYROID NEOPLASM WITH PAPILLARY-LIKE NUCLEAR FEATURES NOMENCLATURE CHANGE AFFECTED THE USEFULNESS OF MOLECULAR TESTS?

The impact of the NIFTP reclassification on the usefulness of these ancillary molecular tests continues to evolve. The 4 commercially available tests discussed herein were developed and validated at a time when noninvasive, encapsulated FVPTCs were generally classified as malignant. Consequently, each of these tests would be expected to flag NIFTPs as abnormal. Along those lines, retrospective studies of institutional experiences with ancillary molecular tests have found NIFTPs among nodules classified as having either a suspicious gene expression profile (by Afirma GEC)[65,113–115] or *RAS* (and *RAS*-like) mutations/fusions by genotyping tests such as ThyroSeq.[87,102,113] Some authors consider these molecular results to represent false-positive outcomes with regard to NIFTP and have advocated a revalidation of these molecular tests in light of the recent NIFTP reclassification.[116] Yet, it remains unclear whether it is appropriate to conflate NIFTPs with nodules demonstrating overtly benign histology. Although the NIFTP nomenclature change underscores their indolent behavior, these tumors may be considered premalignant neoplasms for which a lobectomy is warranted from a diagnostic and therapeutic standpoint.[11,117] From this perspective, the recognition of NIFTPs as abnormal by these molecular tests seems to be compatible with existing recommendations for diagnostic lobectomy for nodules with suspicious Afirma results or *RAS* and *RAS*-like mutations by genotyping tests.

Key Features
NONINVASIVE FOLLICULAR THYROID NEOPLASM WITH PAPILLARY-LIKE NUCLEAR FEATURES

1. A subset of well-circumscribed/encapsulated FV-PTC with no evidence of invasion was recently reclassified as NIFTP.

2. NIFTPs are indolent tumors that may represent precursors to their invasive counterparts (invasive encapsulated FV-PTC).

3. FNA samples of NIFTP are usually classified in one of the 3 indeterminate categories of TBSRTC: AUS/FLUS, FN/SFN, or suspicious for malignancy.

4. Lobectomy is diagnostically necessary and therapeutically sufficient for NIFTP.

5. NIFTP are commonly microfollicular on FNA, lack papillae and psammoma bodies, and only rarely exhibit intranuclear pseudoinclusions. These features help to distinguish NIFTP from cPTC and can be used to minimize falsely malignant cytologic diagnoses for NIFTPs.

SUMMARY

Studies over the past several years have inspired a more nuanced model of thyroid neoplasia. In parallel with this development, there has been growing recognition that conservative therapeutic options may be appropriate for carefully selected low-risk thyroid neoplasms. Both the NIFTP nomenclature change and the increasing use of molecular testing for preoperative risk stratification exemplify this trend toward a more individualized approach to thyroid nodule management.

REFERENCES

1. Rivera M, Ricarte-Filho J, Knauf J, et al. Molecular genotyping of papillary thyroid carcinoma follicular variant according to its histological subtypes (encapsulated vs infiltrative) reveals distinct BRAF and RAS mutation patterns. Mod Pathol 2010; 23(9):1191–200.

2. Zhao L, Dias-Santagata D, Sadow PM, et al. Cytological, molecular, and clinical features of noninvasive follicular thyroid neoplasm with papillary-like nuclear features versus invasive forms of follicular variant of papillary thyroid carcinoma. Cancer Cytopathol 2017;125(5): 323–31.

3. Kim TH, Lee M, Kwon AY, et al. Molecular genotyping of the non-invasive encapsulated follicular variant of papillary thyroid carcinoma. Histopathology 2018;72(4):648–61.

4. Finnerty BM, Kleiman DA, Scognamiglio T, et al. Navigating the management of follicular variant papillary thyroid carcinoma subtypes: a classic PTC comparison. Ann Surg Oncol 2015;22(4): 1200–6.

5. Ghossein R. Encapsulated malignant follicular cell-derived thyroid tumors. Endocr Pathol 2010;21(4): 212–8.

6. Ganly I, Wang L, Tuttle RM, et al. Invasion rather than nuclear features correlates with outcome in encapsulated follicular tumors: further evidence for the reclassification of the encapsulated papillary thyroid carcinoma follicular variant. Hum Pathol 2015;46(5):657–64.

7. Rivera M, Tuttle RM, Patel S, et al. Encapsulated papillary thyroid carcinoma: a clinico-pathologic study of 106 cases with emphasis on its morphologic subtypes (histologic growth pattern). Thyroid 2009;19(2):119–27.

8. Gupta S, Ajise O, Dultz L, et al. Follicular variant of papillary thyroid cancer: encapsulated, nonencapsulated, and diffuse: distinct biologic and clinical entities. Arch Otolaryngol Head Neck Surg 2012; 138(3):227–33.

9. Howitt BE, Jia Y, Sholl LM, et al. Molecular alterations in partially-encapsulated or well-circumscribed follicular variant of papillary thyroid carcinoma. Thyroid 2013;23(10):1256–62.

10. Liu J, Singh B, Tallini G, et al. Follicular variant of papillary thyroid carcinoma: a clinicopathologic study of a problematic entity. Cancer 2006;107(6): 1255–64.

11. Nikiforov YE, Seethala RR, Tallini G, et al. Nomenclature revision for encapsulated follicular variant of papillary thyroid carcinoma: a paradigm shift to reduce overtreatment of indolent tumors. JAMA Oncol 2016;2(8):1023–9.

12. Vivero M, Kraft S, Barletta JA. Risk stratification of follicular variant of papillary thyroid carcinoma. Thyroid 2013;23(3):273–9.

13. Thompson LD. Ninety-four cases of encapsulated follicular variant of papillary thyroid carcinoma: a name change to noninvasive follicular thyroid neoplasm with papillary-like nuclear features would help prevent overtreatment. Mod Pathol 2016; 29(7):698–707.

14. Cancer Genome Atlas Research Network. Integrated genomic characterization of papillary thyroid carcinoma. Cell 2014;159(3):676–90.

15. Nikiforov YE, Nikiforova MN. Molecular genetics and diagnosis of thyroid cancer. Nat Rev Endocrinol 2011;7(10):569–80.

16. Yoo SK, Lee S, Kim SJ, et al. Comprehensive analysis of the transcriptional and mutational landscape of follicular and papillary thyroid cancers. PLoS Genet 2016;12(8):e1006239.

17. Panebianco F, Kelly LM, Liu P, et al. THADA fusion is a mechanism of IGF2BP3 activation and IGF1R signaling in thyroid cancer. Proc Natl Acad Sci U S A 2017;114(9):2307–12.

18. Seethala RR, Baloch ZW, Barletta JA, et al. Noninvasive follicular thyroid neoplasm with papillary-like nuclear features: a review for pathologists. Mod Pathol 2018;31(1):39–55.

19. Maletta F, Massa F, Torregrossa L, et al. Cytological features of "noninvasive follicular thyroid neoplasm with papillary-like nuclear features" and their correlation with tumor histology. Hum Pathol 2016;54:134–42.

20. Brandler TC, Zhou F, Liu CZ, et al. Can noninvasive follicular thyroid neoplasm with papillary-like nuclear features be distinguished from classic papillary thyroid carcinoma and follicular adenomas by fine-needle aspiration? Cancer 2017;125(6):378–88.

21. Strickland KC, Howitt BE, Barletta JA, et al. Suggesting the cytologic diagnosis of noninvasive follicular thyroid neoplasm with papillary-like nuclear features (NIFTP): a retrospective analysis of atypical and suspicious nodules. Cancer Cytopathol 2018;126(2):86–93.

22. Bizzarro T, Martini M, Capodimonti S, et al. Young investigator challenge: the morphologic analysis of noninvasive follicular thyroid neoplasm with papillary-like nuclear features on liquid-based cytology: some insights into their identification. Cancer 2016;124(10):699–710.

23. Strickland KC, Vivero M, Jo VY, et al. Preoperative cytologic diagnosis of noninvasive follicular thyroid neoplasm with papillary-like nuclear features: a prospective analysis. Thyroid 2016;26(10):1466–71.

24. Howitt BE, Chang S, Eszlinger M, et al. Fine-needle aspiration diagnoses of noninvasive follicular variant of papillary thyroid carcinoma. Am J Clin Pathol 2015;144(6):850–7.

25. Mito JK, Alexander EK, Angell TE, et al. A modified reporting approach for thyroid FNA in the NIFTP era: a 1-year institutional experience. Cancer Cytopathol 2017;125(11):854–64.

26. Ibrahim AA, Wu HH. Fine-needle aspiration cytology of noninvasive follicular variant of papillary thyroid carcinoma is cytomorphologically distinct from the invasive counterpart. Am J Clin Pathol 2016;146(3):373–7.

27. Krane JF, Alexander EK, Cibas ES, et al. Coming to terms with NIFTP: a provisional approach for cytologists. Cancer Cytopathol 2016;124(11):767–72.

28. Cibas ES, Ali SZ. The 2017 Bethesda system for reporting thyroid cytopathology. Thyroid 2017;27(11):1341–6.

29. Canberk S, Gunes P, Onenerk M, et al. New Concept of the encapsulated follicular variant of papillary thyroid carcinoma and its impact on The Bethesda System for Reporting Thyroid Cytopathology: a single-institute experience. Acta Cytol 2016;60(3):198–204.

30. Layfield LJ, Baloch ZW, Esebua M, et al. Impact of the reclassification of the non-invasive follicular variant of papillary carcinoma as benign on the malignancy risk of the Bethesda System for Reporting Thyroid Cytopathology: a meta-analysis study. Acta Cytol 2017;61(3):187–93.

31. Zhou H, Baloch ZW, Nayar R, et al. Noninvasive follicular thyroid neoplasm with papillary-like nuclear features (NIFTP): implications for the risk of malignancy (ROM) in the Bethesda system for reporting thyroid cytopathology (TBSRTC). Cancer 2017;126(1):20–6.

32. Strickland KC, Howitt BE, Marqusee E, et al. The impact of noninvasive follicular variant of papillary thyroid carcinoma on rates of malignancy for fine-needle aspiration diagnostic categories. Thyroid 2015;25(9):987–92.

33. Faquin WC, Wong LQ, Afrogheh AH, et al. Impact of reclassifying noninvasive follicular variant of papillary thyroid carcinoma on the risk of malignancy in the Bethesda system for reporting thyroid cytopathology. Cancer Cytopathol 2016;124(3):181–7.

34. Ohori NP, Wolfe J, Carty SE, et al. The influence of the noninvasive follicular thyroid neoplasm with papillary-like nuclear features (NIFTP) resection diagnosis on the false-positive thyroid cytology rate relates to quality assurance thresholds and the application of NIFTP criteria. Cancer Cytopathol 2017;125(9):692–700.

35. Valderrabano P, Khazai L, Thompson ZJ, et al. Cancer risk associated with nuclear atypia in cytologically indeterminate thyroid nodules: a systematic review and meta-analysis. Thyroid 2018;28(2):210–9.

36. American Thyroid Association Guidelines Taskforce on Thyroid Nodules and Differentiated Thyroid Cancer, Cooper DS, Doherty GM, Haugen BR, et al. Revised American Thyroid Association management guidelines for patients with thyroid nodules and differentiated thyroid cancer. Thyroid 2009;19(11):1167–214.

37. Matsuzu K, Sugino K, Masudo K, et al. Thyroid lobectomy for papillary thyroid cancer: long-term follow-up study of 1,088 cases. World J Surg 2014;38(1):68–79.

38. Mendelsohn AH, Elashoff DA, Abemayor E, et al. Surgery for papillary thyroid carcinoma: is lobectomy enough? Arch Otolaryngol Head Neck Surg 2010;136(11):1055–61.

39. Nixon IJ, Ganly I, Patel SG, et al. Thyroid lobectomy for treatment of well differentiated intrathyroid malignancy. Surgery 2012;151(4):571–9.

40. Haugen BR, Alexander EK, Bible KC, et al. 2015 American thyroid association management guidelines for adult patients with thyroid nodules and differentiated thyroid cancer: the American thyroid association guidelines task force on thyroid nodules and differentiated thyroid cancer. Thyroid 2016;26(1):1–133.

41. Bongiovanni M, Spitale A, Faquin WC, et al. The Bethesda system for reporting thyroid cytopathology: a meta-analysis. Acta Cytol 2012;56(4):333–9.

42. Ferris RL, Baloch Z, Bernet V, et al. American thyroid association statement on surgical application of molecular profiling for thyroid nodules: current impact on perioperative decision making. Thyroid 2015;25(7):760–8.

43. Valderrabano P, Leon ME, Centeno BA, et al. Institutional prevalence of malignancy of indeterminate thyroid cytology is necessary but insufficient to accurately interpret molecular marker tests. Eur J Endocrinol 2016;174(5):621–9.

44. Cibas ES, Baloch ZW, Fellegara G, et al. A prospective assessment defining the limitations of thyroid nodule pathologic evaluation. Ann Intern Med 2013;159(5):325–32.

45. Elsheikh TM, Asa SL, Chan JK, et al. Interobserver and intraobserver variation among experts in the diagnosis of thyroid follicular lesions with borderline nuclear features of papillary carcinoma. Am J Clin Pathol 2008;130(5):736–44.

46. Lloyd RV, Erickson LA, Casey MB, et al. Observer variation in the diagnosis of follicular variant of papillary thyroid carcinoma. Am J Surg Pathol 2004;28(10):1336–40.

47. Widder S, Guggisberg K, Khalil M, et al. A pathologic re-review of follicular thyroid neoplasms: the impact of changing the threshold for the diagnosis of the follicular variant of papillary thyroid carcinoma. Surgery 2008;144(1):80–5.

48. Chudova D, Wilde JI, Wang ET, et al. Molecular classification of thyroid nodules using high-dimensionality genomic data. J Clin Endocrinol Metab 2010;95(12):5296–304.

49. Eszlinger M, Krohn K, Frenzel H, et al. Gene expression analysis reveals evidence for inactivation of the TGF-beta signaling cascade in autonomously functioning thyroid nodules. Oncogene 2004;23(3):795–804.

50. Eszlinger M, Wiench M, Jarzab B, et al. Meta- and reanalysis of gene expression profiles of hot and cold thyroid nodules and papillary thyroid carcinoma for gene groups. J Clin Endocrinol Metab 2006;91(5):1934–42.

51. Mazzanti C, Zeiger MA, Costouros NG, et al. Using gene expression profiling to differentiate benign versus malignant thyroid tumors. Cancer Res 2004;64(8):2898–903.

52. Dettmer M, Perren A, Moch H, et al. Comprehensive MicroRNA expression profiling identifies novel markers in follicular variant of papillary thyroid carcinoma. Thyroid 2013;23(11):1383–9.

53. Dettmer M, Vogetseder A, Durso MB, et al. MicroRNA expression array identifies novel diagnostic markers for conventional and oncocytic follicular thyroid carcinomas. J Clin Endocrinol Metab 2013;98(1):E1–7.

54. Dettmer MS, Perren A, Moch H, et al. MicroRNA profile of poorly differentiated thyroid carcinomas: new diagnostic and prognostic insights. J Mol Endocrinol 2014;52(2):181–9.

55. Nikiforova MN, Tseng GC, Steward D, et al. MicroRNA expression profiling of thyroid tumors: biological significance and diagnostic utility. J Clin Endocrinol Metab 2008;93(5):1600–8.

56. Rossi ED, Bizzarro T, Martini M, et al. The evaluation of miRNAs on thyroid FNAC: the promising role of miR-375 in follicular neoplasms. Endocrine 2016;54(3):723–32.

57. Yip L, Kelly L, Shuai Y, et al. MicroRNA signature distinguishes the degree of aggressiveness of papillary thyroid carcinoma. Ann Surg Oncol 2011;18(7):2035–41.

58. Alexander EK, Kennedy GC, Baloch ZW, et al. Preoperative diagnosis of benign thyroid nodules with indeterminate cytology. N Engl J Med 2012;367(8):705–15.

59. Kloos RT, Monroe RJ, Traweek ST, et al. A genomic alternative to identify medullary thyroid cancer preoperatively in thyroid nodules with indeterminate cytology. Thyroid 2016;26(6):785–93.

60. Pankratz DG, Hu Z, Kim SY, et al. Analytical performance of a gene expression classifier for medullary thyroid carcinoma. Thyroid 2016;26(11):1573–80.

61. Wells SA Jr, Asa SL, Dralle H, et al. Revised American Thyroid Association guidelines for the management of medullary thyroid carcinoma. Thyroid 2015;25(6):567–610.

62. Kloos RT, Reynolds JD, Walsh PS, et al. Does addition of BRAF V600E mutation testing modify sensitivity or specificity of the Afirma gene expression classifier in cytologically indeterminate thyroid nodules? J Clin Endocrinol Metab 2013;98(4):E761–8.

63. Pusztaszeri MP, Krane JF, Faquin WC. BRAF testing and thyroid FNA. Cancer Cytopathol 2015; 123(12):689–95.

64. Wu JX, Young S, Hung ML, et al. Clinical factors influencing the performance of gene expression classifier testing in indeterminate thyroid nodules. Thyroid 2016;26(7):916–22.

65. Samulski TD, LiVolsi VA, Wong LQ, et al. Usage trends and performance characteristics of a "gene expression classifier" in the management of thyroid nodules: an institutional experience. Diagn Cytopathol 2016;44(11):867–73.

66. Angell TE, Frates MC, Medici M, et al. Afirma benign thyroid nodules show similar growth to cyto-logically benign nodules during follow-up. J Clin Endocrinol Metab 2015;100(11):E1477–83.

67. Alexander EK, Schorr M, Klopper J, et al. Multi-center clinical experience with the Afirma gene expression classifier. J Clin Endocrinol Metab 2014;99(1):119–25.

68. Chaudhary S, Hou Y, Shen R, et al. Impact of the Afirma gene expression classifier result on the sur-gical management of thyroid nodules with category III/IV cytology and its correlation with surgical outcome. Acta Cytol 2016;60(3):205–10.

69. Marti JL, Avadhani V, Donatelli LA, et al. Wide inter-institutional variation in performance of a molecular classifier for indeterminate thyroid nodules. Ann Surg Oncol 2015;22(12):3996–4001.

70. Harrell RM, Bimston DN. Surgical utility of Afirma: effects of high cancer prevalence and oncocytic cell types in patients with indeterminate thyroid cytology. Endocr Pract 2014;20(4):364–9.

71. Celik B, Whetsell CR, Nassar A. Afirma GEC and thyroid lesions: an institutional experience. Diagn Cytopathol 2015;43(12):966–70.

72. Sacks WL, Bose S, Zumsteg ZS, et al. Impact of Afirma gene expression classifier on cytopathology diagnosis and rate of thyroidectomy. Cancer 2016; 124(10):722–8.

73. McIver B, Castro MR, Morris JC, et al. An indepen-dent study of a gene expression classifier (Afirma) in the evaluation of cytologically indeterminate thy-roid nodules. J Clin Endocrinol Metab 2014;99(11): 4069–77.

74. Brauner E, Holmes BJ, Krane JF, et al. Perfor-mance of the Afirma gene expression classifier in Hurthle cell thyroid nodules differs from other indeterminate thyroid nodules. Thyroid 2015; 25(7):789–96.

75. Villabona CV, Mohan V, Arce KM, et al. Utility of ul-trasound versus gene expression classifier in thy-roid nodules with atypia of undetermined significance. Endocr Pract 2016;22(10):1199–203.

76. Lastra RR, Pramick MR, Crammer CJ, et al. Impli-cations of a suspicious Afirma test result in thyroid fine-needle aspiration cytology: an institutional

experience. Cancer Cytopathol 2014;122(10): 737–44.

77. Harrison G, Sosa JA, Jiang X. Evaluation of the Afirma gene expression classifier in repeat indeter-minate thyroid nodules. Arch Pathol Lab Med 2017; 141(7):985–9.

78. Yang SE, Sullivan PS, Zhang J, et al. Has Afirma gene expression classifier testing refined the inde-terminate thyroid category in cytology? Cancer Cy-topathol 2016;124(2):100–9.

79. Duh QY, Busaidy NL, Rahilly-Tierney C, et al. A systematic review of the methods of diagnostic accuracy studies of the Afirma gene expression classifier. Thyroid 2017;27(10):1215–22.

80. Lithwick-Yanai G, Dromi N, Shtabsky A, et al. Multi-centre validation of a microRNA-based assay for diagnosing indeterminate thyroid nodules utilising fine needle aspirate smears. J Clin Pathol 2017; 70(6):500–7.

81. Nikiforov YE, Steward DL, Robinson-Smith TM, et al. Molecular testing for mutations in improving the fine-needle aspiration diagnosis of thyroid nod-ules. J Clin Endocrinol Metab 2009;94(6):2092–8.

82. Cantara S, Capezzone M, Marchisotta S, et al. Impact of proto-oncogene mutation detection in cytological specimens from thyroid nodules im-proves the diagnostic accuracy of cytology. J Clin Endocrinol Metab 2010;95(3):1365–9.

83. Nikiforov YE, Ohori NP, Hodak SP, et al. Impact of mutational testing on the diagnosis and manage-ment of patients with cytologically indeterminate thyroid nodules: a prospective analysis of 1056 FNA samples. J Clin Endocrinol Metab 2011; 96(11):3390–7.

84. Beaudenon-Huibregtse S, Alexander EK, Guttler RB, et al. Centralized molecular testing for oncogenic gene mutations complements the local cytopathologic diagnosis of thyroid nodules. Thy-roid 2014;24(10):1479–87.

85. Eszlinger M, Piana S, Moll A, et al. Molecular testing of thyroid fine-needle aspirations improves presurgical diagnosis and supports the histologic identification of minimally invasive follicular thyroid carcinomas. Thyroid 2015;25(4):401–9.

86. Labourier E, Shifrin A, Busseniers AE, et al. Molecular testing for miRNA, mRNA, and DNA on fine-needle aspiration improves the preoperative diagnosis of thyroid nodules with indeterminate cytology. J Clin Endocrinol Metab 2015;100(7):2743–50.

87. Paulson VA, Shivdasani P, Angell TE, et al. Noninva-sive follicular thyroid neoplasm with papillary-like nuclear features accounts for more than half of "Carcinomas" harboring RAS mutations. Thyroid 2017;27(4):506–11.

88. Medici M, Kwong N, Angell TE, et al. The variable phenotype and low-risk nature of RAS-positive thy-roid nodules. BMC Med 2015;13:184.

89. Nikiforov YE. Role of molecular markers in thyroid nodule management: then and now. Endocr Pract 2017;23(8):979–88.

90. Eszlinger M, Bohme K, Ullmann M, et al. Evaluation of a two-year routine application of molecular testing of thyroid fine-needle aspirations using a seven-gene panel in a primary referral setting in Germany. Thyroid 2017;27(3):402–11.

91. Armstrong MJ, Yang H, Yip L, et al. PAX8/PPAR-gamma rearrangement in thyroid nodules predicts follicular-pattern carcinomas, in particular the encapsulated follicular variant of papillary carcinoma. Thyroid 2014;24(9):1369–74.

92. Eberhardt NL, Grebe SK, McIver B, et al. The role of the PAX8/PPARgamma fusion oncogene in the pathogenesis of follicular thyroid cancer. Mol Cell Endocrinol 2010;321(1):50–6.

93. Giordano TJ, Beaudenon-Huibregtse S, Shinde R, et al. Molecular testing for oncogenic gene mutations in thyroid lesions: a case-control validation study in 413 postsurgical specimens. Hum Pathol 2014;45(7):1339–47.

94. Krane JF, Cibas ES, Alexander EK, et al. Molecular analysis of residual ThinPrep material from thyroid FNAs increases diagnostic sensitivity. Cancer Cytopathol 2015;123(6):356–61.

95. Najafian A, Noureldine S, Azar F, et al. RAS mutations, and RET/PTC and PAX8/PPAR-gamma chromosomal rearrangements are also prevalent in benign thyroid lesions: implications thereof and a systematic review. Thyroid 2017;27(1):39–48.

96. Nikiforova MN, Lynch RA, Biddinger PW, et al. RAS point mutations and PAX8-PPAR gamma rearrangement in thyroid tumors: evidence for distinct molecular pathways in thyroid follicular carcinoma. J Clin Endocrinol Metab 2003;88(5):2318–26.

97. Eszlinger M, Krogdahl A, Munz S, et al. Impact of molecular screening for point mutations and rearrangements in routine air-dried fine-needle aspiration samples of thyroid nodules. Thyroid 2014; 24(2):305–13.

98. Nikiforov YE, Carty SE, Chiosea SI, et al. Highly accurate diagnosis of cancer in thyroid nodules with follicular neoplasm/suspicious for a follicular neoplasm cytology by ThyroSeq v2 next-generation sequencing assay. Cancer 2014; 120(23):3627–34.

99. Nikiforov YE, Carty SE, Chiosea SI, et al. Impact of the multi-gene ThyroSeq next-generation sequencing assay on cancer diagnosis in thyroid nodules with atypia of undetermined significance/ follicular lesion of undetermined significance cytology. Thyroid 2015;25(11):1217–23.

100. Shrestha RT, Evasovich MR, Amin K, et al. Correlation between histological diagnosis and mutational panel testing of thyroid nodules: a two-year institutional experience. Thyroid 2016;26(8):1068–76.

101. Taye A, Gurciullo D, Miles BA, et al. Clinical performance of a next-generation sequencing assay (ThyroSeq v2) in the evaluation of indeterminate thyroid nodules. Surgery 2018;163(1):97–103.

102. Valderrabano P, Khazai L, Leon ME, et al. Evaluation of ThyroSeq v2 performance in thyroid nodules with indeterminate cytology. Endocr Relat Cancer 2017;24(3):127–36.

103. Karunamurthy A, Panebianco F, S JH, et al. Prevalence and phenotypic correlations of EIF1AX mutations in thyroid nodules. Endocr Relat Cancer 2016; 23(4):295–301.

104. Xu B, Ghossein R. Genomic landscape of poorly differentiated and anaplastic thyroid carcinoma. Endocr Pathol 2016;27(3):205–12.

105. Landa I, Ganly I, Chan TA, et al. Frequent somatic TERT promoter mutations in thyroid cancer: higher prevalence in advanced forms of the disease. J Clin Endocrinol Metab 2013;98(9):E1562–6.

106. Landa I, Ibrahimpasic T, Boucai L, et al. Genomic and transcriptomic hallmarks of poorly differentiated and anaplastic thyroid cancers. J Clin Invest 2016;126(3):1052–66.

107. Liu T, Wang N, Cao J, et al. The age- and shorter telomere-dependent TERT promoter mutation in follicular thyroid cell-derived carcinomas. Oncogene 2014;33(42):4978–84.

108. Melo M, da Rocha AG, Vinagre J, et al. TERT promoter mutations are a major indicator of poor outcome in differentiated thyroid carcinomas. J Clin Endocrinol Metab 2014;99(5):E754–65.

109. Song YS, Lim JA, Choi H, et al. Prognostic effects of TERT promoter mutations are enhanced by coexistence with BRAF or RAS mutations and strengthen the risk prediction by the ATA or TNM staging system in differentiated thyroid cancer patients. Cancer 2016;122(9):1370–9.

110. Xu B, Tuttle RM, Sabra MM, et al. Primary thyroid carcinoma with low-risk histology and distant metastases: clinicopathologic and molecular characteristics. Thyroid 2017;27(5):632–40.

111. Vuong HG, Duong UN, Altibi AM, et al. A meta-analysis of prognostic roles of molecular markers in papillary thyroid carcinoma. Endocr Connect 2017;6(3):R8–17.

112. Nikiforova MN, Mercurio S, Wald AI, et al. Analytical performance of the ThyroSeq v3 genomic classifier for cancer diagnosis in thyroid nodules. Cancer 2018;124(8):1682–90.

113. Jiang XS, Harrison GP, Datto MB. Young investigator challenge: molecular testing in noninvasive follicular thyroid neoplasm with papillary-like nuclear features. Cancer 2016;124(12):893–900.

114. Wong KS, Angell TE, Strickland KC, et al. Noninvasive follicular variant of papillary thyroid carcinoma and the Afirma gene-expression classifier. Thyroid 2016;26(7):911–5.

115. Hang JF, Westra WH, Cooper DS, et al. The impact of noninvasive follicular thyroid neoplasm with papillary-like nuclear features on the performance of the Afirma gene expression classifier. Cancer Cytopathol 2017;125(9):683–91.

116. Sahli ZT, Umbricht CB, Schneider EB, et al. Thyroid nodule diagnostic markers in the face of the new NIFTP category: time for a reset? Thyroid 2017; 27(11):1393–9.

117. Cho U, Mete O, Kim MH, et al. Molecular correlates and rate of lymph node metastasis of non-invasive follicular thyroid neoplasm with papillary-like nuclear features and invasive follicular variant papillary thyroid carcinoma: the impact of rigid criteria to distinguish non-invasive follicular thyroid neoplasm with papillary-like nuclear features. Mod Pathol 2017;30(6):810–25.

Updates in Salivary Gland Fine Needle Aspiration Biopsy
The Use of the Milan System and Ancillary Testing

Edward B. Stelow, MD

KEYWORDS

• Fine needle aspiration biopsy • Salivary gland • Milan System • Ancillary Testing

Key points

• Salivary gland fine needle aspiration biopsies remain common specimens seen by most cytology services.

• The diagnostic diversity and overlap between many of the lesions seen with these biopsies impart many challenges for the cytopathologist, rendering most specific diagnoses impossible with cytology alone.

• Here, the use of the Milan System for the classification of salivary gland fine needle aspiration biopsy is discussed, together with the potential use of ancillary testing in arriving at definitive diagnoses.

ABSTRACT

Salivary gland fine needle aspiration biopsies remain common specimens seen by most cytology services. The diagnostic diversity and overlap between many of the lesions seen with these biopsies impart many challenges for the cytopathologist, rendering most specific diagnoses impossible with cytology alone. Here, the use of the Milan System for the classification of salivary gland fine needle aspiration biopsy FNAB is discussed, together with the potential use of ancillary testing in arriving at definitive diagnoses.

OVERVIEW

The usefulness of fine needle aspiration biopsy (FNAB) varies from site to site. With the thyroid, it is typically used as a screening test to determine whether a patient has surgery for a nodule and what type of surgery he or she will undergo.[1] Pancreatic FNAB is typically used to definitively diagnose mass lesions and, in most cases, diagnosis is required before the initiation of nonsurgical therapy.[2] With lung FNAB, the use is similar; however, the need for extensive ancillary testing to triage toward targeted or immunomodulating therapies typically requires the obtainment of more abundant materials than are required for diagnosis alone.[3]

Fine needle aspiration of salivary gland mass lesions for the triage and treatment of patients has been performed for more than 50 years.[4] At this site, FNAB is used most similarly to FNAB of the thyroid, as a method to direct whether and to what extent surgical therapy is necessary.[5] There are some differences, however.

Department of Pathology, UVA Hospital, University of Virginia, MC 800214, Jefferson Park Avenue, Charlottesville, VA 22908, USA
E-mail address: edstelow@yahoo.com

Surgical Pathology 11 (2018) 489–500
https://doi.org/10.1016/j.path.2018.04.003
1875-9181/18/© 2018 Elsevier Inc. All rights reserved.

Unlike with the thyroid, where most nodules are nonneoplastic and do not require surgery, most salivary gland mass lesions represent neoplasia and require surgery.[1,6–8] Neoplastic thyroid histology, although fret with interobserver variability and morphologic overlap, is relatively straightforward. The World Health Organization classification system for neoplasia of the salivary gland is much more complicated and many of the lesions show marked histologic overlap and/or require the assessment of parameters that can only be seen on histologic sections (eg, vascular invasion) to determine whether the neoplasm is malignant.[9] The World Health Organization currently lists more than 30 benign and malignant epithelial tumors. This is further complicated by the fact that lymph nodes are frequently intimately associated with the parotid gland and that those lymph nodes represent common sites of metastases for cancers of the facial skin or sinonasal tract.[10]

Because of the numerous entities, the frequent histologic overlap between those entities, and the necessity for histology to fully classify some lesions, FNAB of the salivary gland often results in imprecise diagnoses, although there are again notable exceptions (eg, most reactive lymph nodes and pleomorphic adenomas can be diagnosed definitively).[6,7] As such, FNABs of salivary gland masses are often signed out with descriptive diagnoses of recurring categories.

THE MILAN SYSTEM FOR THE CLASSIFICATION OF SALIVARY GLAND FINE NEEDLE ASPIRATION BIOPSY DIAGNOSES

RISK

Because descriptive diagnoses or categories can vary greatly between institutions, there has recently been a movement to systematize salivary gland FNAB sign-out.[7,11–14] The consensus system is now referred to as The Milan System. It uses a 6-tiered classification system akin to that used at other sites (eg, the thyroid gland; **Table 1**). The system itself uses and attempts to codify the most common interpretations seen with salivary gland FNAB.

The categorical system is supposed to allow for risk stratification and treatment, although, similar to the Bethesda System for the classification of Pancreatic Cytologic samples, specific diagnoses or subcategories within the system may be the best predictor of malignancy. For example, an interpretation of suspicious for a high-grade malignancy may function differently than an interpretation of suspicious for low-grade malignancy, and

Table 1
Milan system for the classification of salivary gland fine needle aspiration biopsy

I		Nondiagnostic
II		Nonneoplastic
III		Atypical
IV		Neoplasm
	IVa	Benign neoplasm
	IVb	Neoplasm of unknown malignant potential
V		Suspicious for malignancy
VI		Malignant neoplasm

different surgical treatment may be required for the 2 interpretations.

The data regarding outcomes for the Milan tiered approach are limited at this time.[7,15–17] The risk that a nondiagnostic interpretation will be associated with benign or malignant neoplasia may be up to 44% and 25%, respectively, reports 1 study based on a retrospective study of the literature.[7] This finding likely reflects the overall risks for salivary gland mass lesions that present for biopsy. Included here, too, are aspirates that show only cyst contents, a known proportion of which represent neoplasia, especially low-grade mucoepidermoid carcinoma.

The same retrospective study estimates that aspirates interpreted as nonneoplastic have risks for benign and malignant neoplasia of 13% and 10%, respectively.[7] It is unclear what causes these errors. Interpretative error seems unlikely aside from with low-grade lymphocytic malignancies.[18] Sampling likely plays a role, and it may be that some changes seen with salivary gland histology adjacent to neoplasia may lead to the false judgment that they represent the mass lesion itself. This would be akin to a diagnosis of chronic pancreatitis for an aspirate of a pancreatic mass, where the chronic pancreatitis has developed secondary to an unsampled adenocarcinoma.[19] It may also be that some samples showing only normal salivary gland have been included here.

Two recent studies have looked at the more subjective interpretations of atypical and suspicious by accumulating data retrospectively from multiple institutions.[16,17] In 1 study, the authors found that approximately 4% of salivary gland FNABs were interpreted as atypical, and that the risks for benign and malignant neoplasia were 7% and 19%, respectively.[16] It should be noted, however, that only 01% of cases had follow-up. The authors of the other article found that 2.2% of salivary gland FNABs were interpreted as suspicious, and that the risks for benign and malignant neoplasia for this interpretation were 13% and 83%, respectively.[17] This finding is at variance with another study that showed rates of benign and malignant neoplasia at 36% and 59%, respectively.[7] The high rate of malignancy for such a diagnosis suggests that the suspicious category may be used for tumors showing obvious cytologic atypia, something not usually seen with the lower grade malignancies. The variance with outcomes suggests some variability in how the diagnosis is used with some cytologic specimens.

Of salivary gland FNABs interpreted as benign neoplasm, 95% have been from benign neoplasms and 3% have been from malignancies.[7] This finding likely has to do with the facts that (1) the definite diagnosis of benign neoplasia is usually made when the prototypical cytologic features of pleomorphic adenoma or Warthin tumor are seen, (2) pleomorphic adenoma and Warthin tumors are much more common than other salivary gland tumors, and (3) the prototypical cytologic features seen with the 2 tumors do not overlap with any other common tumors.[20] Undoubtedly, some pleomorphic adenomas will have unsampled malignancies (carcinoma ex pleomorphic adenoma) and some uncommon malignancies may show cytomorphologies almost identical to those of Warthin tumor (eg, oncocytic mucoepidermoid carcinoma).[21,22]

Samples interpreted as showing neoplasia of unknown malignant potential show follow-up rates of benign and malignant neoplasia of 48% and 38%, respectively.[7] Thus, a slight majority the neoplasms interpreted within this category are benign. As with the diagnosis of suspicious, there may be some variability as to whether one categorizes an aspirate here or not. Stated elsewhere in this article, this category is for aspirates that are diagnostic but for which either resection or additional material is required to make a more specific diagnosis. In addition, some recurring subpatterns may be seen within this category, such as those from a basaloid neoplasm or oncocytic neoplasm.[12,23] These subcategories may be actually associated with different risks for benign and malignant neoplasia. Indeed, even further divisions of these groups may be possible and may allow for further risk stratification.[12]

Definitive diagnosis as malignancy should carry with it a very high positive predictive value, at or near 100%.[15] This is because the diagnosis will potentially be used to justify nonsurgical oncologic treatment in some cases, such as radiation therapy. Although some authors have shown such follow-up, larger syntheses of the literature have suggested a positive predictive value for this diagnosis closer to 90%.[6,7] Benign tumors should only rarely be diagnosed as malignant on FNAB and should include some anticipated pitfalls. For example, uncommonly Warthin tumors can occur with squamous metaplasia and have such a degree of cytologic atypia as to be interpreted as malignant.[24]

NONDIAGNOSTIC SAMPLES

Nondiagnostic samples are seen with 10% to 20% of FNABs at many sites. However, FNAB of the salivary glands seems to have yielded somewhat lower rates for this interpretation.[7,15] This may be because many include aspirates showing only normal salivary tissue as benign rather than as nondiagnostic, as they truly are in the face of a sampled mass lesion. Preparations typically show nothing except blood, bland benign mesenchymal tissue, or normal appearing salivary gland tissue. Preparations that are poorly prepared and, thus, cannot be interpreted are also to be placed in the category.[14] Smears of normal salivary gland usually show bland adipose tissue with occasional sheets of bland ductal cells admixed with fragments of tissue containing normal acinar structures, typically 3-dimensional, grapelike clusters of bland cells with abundant cytoplasm and small uniform nuclei.

As with the thyroid, aspirates that show features of cyst material only are also nondiagnostic.[14] Such smears may contain macrophages, siderophages, acellular debris, and even bland epithelial cells. With the thyroid, such samples may sometimes be seen with poorly sampled papillary thyroid carcinomas.[25] With salivary gland FNAB, such samples can sometimes be seen with low-grade mucoepidermoid carcinomas, or, much less commonly, other neoplasms.[26]

NONNEOPLASTIC LESIONS

Nonneoplastic mass lesions of the salivary glands include sialadenitis, reactive lymph nodes, and mucoceles, among other less common entities. As mentioned above, cyst change only should be reported as nondiagnostic. It is unclear that a sample from a mucocele or mucous retention cyst would seem to be different and how one would distinguish such a lesion from a sample of low-grade mucoepidermoid carcinoma.

Sialadenitis often presents as a mass lesion. Acute and chronic sialadenitis may be seen with obstruction or injury such as that seen after radiation therapy for head and neck squamous cell carcinoma or after radioiodine therapy for thyroid cancer.[27,28] Some cases may, thus, be more clinically obvious, occurring after therapy and therefore are not sampled by more knowing physicians. Two variants of sialadenitis, however, typically present as mass lesions without any obvious clinically relevant history. These are chronic sclerosing sialadenitis and lymphoepithelial sialadenitis.

Chronic sclerosing sialadenitis (ie, Kuttner tumor) is a member of the immunoglobulin (Ig) G4-sclerosing diseases.[29] It almost exclusively involves the submandibular glands, affects older individuals of either sex and is usually unilateral. As with IgG4-sclerosing disease at other sites, the lesions are histologically composed of storiform fibrosis with lymphoplasmacytic inflammation with phlebitis. Increased numbers and percentages of IgG4-expressing plasma cells typify the disease. Aspirates thus show chronic inflammatory cells admixed with salivary gland showing variable degrees of fibrosis.[30] Not surprisingly, preparations often have low cellularity. In the absence of cell block or core needle histology with definitive diagnostic findings or known serology studies (ie, high serum concentrations of IgG4), a diagnosis is likely impossible.

Lymphoepithelial sialadenitis usually involves the parotid gland and describes a histologic entity most often associated with Sjogren syndrome.[31] The disease is more common in older women and usually affects both glands (although often asymmetrically). Histologically, the disease is associated with a dense lymphocytic infiltrate, usually with numerous germinal centers, and gland atrophy. Lymphoepithelial lesions, that is, lymphocytes infiltrating residual epithelial structures, are easy to find and lend the disease its moniker. With cytology samples, numerous polymorphous lymphocytes are seen with occasional bland sheets of epithelial cells.[32] Often ancillary testing (eg, flow cytometry) is required to exclude a low-grade lymphoma.[18] As with chronic sclerosing sialadenitis, it is unclear if cytology alone, outside the context of a patient with known Sjogren disease or a more ample core biopsy or cell block, can make a definitive diagnose of the disease.

Because the parotid gland contains lymph nodes, reactive nodal hyperplasia can present as a mass lesion of the parotid gland.[33] An aspirate of the parotid gland mass showing only polymorphous lymphocytes can generally be diagnosed as nonneoplastic and ancillary testing is seldom needed to exclude lymphoma.

ATYPICAL LESIONS

Because some aspirates show features that seems to be abnormal and show features that may or may not represent neoplasia, the diagnostic category atypical was included with the Milan system. As with Pap tests, thyroid aspirates, and others, the category is difficult to define.[34] The identification of mildly atypical epithelial cells in an aspirate that otherwise shows features of a cyst or sialadenitis may be an example of a case that could be placed within this category. As with the thyroid, it is believed that such an interpretation would most likely result in further sampling of the lesion.

BENIGN NEOPLASM AND NEOPLASM OF UNKNOWN MALIGNANT POTENTIAL

The Milan system groups together into a single category aspirates interpreted as definitively benign neoplasms (eg, pleomorphic adenoma) and those interpreted as showing features of a neoplasm that may be benign or malignant. This category is then subcategorized as benign neoplasm and neoplasm of uncertain malignant potential. Further subclassification of the latter is also suggested based on frequently used pattern descriptors (eg, basaloid neoplasm).[12,23]

Benign Neoplasm

The most commonly diagnosed benign neoplasms of the salivary gland are pleomorphic adenoma and Warthin tumor.[14,35] Both lesions have a typical cytomorphology in the majority of cases and both show histologic and cytologic overlap with other benign and malignant salivary gland neoplasms, even when they exhibit typical features.[24,26,36]

Pleomorphic adenoma represents more than one-half of all benign salivary gland neoplasia.[35] Tumors are typically well-circumscribed and composed of bland ductal and myoepithelial cells and stromal tissue. Aspirates of typical cases show an admixture of these features with sheets of bland ductal cells and single myoepithelial cells with fibrillary extracellular material (**Fig. 1**).[37] Because pleomorphic adenoma is so much more common than other salivary gland tumors and because its cytologic features of a typical tumor are only uncommonly seen with a malignant neoplasm (eg, carcinoma ex pleomorphic adenoma), the definite diagnosis of pleomorphic adenoma by cytologic sampling is very predictive of benign neoplasia (almost always pleomorphic adenoma at resection).[23] Because pleomorphic adenomas can contain only minimal stroma or can have squamous and mucinous metaplasia, they may sometimes be interpreted within other diagnostic categories with cytologic sampling (eg, many stromal-poor tumors may be classified as

Fig. 1. Prototypical cyto-logic features of pleo-morphic adenoma. The presence of fibrillary extra-cellular material with bland single (myoepithe-lial) cells and/or bland sheets of ductal cells is pre-dictive of this benign neoplasm (Papanicolaou stain, original magnifica-tion ×100).

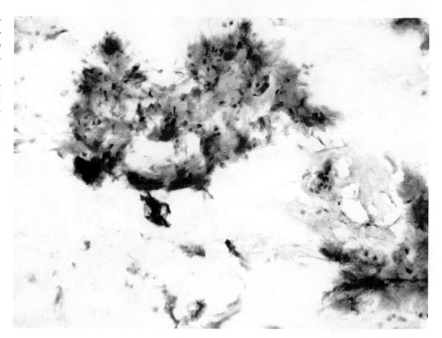

basaloid neoplasms within the neoplasm of un-known malignant potential category).[23]

Warthin tumors almost always involve the pa-rotid glands of smokers.[38] They are typically composed of ribbons, cysts, and papillary struc-tures lined by a double layer of bland oncocytic cells and surrounded polymorphous lympho-cytes. Typical aspirates then show sheets of bland oncocytes admixed with lymphocyte and variable amounts of degenerating cystic debris.[37] Because oncocytes and lymphocytes may be seen with other salivary gland tumors, there is a low but definite risk for cases diag-nosed definitively as Warthin tumor on aspiration biopsy to be found to be a different oncocytic neoplasm at resection (eg, oncocytic mucoepi-dermoid carcinoma may show aspirate findings indistinguishable from those of a typical Warthin tumor).[24,26] In addition, Warthin tumors may show squamous and mucinous metaplasia with reactive cytologic atypia and, thus, may be categorized outside of benign with cytologic sampling.

Other definitive benign diagnoses based on cytologic sampling or even limited core sampling are problematic. The diagnoses of basal cell adenoma, oncocytoma, and myoepithelioma all require assessment of a resected specimen to distinguish these lesions from their respective ma-lignant counterparts, and there are no known mo-lecular changes that have been shown to predict such lesions as benign.

Neoplasm of Unknown Malignant Potential

The World Health Organization system for the classification system of tumors of the salivary glands classifies only 1 tumor as having unknown malignant potential, sialoblastoma.[9] The Milan system uses this term differently for cytologic specimens for the classification of aspirates that show features of neoplasia that may be seen with both benign and malignant neoplasms.[14] Such aspirates include those from some pleomor-phic adenomas, basal cell adenomas and adeno-carcinoma, myoepithelioma, myoepithelial carcinoma, epithelial-myoepithelial carcinoma, clear cell carcinoma, oncocytoma, oncocytic car-cinoma, acinic cell carcinoma, and secretory car-cinoma, among other rarer tumors. By definition, they do not include most tumors that are high-grade malignancies (it should be noted that some pathologists and clinicians do consider adenoid cystic carcinoma an intermediate or high-grade malignancy).[12]

The majority of basaloid tumors produce cellular aspirates composed of a mixture of small, bland, single cells; clusters of cells; and larger sheets of cells. Some background acellular material may be present, but it is not the abundant fibrillary ma-terial seen with a typical pleomorphic adenoma (**Fig. 2**). Mitotic figures are uncommon, and cyto-logic pleomorphism and necrosis are not seen. The cells have a small amount of delicate cyto-plasm and uniform nuclei. Most have categorized

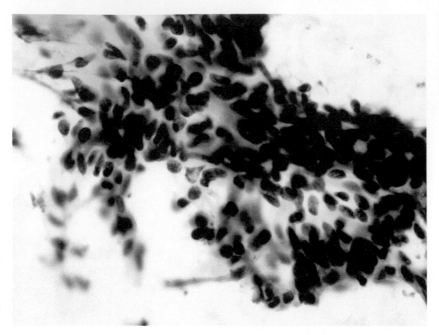

Fig. 2. Basaloid/basal cell neoplasm. Aspirates showing only bland basaloid cells may range from benign (eg, pleomorphic adenoma and basal cell adenoma) or malignant (eg, basal cell adenocarcinoma or adenoid cystic carcinoma) tumors (Papanicolaou stain, original magnification ×400).

such smears as basaloid or basal cell neoplasm, or some similar appellation.[39–43] Such aspirates typically are from cellular pleomorphic adenomas, basal cell adenoma or adenocarcinomas, adenoid cystic carcinomas, epithelial-myoepithelial carcinomas, and clear cell carcinomas.[23]

Certain cytologic features may lead one favor one lesion over another. For example, the identification of prototypical acellular cylinders may lead one to favor a diagnosis of adenoid cystic carcinoma (**Fig. 3**), and as such use the diagnostic category of suspicious for malignancy or even malignancy.[41] Furthermore, the use of ancillary testing may allow for one to better categorize such aspirates (**Box 1**).[18,29,33,39,44–64] β-Catenin nuclear immunoreactivity or LEF-1 expression would be consistent with a basal cell adenoma or adenocarcinoma. The identification of specific cytogenetic abnormalities could help one to make a definitive diagnosis (eg, confirmation of

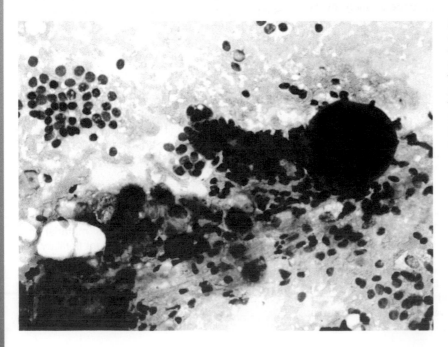

Fig. 3. The presence of acellular metachromatic cylinders in an aspirate otherwise showing features of a basaloid neoplasm is very predictive of adenoid cystic carcinoma (Diff-Quick stain, original magnification ×200).

Box 1
Ancillary testing[a] with salivary gland biopsies for specific diagnoses

Diagnosis	Ancillary Test	Notes
Reactive lymph node and lymphoepithelial lesion	Flow cytometry	Although not needed with all cases, flow cytometry is a powerful tool for excluding low-grade lymphoma
Chronic sclerosing sialadenitis	IgG4 IHC	The use and specificity with biopsy samples is not known
Pleomorphic adenoma	PLAG1 or HMGA2 IHC; *PLAG1* or *HMGA2* FISH	Approximately 30% of cases will not have either translocation; cannot exclude carcinoma ex pleomorphic adenoma or salivary duct carcinoma
Basal cell adenoma	β-Catenin IHC	The use with small biopsies seems to be limited; cannot exclude basal cell adenocarcinoma
Basal cell adenocarcinoma	β-Catenin IHC	The use with small biopsies seems to be limited; cannot exclude basal cell adenoma
Adenoid cystic carcinoma	MYB IHC *MYB* FISH	At least 20% of cases do not have translocation; IHC for MYB may not be helpful
Clear cell carcinoma	*EWSR1* FISH	Tumors more common in the mouth; translocations with *EWSR1* rarely also seen with clear cell myoepithelial tumors
Secretory carcinoma	S-100 and mammaglobin IHC coexpression *ETV6* FISH	Translocation present by definition
Mucoepidermoid carcinoma	*MAML2* FISH	At least 20% of cases do not have the translocation
Intraductal carcinoma	*RET* FISH	Tumors are very uncommon and usually not sampled by FNAB. RET translocation may not be visible.
Carcinoma ex pleomorphic adenoma	PLAG1 or HMGA IHC; *PLAG1* or *HMGA2* FISH	Present in only a subset of these tumors
Salivary duct carcinoma	AR IHC, HER2 IHC or ISH; PLAG1 or HMGA IHC; *PLAG1* or *HMGA2* FISH	*PLAG1* and *HMGA2* rearrangements suggest development from pleomorphic adenoma
Undifferentiated (lymphoepithelial) carcinoma	EBV ISH	Keratin IHC should also be performed
Lymphoma	IHC, flow cytometry, etc	Immunophenotyping should be attempted with any case suspected of being lymphoma

Abbreviations: EBV, Epstein-Barr virus; FISH/ISH, fluorescent in situ hybridization; FNAB, fine needle aspiration biopsy; IgG4, immunoglobulin G4; IHC, immunohistochemistry.
[a] IHC, FISH/ISH, and flow cytometry are common enough methods used with material obtained by FNAB. More advanced molecular methods may come to be used to identify specific genetic alterations but are not widely used in diagnostics with salivary gland tumors at this time.

PLAG, *MYB*, or *EWSR1* gene rearrangement by fluorescent in situ hybridization are relatively specific for pleomorphic adenoma, adenoid cystic carcinoma and clear cell carcinoma, respectively).

Another potential grouping with the Milan system category of neoplasm of unknown malignant potential contains aspirates of neoplasms composed of larger epithelial cells with relatively bland cytology (large or oncocytic cell epithelial neoplasm).[7,12,14,23] These would include aspirates from some lower grade mucoepidermoid carcinomas, acinic cell carcinomas, secretory carcinomas (mammary analogue secretory carcinomas), oncocytic neoplasms, Warthin tumors, and rare pleomorphic adenomas and myoepithelial neoplasms (**Fig. 4**). As with basaloid neoplasms, certain cytologic features may lead one to strongly favor a specific lesion (eg, the presence of abundant extracellular mucus).[12,23] Again, the identification of specific molecular abnormalities or protein

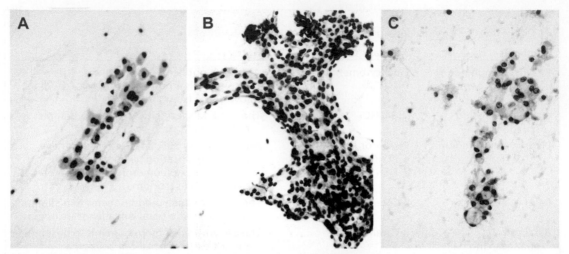

Fig. 4. Three aspirates showing features of a low-grade epithelial/oncocytic neoplasm. (*A*) Low-grade mucoepidermoid carcinoma, (*B*) acinic cell carcinoma, and (*C*) secretory carcinoma. Cytologic features can help to predict the specific diagnosis but ancillary testing is likely required for a definitive diagnosis (Papanicolaou stain, original magnification ×200).

expression could enable the pathologist to make definitive diagnoses (eg, detection of *MAML2* or *ETV6* rearrangement by fluorescent in situ hybridization are specific for mucoepidermoid carcinoma and secretory carcinoma, respectively; see **Box 1**).

Other patterns may be seen within this category, but they are less common and less likely to be well-defined and reproducible. Distinguishing basaloid neoplasms from large cell neoplasms may be helpful as the rate of follow-up malignancy may differ.[12] Because the description basaloid neoplasm could be used to describe most stromal-poor pleomorphic adenomas, the category may have a higher percentage of benign follow-up when compared with large cell epithelial neoplasms.[12]

SUSPICIOUS FOR MALIGNANCY

As with the atypical category, this category is difficult to define. In essence, the pathologist must believe the cytologic features seen to be those most likely but not definitively for a malignancy. These could be from either low- or high-grade malignancies, but one would imagine it would more likely be used with tumors suspicious for high-grade malignancies.

With the case of high-grade malignancy, the pathologist is most likely to be constrained by sample quantity. That is to say, the cytologic features are those of a typical epithelial malignancy but there are simply too few cells present for the cytopathologist to feel comfortable with a definitive malignancy.[11] With low-grade malignancies, the diagnostic dilemmas may be more indicative of the overlap of histologic features or need for

ancillary testing for a definitive diagnosis. Basaloid epithelial cells with acellular cylinders of extracellular material may be present, but the pathologist might not believe that a definitive diagnosis of adenoid cystic carcinoma can be made. A preparation may include low-grade large cells present in sheets with granular or vacuolated cytoplasm unlikely to be from a benign neoplasm, yet the pathologist may believe a definite diagnosis of malignancy cannot be made. It is unclear why FNABs from such lesions should instead be interpreted as neoplasm of unknown malignant potential.

MALIGNANCY

As noted, the positive predictive rate of a malignant cytologic diagnosis should approach 100%. For this reason, cytologic samples that show overlapping features with a benign or malignant neoplasm will typically not be diagnosed within this category. Instead, when cytologic material only is obtained, this interpretation must primarily be restricted to high-grade malignancies (eg, salivary duct carcinoma and high-grade mucoepidermoid carcinoma) or known metastases.

Most high-grade carcinomas of the salivary gland retain an obvious epithelioid phenotype.[9] As such, the cytologic features are akin to those of sampled carcinomas at other sites of the body. Nuclear and cytologic atypia will be moderate to severe and mitotic activity and necrosis are often present (**Fig. 5**).[65,66] Variable degrees of intracytoplasmic and extracellular mucous can be present and its presence may lead one to favor a diagnosis of high-grade mucoepidermoid

Fig. 5. Salivary duct carcinoma. Cytologic features of high-grade epithelial malignancy are present, allowing for this aspirate to be definitively classified as malignant. A specific malignant diagnosis, however, would likely require ancillary testing (Papanicolaou stain, original magnification ×400).

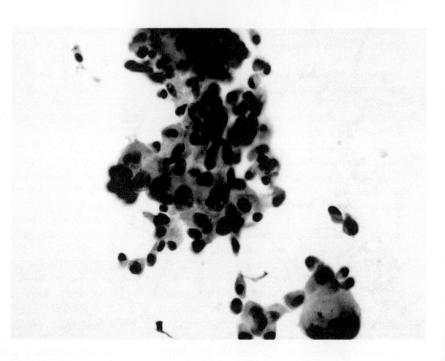

carcinoma.[67,68] Neuroendocrine features, including a small cell phenotype, are only rarely seen as primary salivary gland neoplasia.[69] Definitive keratinization, somewhat ironically, is also rarely seen with primary salivary gland neoplasia, including with high-grade mucoepidermoid carcinoma, although other squamous features (eg, larger, more polygonal cells) may be seen.

Immunohistochemistry and other ancillary testing can be of assistance with high-grade malignancies to assist in making precise diagnoses (see **Box 1**). Histochemical stains to identify mucus or the identification of a *MAML2* abnormality would point to a diagnosis of mucoepidermoid carcinoma.[53] Expression of androgen receptor or HER2 would support salivary duct carcinoma.[60,61] The identification of genetic abnormalities typical of lower grade neoplasms (eg, *MYB* rearrangement) would suggest high-grade transformation of a lower grade tumor.[70]

The definitive diagnoses of low-grade malignancies typically require ancillary testing and, in most cases, cannot be accomplished with cytologic material only (see **Box 1**). Many of these tumors have genetic abnormalities that are entirely or almost entirely specific. For example, the identification of a *MAML2* rearrangement would be diagnostic of mucoepidermoid carcinoma, whereas an *EWSR1* rearrangement would be highly suggestive of clear cell carcinoma (although some have described *EWSR1* rearrangement uncommonly in other in other clear cell malignancies and mimics).[47–49,53,54]

SUMMARY

FNAB of the salivary glands is a powerful tool for assisting with the management of salivary gland masses. Fortunately, the most common benign neoplasm—pleomorphic adenoma—can be diagnosed accurately in most cases with cytology alone. Almost all other diagnoses, however, require ancillary testing if a definitive diagnosis is going to be made (even benign lymph nodes often require flow cytometry for a correct diagnosis). The Milan System for the reporting of salivary gland FNAB specimens attempts to codify diagnostic categories for the reporting these specimens.

REFERENCES

1. Jo VY, Stelow EB, Dustin SM, et al. Malignancy risk for fine-needle aspiration of thyroid lesions according to the Bethesda system for reporting thyroid cytopathology. Am J Clin Pathol 2010;134:450–6.

2. Bellizzi AM, Stelow EB. Pancreatic cytopathology: a practical approach and review. Arch Pathol Lab Med 2009;133:388–404.

3. Osmani L, Askin F, Gabrielson E, et al. Current WHO guidelines and the critical role of immunohistochemical markers in the subclassification of non-small cell lung carcinoma (NSCLC): moving from targeted therapy to immunotherapy. Semin Cancer Biol 2017. https://doi.org/10.1016/j.semcancer.2017.11.019.

4. Mavec P, Eneroth CM, Franzen S, et al. Aspiration biopsy of salivary gland tumours. I. Correlation of

cytologic reports from 652 aspiration biopsies with clinical and histologic findings. Acta Otolaryngol 1964;58:471–84.

5. Lombardi D, McGurk M, Vander Poorten V, et al. Surgical treatment of salivary malignant tumors. Oral Oncol 2017;65:102–13.

6. Schmidt RL, Hall BJ, Wilson AR, et al. A systematic review and meta-analysis of the diagnostic accuracy of fine-needle aspiration cytology for parotid gland lesions. Am J Clin Pathol 2011;136:45–59.

7. Wei S, Layfield LJ, LiVolsi VA, et al. Reporting of fine needle aspiration (FNA) specimens of salivary gland lesions: a comprehensive review. Diagn Cytopathol 2017;45:820–7.

8. Eneroth CM, Franzen S, Zajicek J. Aspiration biopsy of salivary gland tumors. A critical review of 910 biopsies. Acta Cytol 1967;11:470–2.

9. Tumours of salivary glands. In: El-Naggar AK, Chan JKC, Grandis JR, et al, editors. WHO classification of head and neck tumours. Lyon (France): IARC; 2017. p. 159–202.

10. Chute DJ, Stelow EB. Cytology of head and neck squamous cell carcinoma variants. Diagn Cytopathol 2010;38:65–80.

11. Baloch ZW, Faquin WC, Layfield LJ. Is it time to develop a tiered classification scheme for salivary gland fine-needle aspiration specimens? Diagn Cytopathol 2017;45:285–6.

12. Griffith CC, Schmitt AC, Pantanowitz L, et al. A pattern-based risk-stratification scheme for salivary gland cytology: a multi-institutional, interobserver variability study to determine applicability. Cancer Cytopathol 2017;125:776–85.

13. Pusztaszeri M, Baloch Z, Vielh P, et al. Application of the Milan system for reporting risk stratification in salivary gland cytopathology. Cancer 2018;126: 69–70.

14. Rossi ED, Faquin WC, Baloch Z, et al. The Milan system for reporting salivary gland cytopathology: analysis and suggestions of initial survey. Cancer Cytopathol 2017;125:757–66.

15. Rohilla M, Singh P, Rajwanshi A, et al. Three-year cytohistological correlation of salivary gland FNA cytology at a tertiary center with the application of the Milan system for risk stratification. Cancer Cytopathol 2017;125:767–75.

16. Wang H, Malik A, Maleki Z, et al. "Atypical" salivary gland fine needle aspiration: risk of malignancy and interinstitutional variability. Diagn Cytopathol 2017; 45:1088–94.

17. Maleki Z, Miller JA, Arab SE, et al. "Suspicious" salivary gland FNA: risk of malignancy and interinstitutional variability. Cancer Cytopathol 2018;126(2): 94–100.

18. Stacchini A, Aliberti S, Pacchioni D, et al. Flow cytometry significantly improves the diagnostic value of fine needle aspiration cytology of lymphoproliferative lesions of salivary glands. Cytopathology 2014;25:231–40.

19. Stelow EB, Bardales RH, Lai R, et al. The cytological spectrum of chronic pancreatitis. Diagn Cytopathol 2005;32:65–9.

20. Ellis GL, Auclair PL. Tumors of the salivary glands. Washington, DC: American Registry of Pathology; 2008.

21. Al-Khafaji BM, Nestok BR, Katz RL. Fine-needle aspiration of 154 parotid masses with histologic correlation: ten-year experience at the University of Texas M. D. Anderson Cancer Center. Cancer 1998;84:153–9.

22. Jahan-Parwar B, Huberman RM, Donovan DT, et al. Oncocytic mucoepidermoid carcinoma of the salivary glands. Am J Surg Pathol 1999;23:523–9.

23. Griffith CC, Pai RK, Schneider F, et al. Salivary gland tumor fine-needle aspiration cytology: a proposal for a risk stratification classification. Am J Clin Pathol 2015;143:839–53.

24. Daneshbod Y, Daneshbod K, Khademi B. Diagnostic difficulties in the interpretation of fine needle aspirate samples in salivary lesions: diagnostic pitfalls revisited. Acta Cytol 2009;53:53–70.

25. Jaragh M, Carydis VB, MacMillan C, et al. Predictors of malignancy in thyroid fine-needle aspirates "cyst fluid only" cases: can potential clues of malignancy be identified? Cancer 2009;117:305–10.

26. MacLeod CB, Frable WJ. Fine-needle aspiration biopsy of the salivary gland: problem cases. Diagn Cytopathol 1993;9:216–24, [discussion: 224–5].

27. Allweiss P, Braunstein GD, Katz A, et al. Sialadenitis following I-131 therapy for thyroid carcinoma: concise communication. J Nucl Med 1984;25:755–8.

28. Porter SR, Scully C, Hegarty AM. An update of the etiology and management of xerostomia. Oral Surg Oral Med Oral Pathol Oral Radiol Endod 2004;97: 28–46.

29. Bhatti RM, Stelow EB. IgG4-related disease of the head and neck. Adv Anat Pathol 2013;20:10–6.

30. Kaba S, Kojima M, Matsuda H, et al. Kuttner's tumor of the submandibular glands: report of five cases with fine-needle aspiration cytology. Diagn Cytopathol 2006;34:631–5.

31. Morgan WS, Castleman B. A clinicopathologic study of Mikulicz's disease. Am J Pathol 1953;29:471–503.

32. Gunhan O, Celasun B, Dogan N, et al. Fine needle aspiration cytologic findings in a benign lymphoepithelial lesion with microcalcifications. A case report. Acta Cytol 1992;36:744–7.

33. Allen EA, Ali SZ, Mathew S. Lymphoid lesions of the parotid. Diagn Cytopathol 1999;21:170–3.

34. Bongiovanni M, Krane JF, Cibas ES, et al. The atypical thyroid fine-needle aspiration: past, present, and future. Cancer Cytopathol 2012;120:73–86.

35. Stewart CJ, MacKenzie K, McGarry GW, et al. Fine-needle aspiration cytology of salivary gland: a

review of 341 cases. Diagn Cytopathol 2000;22:
139–46.

36. Mukunyadzi P. Review of fine-needle aspiration cytology of salivary gland neoplasms, with emphasis on differential diagnosis. Am J Clin Pathol 2002;118(Suppl):S100–15.

37. Kline TS, Merriam JM, Shapshay SM. Aspiration biopsy cytology of the salivary gland. Am J Clin Pathol 1981;76:263–9.

38. Chaudhry AP, Gorlin RJ. Papillary cystadenoma lymphomatosum (adenolymphoma); a review of the literature. Am J Surg 1958;95:923–31.

39. Avadhani V, Cohen C, Siddiqui MT. PLAG1: an immunohistochemical marker with limited utility in separating pleomorphic adenoma from other basaloid salivary gland tumors. Acta Cytol 2016;60: 240–5.

40. Griffith CC, Siddiqui MT, Schmitt AC. Ancillary testing strategies in salivary gland aspiration cytology: a practical pattern-based approach. Diagn Cytopathol 2017;45:808–19.

41. Kapadia SB, Dusenbery D, Dekker A. Fine needle aspiration of pleomorphic adenoma and adenoid cystic carcinoma of salivary gland origin. Acta Cytol 1997;41:487–92.

42. Molnar SL, Zarka MA, De Las Casas LE. Going beyond "basaloid neoplasm": fine needle aspiration cytology of epithelial-myoepithelial carcinoma of the parotid gland. Diagn Cytopathol 2016;44:422–5.

43. Tawfik O, Tsue T, Pantazis C, et al. Salivary gland neoplasms with basaloid cell features: report of two cases diagnosed by fine-needle aspiration cytology. Diagn Cytopathol 1999;21:46–50.

44. Brill LB 2nd, Kanner WA, Fehr A, et al. Analysis of MYB expression and MYB-NFIB gene fusions in adenoid cystic carcinoma and other salivary neoplasms. Mod Pathol 2011;24:1169–76.

45. Foo WC, Jo VY, Krane JF. Usefulness of translocation-associated immunohistochemical stains in the fine-needle aspiration diagnosis of salivary gland neoplasms. Cancer Cytopathol 2016;124:397–405.

46. Jo VY, Sholl LM, Krane JF. Distinctive patterns of CTNNB1 (beta-catenin) alterations in salivary gland basal cell adenoma and basal cell adenocarcinoma. Am J Surg Pathol 2016;40:1143–50.

47. Antonescu CR, Katabi N, Zhang L, et al. EWSR1-ATF1 fusion is a novel and consistent finding in hyalinizing clear-cell carcinoma of salivary gland. Genes Chromosomes Cancer 2011;50:559–70.

48. Shah AA, LeGallo RD, van Zante A, et al. EWSR1 genetic rearrangements in salivary gland tumors: a specific and very common feature of hyalinizing clear cell carcinoma. Am J Surg Pathol 2013;37: 571–8.

49. Skalova A, Weinreb I, Hyrcza M, et al. Clear cell myoepithelial carcinoma of salivary glands showing EWSR1 rearrangement: molecular analysis of 94 salivary gland carcinomas with prominent clear cell component. Am J Surg Pathol 2015;39:338–48.

50. Griffith CC, Stelow EB, Saqi A, et al. The cytological features of mammary analogue secretory carcinoma: a series of 6 molecularly confirmed cases. Cancer Cytopathol 2013;121:234–41.

51. Shah AA, Wenig BM, LeGallo RD, et al. Morphology in conjunction with immunohistochemistry is sufficient for the diagnosis of mammary analogue secretory carcinoma. Head Neck Pathol 2015;9:85–95.

52. Skalova A, Vanecek T, Sima R, et al. Mammary analogue secretory carcinoma of salivary glands, containing the ETV6-NTRK3 fusion gene: a hitherto undescribed salivary gland tumor entity. Am J Surg Pathol 2010;34:599–608.

53. Seethala RR, Chiosea SI. MAML2 status in mucoepidermoid carcinoma can no longer be considered a prognostic marker. Am J Surg Pathol 2016;40: 1151–3.

54. Seethala RR, Dacic S, Cieply K, et al. A reappraisal of the MECT1/MAML2 translocation in salivary mucoepidermoid carcinomas. Am J Surg Pathol 2010; 34:1106–21.

55. Weinreb I, Bishop JA, Chiosea SI, et al. Recurrent RET gene rearrangements in intraductal carcinomas of salivary gland. Am J Surg Pathol 2018;42(4): 442–52.

56. Andreasen S, von Holstein SL, Homoe P, et al. Recurrent rearrangements of the PLAG1 and HMGA2 genes in lacrimal gland pleomorphic adenoma and carcinoma ex pleomorphic adenoma. Acta Ophthalmol 2018. https://doi.org/10.1111/aos. 13667.

57. Chiosea SI, Thompson LD, Weinreb I, et al. Subsets of salivary duct carcinoma defined by morphologic evidence of pleomorphic adenoma, PLAG1 or HMGA2 rearrangements, and common genetic alterations. Cancer 2016;122:3136–44.

58. Katabi N, Ghossein R, Ho A, et al. Consistent PLAG1 and HMGA2 abnormalities distinguish carcinoma ex-pleomorphic adenoma from its de novo counterparts. Hum Pathol 2015;46:26–33.

59. Bahrami A, Perez-Ordonez B, Dalton JD, et al. An analysis of PLAG1 and HMGA2 rearrangements in salivary duct carcinoma and examination of the role of precursor lesions. Histopathology 2013;63: 250–62.

60. Cornolti G, Ungari M, Morassi ML, et al. Amplification and overexpression of HER2/neu gene and HER2/neu protein in salivary duct carcinoma of the parotid gland. Arch Otolaryngol Head Neck Surg 2007;133:1031–6.

61. Glisson B, Colevas AD, Haddad R, et al. HER2 expression in salivary gland carcinomas: dependence on histological subtype. Clin Cancer Res 2004;10:944–6.

62. Huang DP, Ng HK, Ho YH, et al. Epstein-Barr virus (EBV)-associated undifferentiated carcinoma of the parotid gland. Histopathology 1988;13:509–17.

63. Saemundsen AK, Albeck H, Hansen JP, et al. Epstein-Barr virus in nasopharyngeal and salivary gland carcinomas of Greenland Eskimoes. Br J Cancer 1982;46:721–8.

64. Schmitt AC, Griffith CC, Cohen C, et al. LEF-1: diagnostic utility in distinguishing basaloid neoplasms of the salivary gland. Diagn Cytopathol 2017;45:1078–83.

65. Fyrat P, Cramer H, Feczko JD, et al. Fine-needle aspiration biopsy of salivary duct carcinoma: report of five cases. Diagn Cytopathol 1997;16:526–30.

66. Moriki T, Ueta S, Takahashi T, et al. Salivary duct carcinoma: cytologic characteristics and application of androgen receptor immunostaining for diagnosis. Cancer 2001;93:344–50.

67. Cohen MB, Fisher PE, Holly EA, et al. Fine needle aspiration biopsy diagnosis of mucoepidermoid carcinoma. Statistical analysis. Acta Cytol 1990;34:43–9.

68. Stanley MW, Bardales RH, Farmer CE, et al. Primary and metastatic high-grade carcinomas of the salivary glands: a cytologic-histologic correlation study of twenty cases. Diagn Cytopathol 1995;13:37–43.

69. Mair S, Phillips JI, Cohen R. Small cell undifferentiated carcinoma of the parotid gland. Cytologic, histologic, immunohistochemical and ultrastructural features of a neuroendocrine variant. Acta Cytol 1989;33:164–8.

70. Costa AF, Altemani A, Garcia-Inclan C, et al. Analysis of MYB oncogene in transformed adenoid cystic carcinomas reveals distinct pathways of tumor progression. Lab Invest 2014;94:692–702.

Head and Neck Cytopathology
Human Papillomavirus-Positive Carcinomas, Including Diagnostic Updates, Testing Modalities, and Recommendations

Emilio Madrigal, DO[a], Justin A. Bishop, MD[b],
William C. Faquin, MD, PhD[a],*

KEYWORDS

- Head and neck cytopathology • Human papillomavirus • Head and neck squamous cell carcinoma
- FNA

ABSTRACT

Oropharyngeal squamous cell carcinoma caused by transcriptionally active human papillomavirus (HPV) is now well established as a unique form of head and neck cancer. Given the high frequency of metastasis to cervical lymph nodes by HPV-positive oropharyngeal squamous cell carcinomas, fine-needle aspiration (FNA) represents a widely accepted method for the sampling and diagnosis of these cancers. The recently published College of American Pathologists Guideline (2017) provides recommendations for the effective performance and interpretation of high-risk (HR) HPV testing in head and neck squamous cell carcinoma (HNSCC), including testing on FNA samples of metastatic HNSCC to cervical lymph nodes. There is a wide range of options available for HR-HPV testing in cytologic specimens.

OVERVIEW TO HUMAN PAPILLOMAVIRUS-POSITIVE HEAD AND NECK SQUAMOUS CELL CARCINOMA

Oropharyngeal squamous cell carcinoma (OPSCC) caused by transcriptionally active human papillomavirus (HPV) is now well established as a unique form of head and neck cancer.[1–5] The 1980s saw the beginning of sharply differing incidences between the 2 leading pathways to head and neck cancer, with a significant increase in HPV-positive OPSCC and a contrasting decrease in conventional alcohol and tobacco–related head and neck squamous cell carcinoma (HNSCC). In the United States, the incidence of OPSCC has already surpassed that of cervical squamous cell carcinoma, with more than 16,000 cases occurring annually.[2]

The specialized, reticulated tonsillar crypt epithelium of the oropharynx, characteristic of the palatine tonsils and lingual tonsillar subsites, appears to be especially susceptible to high-risk (HR)-HPV infection and subsequent malignant transformation.[6] This pattern contrasts with traditional alcohol and tobacco–related HNSCC that typically arises from surface squamous epithelium. HR-HPV, a small, nonenveloped, double-stranded DNA virus, drives malignancies through the continued function of its E6 and E7 oncoproteins that target several critical cellular pathways, leading to deregulation of proliferation and evasion of apoptosis as well as overexpression of p16.[7] Approximately 200 HPV types have been identified, and the HR-HPV type 16 is most commonly associated with HNSCC, although it is not uniformly distributed in the head and neck.

None of the authors have any disclosures.

[a] Department of Pathology, Massachusetts General Hospital, 55 Fruit Street, Warren 219, Boston, MA 02114, USA; [b] Department of Pathology, The University of Texas Southwestern Medical Center, 5323 Harry Hines Boulevard, Dallas, TX 75390–9072, USA
* Corresponding author.
E-mail address: wfaquin@mgh.harvard.edu

Surgical Pathology 11 (2018) 501–514
https://doi.org/10.1016/j.path.2018.04.002

HR-HPV is associated with 80% to 90% of cancers of the oropharynx, while it is only responsible for less than 5% of oral cavity, hypopharyngeal, and laryngeal carcinomas.[8] Furthermore, there is an uneven distribution of HR-HPV in OPSCC with 92% of the palatine and lingual tonsillar carcinomas being HPV-positive, whereas only 3% of nontonsillar oropharyngeal cancers are HPV-positive.[6]

HPV-positive OPSCC displays a characteristic clinical profile distinct from conventional HPV-negative HNSCC, in that it affects younger patients that often lack traditional risk factors, namely, tobacco and alcohol abuse. Instead, patients are predominantly men (3:1–8:1, male:female ratio) who typically have social histories of certain sexual practices, including a high number of lifetime sex partners and histories of oral-genital and/or oral-anal sex.[4,9–11] Although patients with HPV-positive OPSCC often present with metastatic squamous cell carcinoma (SCC) to level II or level III cervical lymph nodes, it somewhat paradoxically carries an improved prognosis relative to HPV-negative HNSCC, and these patients may be candidates for less aggressive treatment in the context of a clinical trial.[12,13] Retrospective analyses of clinical trials indicate that there is a survival benefit for patients with HPV-positive OPSCC, with meta-analysis data reporting a 53% better overall and 74% better disease-specific survival.[12] Consequently, accurate assessment of tumor HR-HPV status is critical. Given these differences between HPV-positive OPSCC and HPV-negative OPSCC, the 8th Edition of the American Joint Committee on Cancer (AJCC) Cancer Staging Manual includes a separate set of criteria for these 2 groups of OPSCC.[14]

CYTOLOGIC EVALUATION OF HUMAN PAPILLOMAVIRUS-POSITIVE HEAD AND NECK SQUAMOUS CELL CARCINOMA

Metastatic head and neck carcinomas to cervical lymph nodes are frequently diagnosed by fine-needle aspiration (FNA), which is often done in conjunction with ultrasound guidance.[15–18] Even though HPV-positive OPSCC may occur as a relatively small primary lesion (low T stage) within the tonsillar crypts where it is difficult to detect except by tissue biopsy, it often presents with early cervical nodal metastases (high N stage). The frequent presentation as metastatic carcinoma has led to an important diagnostic role for cytology in the initial detection and diagnosis of these cancers. The role of FNA in the initial evaluation of metastatic HPV-positive OPSCC cannot be overemphasized; in many cases, the cytologic material is the first sample (and may be the only tumor specimen) available for diagnostic workup. In a subset of cases, a primary site of origin will not be identified even after exhaustive clinical and radiologic evaluation resulting in a metastatic SCC of unknown primary.[19] The material obtained by FNA can be tested for HR-HPV and used to classify the metastatic HNSCC as HPV-positive (and distinct from Epstein-Barr virus–related HNSCC), and thus indicative of an origin from the oropharynx.[20]

Metastatic HPV-positive OPSCCs have a typical cytologic appearance characterized by cohesive clusters of oval to somewhat elongate basaloid epithelial cells often in a cystic background of macrophages and cellular debris (**Fig. 1**). The basaloid appearance of the cells reflects the non-keratinizing nature of these cancers. Nuclei are hyperchromatic; nucleoli are absent or indistinct, and cytoplasm is scant and dense. Mitoses and apoptotic cells are frequently present. This cytologic pattern differs from conventional alcohol and tobacco–related HNSCC that frequently display keratinization and contain cells (including dyskeratotic forms) that are easily recognizable as squamous in both air-dried and alcohol-fixed cytologic preparations. For FNA cases of HPV-positive OPSCC where the differentiation of the basaloid cells as "squamous" is uncertain, immunohistochemical markers applied to cell block material can be helpful. All HNSCCs (HPV-positive as well as HPV-negative) are immunoreactive for the usual squamous cell markers, including p63, p40, and keratin 5/6.

The FNA appearance of these cancers is so distinctive that the diagnosis of nonkeratinizing HNSCC is usually straightforward. However, in a subset of cases, the diagnosis is not obvious, and there is a differential diagnosis that includes benign developmental cysts, such as a branchial cleft cyst or duplication cyst, as well as other metastatic carcinomas with basaloid features, such as basaloid SCC, nasopharyngeal carcinoma, small cell neuroendocrine carcinoma, and adenoid cystic carcinoma. In addition to a role for testing for HR-HPV, cytomorphologic and immunocytochemical features can usually readily distinguish between these differential diagnostic entities.

HISTOLOGIC FEATURES OF HUMAN PAPILLOMAVIRUS-POSITIVE HEAD AND NECK SQUAMOUS CELL CARCINOMA

When encountered in surgical pathology material, HPV-positive OPSCC also exhibits a characteristic

Fig. 1. FNA of HPV-positive OPSCC. (*A*) The aspirate shows cohesive groups of tumor cells with the characteristic basaloid features of the nonkeratinizing SCC (smear, Diff-Quik stain, original magnification ×600). (*B*) This aspirate shows cyst contents with many degenerate cells from a metastatic HPV-positive OPSCC to a level III cervical lymph node (Thin-Prep, Papanicolaou stain, original magnification ×400).

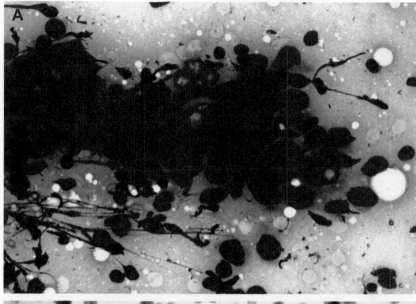

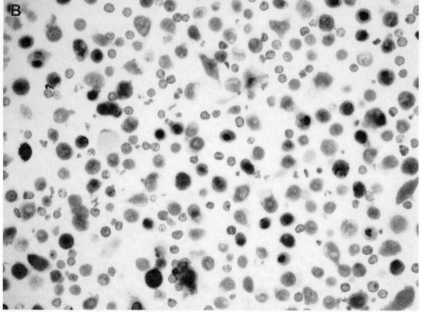

histomorphologic appearance that departs from that of conventional HNSCC in many ways.[21–23] Although conventional HNSCC typically arises from surface squamous dysplasia as cords and nests of keratinizing cells with an associated desmoplastic stromal reaction, HPV-positive OPSCC arises from the specialized oropharyngeal crypt epithelium as cohesive lobules and sheets of cells with little or no keratinization, without a desmoplastic response, and without a defined precursor lesion (**Fig. 2**).[24] HPV-positive OPSCC has a histologic appearance that some might interpret as "poorly differentiated"; however, it also closely mimics the benign crypt lining oropharyngeal epithelium, with scant cytoplasm, indistinct cell borders, and round to oval nuclei with inconspicuous nucleoli. Given the improved prognosis associated with these cancers, HPV-positive OPSCCs might best be conceptually considered well-differentiated carcinomas. The recent College of American Pathologists (CAP) Guideline now recommends that pathologists not provide a tumor grade or differentiation status for HPV-positive OPSCC. Also, similar to normal tonsillar crypts, HPV-positive OPSCC is accompanied by stromal and/or intratumoral lymphocytes, and it typically

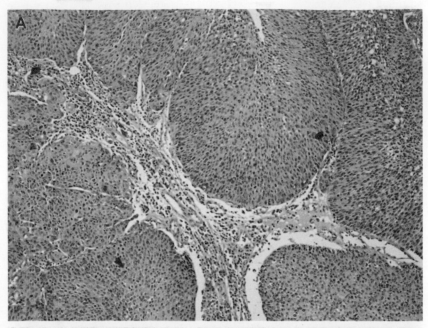

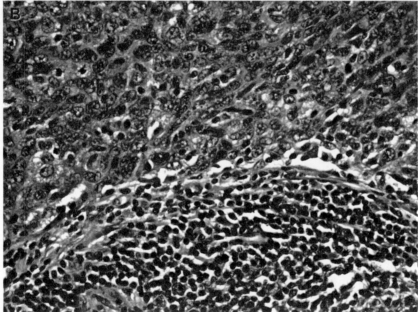

Fig. 2. Histologic features of HPV-positive OPSCC. (*A*) The SCC is nonkeratinizing and grows in cohesive lobular nests lacking a desmoplastic stromal response (H&E, original magnification ×100). (*B*) Syncytial group of OPSCC in a lymphoid background (H&E, original magnification ×400).

is mitotically active. When HPV-positive OPSCC metastasizes to cervical lymph nodes or distant sites such as lung, it maintains its characteristic basaloid appearance and its HPV-positive phenotype, except that cystic degeneration becomes more common, especially in lymph nodes.[23,25,26] The latter feature can be a pitfall for FNA. In addition to its classical appearance, HPV-positive OPSCC can also exhibit a lymphoepithelial morphology resembling nasopharyngeal carcinoma, or a pattern with comedonecrosis resembling basaloid SCC.[27]

OTHER FORMS OF HUMAN PAPILLOMAVIRUS POSITIVE HEAD AND NECK SQUAMOUS CELL CARCINOMA

As previously described, the prototypical HPV-positive HNSCC arises in the oropharynx, but there are other forms of HPV-positive head and neck carcinoma, including those that arise in the oropharynx and the sinonasal cavity. These other forms of HPV-positive carcinomas are less likely to be sampled by FNA but instead are typically detected by tissue biopsy. To date, only HPV-positive OPSCC and its SCC subtypes are strongly linked by evidence-based data to improved patient outcome relative to HPV-negative HNSCC.

PAPILLARY SQUAMOUS CELL CARCINOMA

Papillary SCC is a particularly well-differentiated exophytic form of SCC characterized by prominent elongate fibrovascular cores lined by squamous cells with a high nuclear-cytoplasmic ratio resembling SCC in situ (**Fig. 3**).[28] These tumors represent a subset of HPV-positive SCC in the oropharynx, but they also occur in other subsites of the head and neck where they generally have a good prognosis regardless of HPV status.[29]

HUMAN PAPILLOMAVIRUS-POSITIVE ADENOCARCINOMA OF THE OROPHARYNX

Rare examples of adenocarcinomas arising in the oropharynx, particularly the base of tongue, have been described that show overexpression of p16 and are positive for HR-HPV. These HPV-positive adenocarcinomas display a negative immunohistochemical profile for p63, high-molecular-weight keratins, and neuroendocrine

markers. The differential diagnosis for these tumors would include salivary gland adenocarcinomas and metastatic carcinoma. To date, the prognostic relevance of HPV-positive primary adenocarcinomas of the oropharynx remains unknown due to the small number of reported cases with limited clinical follow-up.[30]

HUMAN PAPILLOMAVIRUS-POSITIVE ADENOSQUAMOUS CARCINOMA

Adenosquamous carcinoma (ADSC) of the upper aerodigestive tract is an uncommon neoplasm composed of a combination of malignant glandular and squamous elements. It is usually associated with an aggressive clinical course. Occasional HPV-positive ADSCs have been reported in the oropharynx and the sinonasal tract, although the significance of HPV-positivity in this subset of carcinomas is uncertain.[31,32] Although these carcinomas have morphologic similarities to mucoepidermoid carcinomas, they are derived from the mucosal epithelium rather than being of salivary gland origin, and they are negative for MAML2 gene rearrangements.[33,34]

A subset of ADSCs with relatively bland histomorphology, predominantly nonkeratinizing squamous differentiation, and ciliated malignant glandular cells has been described (**Fig. 4**).[34] These examples have mainly originated in the oropharynx or have been metastatic to cervical lymph nodes (unknown primary site). This novel subset of ciliated ADSCs

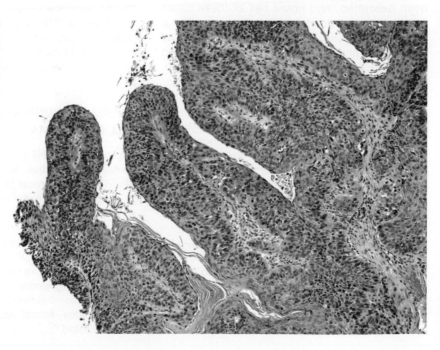

Fig. 3. Histologic features of papillary SCC. This HPV-positive papillary SCC of the oropharynx has an exophytic growth pattern with prominent fibrovascular cores (H&E, original magnification ×100).

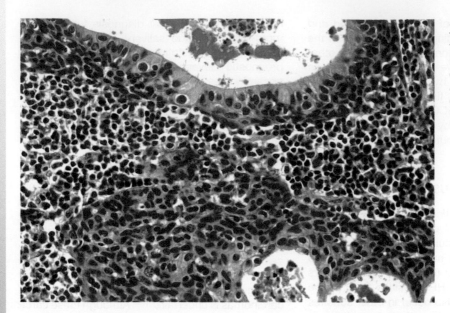

Fig. 4. Histologic features of ciliated ADSC. This HPV-positive carcinoma of the oropharynx contains both squamous and a ciliated glandular component (H&E, original magnification ×400).

are HPV-positive carcinomas that can pose potential diagnostic pitfalls given their resemblance to MEC and by defying conventional wisdom regarding the benignity of ciliated epithelium.[34]

HUMAN PAPILLOMAVIRUS-POSITIVE SMALL CELL CARCINOMA OF THE OROPHARYNX

Oropharyngeal carcinomas showing histomorphologic features of small cell carcinoma have been described, and about half of these cases contained a component of more conventional HPV-positive OPSCC. Both the small cell component and the SCC component harbored HPV by HPV-specific testing.[35] As expected, the small cell carcinomas show immunohistochemical evidence of neuroendocrine differentiation and typically show loss of the squamous markers keratin 5/6 and p63. Despite being HPV-positive, these small cell carcinomas of the oropharynx tend to follow an aggressive clinical course overriding any perceived prognostic benefit that might be suggested by the positive HPV status.[30]

HUMAN PAPILLOMAVIRUS-RELATED MULTIPHENOTYPIC SINONASAL CARCINOMA

Bishop and colleagues[36] have described a subset of sinonasal carcinomas that exhibit histologic features of salivary gland carcinomas (most often adenoid cystic carcinoma), including a biphasic proliferation of ducts and basaloid myoepithelial cells arranged in nests and solid areas with cribriform and microcystic architecture (**Fig. 5**). However, in contrast to true adenoid cystic carcinoma of minor salivary gland origin, these HPV-positive carcinomas are associated with squamous dysplasia or SCC of the overlying surface mucosa and a lack of *MYB* gene rearrangements.[36] They show diffuse expression of p16 and are positive for HR-HPV by HPV-specific tests. Of note, the most commonly identified HR-HPV subtype in HPV-related multiphenotypic sinonasal carcinoma is HPV type 33.[30] With approximately 50 published cases, this tumor appears to behave in a somewhat indolent manner, with frequent recurrences but rare metastases and no reported tumor deaths.[36]

SINONASAL NONKERATINIZING SQUAMOUS CELL CARCINOMA

Approximately 20% to 25% of all sinonasal carcinomas are positive for transcriptionally active HR-HPV, and the most common HPV-positive carcinoma in the sinonasal cavity is sinonasal nonkeratinizing SCC (**Fig. 6**).[31] The carcinoma often displays an inverted ribbonlike growth pattern resembling the histologic growth pattern seen in inverted papillomas of the sinonasal cavity. Overall, these carcinomas tend to have an indolent, but locally aggressive behavior, and a difference in prognosis between the HPV-positive and HPV-negative forms has not been definitively demonstrated.[37]

Fig. 5. Histologic features of HPV-related multiphenotypic sinonasal carcinoma. The carcinoma shows a cribriform growth pattern reminiscent of adenoid cystic carcinoma (H&E, original magnification ×100).

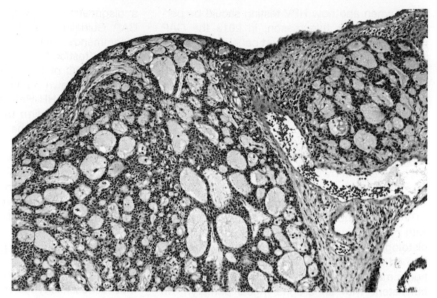

THE ROLE OF HUMAN PAPILLOMAVIRUS TESTING IN HEAD AND NECK SQUAMOUS CELL CARCINOMA

Performing testing for HR-HPV in HNSCC is important for many reasons. Aside from its prominent role as a prognostic marker, determining HPV status can grant a patient eligibility for clinical trials investigating novel treatment options (eg, radiotherapy deescalation or vaccine-based therapies),

and it is now integrated into the recently updated 8th Edition of the AJCC staging manual.[12,13] In addition, the site specificity of HPV-positive SCC can be exploited such that demonstrating HR-HPV in a cervical neck lymph node with metastatic SCC of unknown primary points to the ipsilateral oropharynx as the primary site of tumor origin with a high degree of accuracy.[20] Although the importance of HR-HPV testing in OPSCC is well recognized, there remains considerable confusion

Fig. 6. Histologic features of sinonasal nonkeratinizing SCC. This carcinoma has a ribbonlike inverted growth pattern reminiscent of inverted sinonasal papillomas (H&E, original magnification ×100).

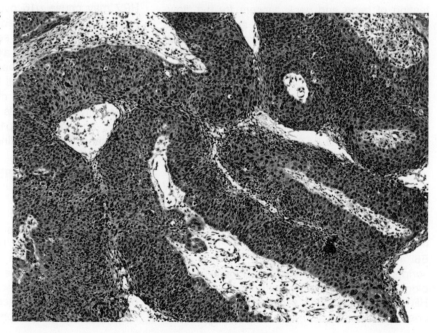

about when and how HPV testing should be performed.[38–40] For this reason, in 2013 the CAP appointed an 11-person expert panel and a 9-person advisory panel to formulate a comprehensive set of evidence-based recommendations, which have recently been published.[41]

Up to 80% to 90% of OPSCC contain transcriptionally active HR types of HPV. Although HPV DNA can be detected in certain nonoropharyngeal head and neck cancers, it is sometimes not a transcriptionally active virus, and its presence has not yet been shown by evidence in the literature to be clinically or biologically relevant.[22,42–44] As a result, the current CAP Guideline recommends that HR-HPV testing should be performed on all patients with newly diagnosed OPSCC, including all SCC histologic subtypes.[41] This testing may be performed on the primary tumor or a regional lymph node metastasis when the clinical findings are consistent with an oropharyngeal primary.[41] In addition, testing should not routinely be performed on patients with nonoropharyngeal primary tumors of the head and neck. Similar recommendations have also been endorsed by the Royal College of Pathologists and Cancer Care Ontario.[45,46]

Ninety percent to 95% of HPV-positive OPSCC are caused by HPV type 16, and as a result, detection of at least this type is mandatory for any head and neck cancer HPV detection strategy.[8] The remaining HPV-positive OPSCCs are caused by other "high-risk" HPV types, including 18, 31, 33, 35, 39, 45, 51, 52, 56, 58, 59, 68, 69, 73, and 82. Therefore, HPV-specific testing of OPSCC usually includes these other HR viral types in the form of a "cocktail." Notably, there is no role for the routine testing of head and neck cancers for the "low-risk" types of HPV (ie, types 6 and 11). These HPV types cause squamous and respiratory papillomas in the upper and lower aerodigestive tracts but do not cause OPSCC.

CONVENTIONAL METHODS FOR HIGH-RISK–HUMAN PAPILLOMAVIRUS TESTING USING FORMALIN-FIXED PARAFFIN-EMBEDDED MATERIAL

There are many methods available for HR-HPV testing in HNSCC, including p16 immunohistochemistry (IHC),[47–50] in situ hybridization (ISH) for HR-HPV DNA,[51] polymerase chain reaction (PCR) for the E6 and E7 proteins,[52,53] ISH for the E6 and E7 messenger RNA (mRNA) transcripts,[42,54,55] and combinations of these methodologies. These and other methods of testing for HR-HPV differ in their sensitivities, specificities, cost, technical requirements, and applicability to a diagnostic laboratory. The recently published CAP Guideline for HR-HPV testing in HNSCC recommends that pathologists should perform HR-HPV testing by surrogate marker p16 IHC for primary SCC of the oropharynx and metastatic SCC of unknown primary to level II or III cervical lymph nodes. HR-HPV–specific tests would be performed to confirm the p16 result in selected circumstances or at the discretion of the pathologist.[41] Primary OPSCCs that test positive for HR-HPV or its surrogate marker p16 are reported as HPV-positive or p16-positive without a tumor grade or differentiation status.[30] The authors briefly describe some of the available testing methodologies in later discussion.

P16 IMMUNOHISTOCHEMISTRY

Among the simplest, most cost-effective, and most accessible types of HPV testing is the surrogate immunohistochemical marker, p16. A consequence of the HPV viral oncoprotein E7 binding to and degrading the retinoblastoma protein is the cellular accumulation of p16, which in turn can easily be detected by IHC.[48] There are many advantages to using p16 IHC for HPV testing, including that it is easy to perform on paraffin-embedded tissues, including cell blocks, that it is very sensitive for the presence of transcriptionally active HPV (approaching 100%), and that it shows high specificity when used in the setting of a non-keratinizing SCC of the oropharynx.[47,49,50] In contrast, in head and neck sites outside the oropharynx, p16 is not entirely specific because other molecular mechanisms independent of HR-HPV may cause p16 overexpression.[42,43,56] For p16 IHC to be interpreted as positive, p16 immunoexpression must be seen in at least 70% of tumor cells in a nuclear and cytoplasmic distribution (**Fig. 7**). For FNA specimens, quantifying p16 IHC positivity in a cell block can be difficult because criteria for a minimum percentage of p16-positive tumor cells have not been established, and because p16 expression may be diminished in degenerating tumor cells.[57]

POLYMERASE CHAIN REACTION–BASED TECHNIQUES

PCR-based techniques are commonly used to identify HPV DNA in tissue. These methods have the advantage of very high sensitivity because PCR can amplify even very small amounts of HPV DNA. However, this sensitivity comes at the expense of specificity because the mere presence of HR-HPV does not necessarily convey whether the virus is transcriptionally active or simply a

Fig. 7. IHC for p16. HPV-positive OPSCC is characterized by having diffuse cytoplasmic and nuclear staining for p16 (IHC stain, original magnification ×400).

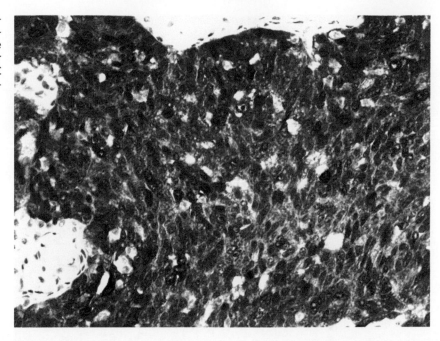

"passenger" and possibly biologically insignificant.[50,58] Also, PCR-based testing does not indicate whether the HPV is present within the tumor cells or nonspecifically within background nonneoplastic tissue. The latter is an important issue given the significant proportion of the population harboring HR-HPV within nonneoplastic tissues of the upper aerodigestive tract. Detection of the HPV E6 and E7 mRNA transcripts by PCR, on the other hand, is regarded by many investigators as the "gold standard" of HPV detection because it confirms that the virus is not only present, but transcriptionally active.[59,60] Unfortunately, at this time PCR for E6/E7 mRNA is technically demanding and impractical to implement for most diagnostic laboratories, although this may change in the future.

DNA IN SITU HYBRIDIZATION

DNA ISH for HR-HPV offers the advantages of visualizing the viral DNA in the context of the tumor histology, and it is relatively simple to integrate into the diagnostic pathology workflow. The presence of punctate hybridization signals in tumor nuclei is a very specific pattern for integration of HPV DNA into the host genome. However, at low viral copy levels, HPV DNA may be difficult to detect by ISH, limiting the sensitivity of this method.[41] In addition, the interpretation of HPV DNA ISH can be challenging in cases whereby hybridization signals are scant, focal, or unusually faint or small. Last, because it detects DNA, this method does not directly inform the clinician about the transcriptional activity of the virus.

RNA IN SITU HYBRIDIZATION

Recently, several commercially available platforms for ISH that detect HPV E6/E7 mRNA transcripts in formalin-fixed paraffin-embedded (FFPE) tumor tissues have been introduced (**Fig. 8**).[42,54,61] RNA ISH is an exciting advance because this method combines the histologic context of ISH with the specificity for transcriptionally active HPV of mRNA PCR. Also, RNA ISH appears to be much more sensitive than DNA ISH because at low viral copy numbers, where DNA ISH signals are absent or equivocal, RNA ISH signals are consistently robust.[42] With optimization of automated IHC platforms on the horizon, widespread implementation of this promising HPV detection method may be imminent.

TESTING METHODS USED IN COMBINATION

For selected situations as outlined in the recent CAP Guideline, use of p16 IHC followed by an HPV-specific test can be considered.[49,50,62] The most common strategy uses the very high sensitivity of p16 IHC paired with a more specific ISH or PCR-based HR-HPV test. The 2 tests can be performed in a manner whereby only a p16-positive result leads to the second HPV-specific test.

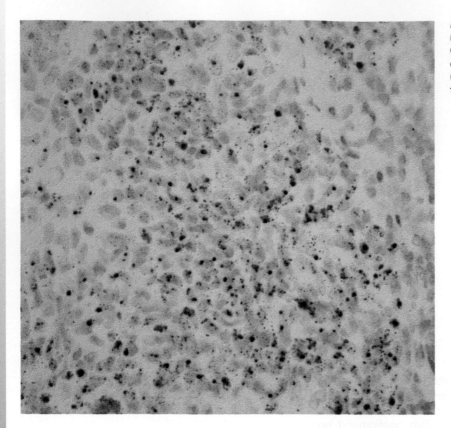

Fig. 8. ISH for HPV E6/E7 mRNA. This HPV-positive OPSCC shows a diffuse dotlike positive result (RNA ISH, original magnification ×400).

HIGH-RISK–HUMAN PAPILLOMAVIRUS TESTING APPLIED TO FINE-NEEDLE ASPIRATION SAMPLES OF HEAD AND NECK SQUAMOUS CELL CARCINOMA

Approximately 80% to 85% of HPV-positive OPSCCs present with early cervical nodal metastases, which can be easily sampled and diagnosed using FNA.[9,47] Cytologic evaluation has become an essential method for the early detection of metastatic HNSCC, and FNA biopsies can provide adequate material to determine HR-HPV status, leading to overall improved patient care. The current CAP Guideline recommends HR-HPV testing be performed on HNSCC FNA samples from all patients with known OPSCC not previously tested for HR-HPV, with suspected OPSCC, or with metastatic SCC of unknown primary.[41] Any of the aforementioned testing methods for HR-HPV can be applied to classify the metastatic HNSCC as HPV-positive or HPV-negative and help define the malignancy as a primary SCC of the oropharynx. The CAP Guideline further explains that if the result of HR-HPV testing is negative, testing should be repeated on tissue if it becomes available.

HR-HPV testing on cytologic specimens has been performed using FFPE FNA samples in cell blocks, liquid-based specimens (SurePath, Becton, Dickinson and Co, Franklin Lakes, NJ, USA, and ThinPrep, Hologic, Marlborough, MA, USA), and scrapes from air-dried or alcohol-fixed smears.[41] There is sufficient evidence to support the use of FNA as a valid method to obtain material for HR-HPV testing. The sensitivities and specificities of HPV assays for detecting HR-HPV using FNA material are reported to be greater than 90%, but the accuracy of any particular HPV testing modality remains largely unknown because of insufficient evidence-based literature.[41] Because no recommendation is made regarding the use of any specific testing methodology for FNA samples, the CAP Guideline statement provides laboratories with the autonomy to select the methodology most suitable for the particular laboratory.

Cytologic specimens are suitable for all standard tissue-based methods of HR-HPV detection because a corresponding cell block composed of FFPE tissue can usually be prepared from the FNA. There are caveats, however, to HR-HPV testing in FNA cell block material. The use of p16

IHC alone for the FNA evaluation of a squamous cyst in the neck is not recommended for cases where the cytologic differential diagnosis includes a branchial cleft cyst because the squamous epithelial lining of branchial cleft cysts can be positive.[48] Depending on the cellularity of the corresponding cell block or FNA sample, it may not be possible to assess the extent of p16 positivity. In addition, minimum thresholds for the percentage of positive cells needed to interpret a cell block as p16-positive have not been defined. In traditional biopsies, a positive p16 IHC result requires that at least 70% of the squamous cells show strong cytoplasmic and nuclear reactivity. The CAP Guideline recommends that if a laboratory uses cytology samples for p16 IHC testing, it should validate the criteria (ie, cutoff) for a positive result.[41]

When applied to primary nonkeratinizing SCC of the oropharynx, p16 is considered an acceptable surrogate marker for HR-HPV infection. Although p16 IHC is highly sensitive (approaching 100%) for the presence of HR-HPV when correctly interpreted, the specificity depends upon the context in which p16 IHC is used. It is important to keep in mind that overexpression of p16 can occur independently of HR-HPV in several malignancies that may be in the differential diagnosis of HPV-related HNSCC.[54,63] In addition to p16 IHC, standard PCR-based methods and ISH for HR-HPV DNA or mRNA can be applied to FNA material in the FFPE cell block.[1,2,5,9–11,57,58,60]

In the authors' experience, an effective method for assessing HR-HPV in an FNA specimen of metastatic HNSCC is to perform testing for HR-HPV directly on the liquid-based FNA sample.[49] Techniques already in use for HPV detection in liquid-based cervical cytology, such as the Roche cobas platform,[49] Cervista,[50] and Hybrid Capture,[47] can also be applied for HR-HPV detection in FNA of metastatic HNSCC. These detection methods have the advantage that several of them are already approved by the US Food and Drug Administration, they are widely implemented and validated in laboratories, they provide a clear-cut objective result, and some of the testing platforms can be automated. As the CAP Guideline points out, cytology laboratories that process FNA samples are most likely already equipped to provide HR-HPV testing because it is commonly performed on cervical cytology specimens. However, if this practice is implemented, a proper validation for liquid-based FNA samples is required.[41]

SUMMARY

In summary, the recent CAP Guideline provides recommendations for the effective performance and interpretation of HR-HPV testing in HNSCC. Among the 14 recommendations, one states that HR-HPV testing should be performed on FNA samples of metastatic HNSCC to cervical lymph nodes. Given the high frequency of metastasis to cervical lymph nodes by HPV-positive OPSCCs, FNA represents a simple and effective method to sample and diagnose these cancers. There is a wide range of options for HR-HPV testing, and it will be important for laboratories handling these FNA specimens to select the method that they deem most suitable.

REFERENCES

1. Adelstein DJ, Ridge JA, Gillison ML, et al. Head and neck squamous cell cancer and the human papillomavirus: summary of a National Cancer Institute State of the Science Meeting, November 9-10, 2008, Washington, D.C. Head Neck 2009;31:1393–422.
2. Chaturvedi AK, Engels EA, Pfeiffer RM, et al. Human papillomavirus and rising oropharyngeal cancer incidence in the United States. J Clin Oncol 2011;29:4294–301.
3. D'Souza G, Kreimer AR, Viscidi R, et al. Case-control study of human papillomavirus and oropharyngeal cancer. N Engl J Med 2007;356:1944–56.
4. Gillison ML, Koch WM, Capone RB, et al. Evidence for a causal association between human papillomavirus and a subset of head and neck cancers. J Natl Cancer Inst 2000;92:709–20.
5. Marur S, D'Souza G, Westra WH, et al. HPV-associated head and neck cancer: a virus-related cancer epidemic. Lancet Oncol 2010;11:781–9.
6. Gelwan E, Malm IJ, Khararjian A, et al. Nonuniform distribution of high-risk human papillomavirus in squamous cell carcinomas of the oropharynx: rethinking the anatomic boundaries of oral and oropharyngeal carcinoma from an oncologic HPV perspective. Am J Surg Pathol 2017;41:1722–8.
7. Doorbar J, Egawa N, Griffin H, et al. Human papillomavirus molecular biology and disease association. Rev Med Virol 2015;25(Suppl 1):2–23.
8. Kreimer AR, Clifford GM, Boyle P, et al. Human papillomavirus types in head and neck squamous cell carcinomas worldwide: a systematic review. Cancer Epidemiol Biomarkers Prev 2005;14:467–75.
9. Ang KK, Harris J, Wheeler R, et al. Human papillomavirus and survival of patients with oropharyngeal cancer. N Engl J Med 2010;363:24–35.
10. Fakhry C, Westra WH, Li S, et al. Improved survival of patients with human papillomavirus-positive head and neck squamous cell carcinoma in a prospective clinical trial. J Natl Cancer Inst 2008;100:261–9.

11. Ragin CC, Taioli E. Survival of squamous cell carcinoma of the head and neck in relation to human papillomavirus infection: review and meta-analysis. Int J Cancer 2007;121:1813–20.

12. Bonilla-Velez J, Mroz EA, Hammon RJ, et al. Impact of human papillomavirus on oropharyngeal cancer biology and response to therapy: implications for treatment. Otolaryngol Clin North Am 2013;46: 521–43.

13. Mirghani H, Amen F, Blanchard P, et al. Treatment de-escalation in HPV-positive oropharyngeal carcinoma: ongoing trials, critical issues and perspectives. Int J Cancer 2015;136:1494–503.

14. Lydiatt WM, Patel SG, O'Sullivan B, et al. Head and neck cancers—major changes in the American Joint Committee on Cancer Eighth Edition Cancer Staging Manual. CA Cancer J Clin 2017; 67:122–37.

15. Allsion DB, Miller JA, Coquia SF, et al. Ultrasonography-guided fine-needle aspiration with concurrent small core biopsy of neck masses and lymph nodes yields adequate material for HPV testing in head and neck squamous cell carcinomas. J Am Soc Cytopathol 2016;5:22–30.

16. Holmes BJ, Westra WH. The expanding role of cytopathology in the diagnosis of HPV-related squamous cell carcinoma of the head and neck. Diagn Cytopathol 2014;42:85–93.

17. Krane JF. Role of cytology in the diagnosis and management of HPV-associated head and neck carcinoma. Acta Cytol 2013;57:117–26.

18. Pusztaszeri MP, Faquin WC. Cytologic evaluation of cervical lymph node metastases from cancers of unknown primary origin. Semin Diagn Pathol 2015;32: 32–41.

19. Chernock RD, Lewis JS. Approach to metastatic carcinoma of unknown primary in the head and neck: squamous cell carcinoma and beyond. Head Neck Pathol 2015;9:6–15.

20. Begum S, Gillison ML, Ansari-Lari MA, et al. Detection of human papillomavirus in cervical lymph nodes: a highly effective strategy for localizing site of tumor origin. Clin Cancer Res 2003;9:6469–75.

21. Chernock RD, El-Mofty SK, Thorstad WL, et al. HPV-related nonkeratinizing squamous cell carcinoma of the oropharynx: utility of microscopic features in predicting patient outcome. Head Neck Pathol 2009;3: 186–94.

22. Lewis JS Jr, Khan RA, Masand RP, et al. Recognition of nonkeratinizing morphology in oropharyngeal squamous cell carcinoma - a prospective cohort and interobserver variability study. Histopathology 2012;60:427–36.

23. Westra WH. The morphologic profile of HPV-related head and neck squamous carcinoma: implications for diagnosis, prognosis, and clinical management. Head Neck Pathol 2012;6(Suppl 1):S48–54.

24. Westra WH. The pathology of HPV-related head and neck cancer: implications for the diagnostic pathologist. Semin Diagn Pathol 2015;32:42–53.

25. Goldenberg D, Begum S, Westra WH, et al. Cystic lymph node metastasis in patients with head and neck cancer: an HPV-associated phenomenon. Head Neck 2008;30:898–903.

26. Mehrad M, Zhao H, Gao G, et al. Transcriptionally-active human papillomavirus is consistently retained in the distant metastases of primary oropharyngeal carcinomas. Head Neck Pathol 2014;8: 157–63.

27. El-Mofty SK. Histopathologic risk factors in oral and oropharyngeal squamous cell carcinoma variants: an update with special reference to HPV-related carcinomas. Med Oral Patol Oral Cir Bucal 2014;19: e377–85.

28. Mehrad M, Carpenter DH, Chernock RD, et al. Papillary squamous cell carcinoma of the head and neck: clinicopathologic and molecular features with special reference to human papillomavirus. Am J Surg Pathol 2013;37:1349–56.

29. Lewis JS Jr, Thorstad WL, Chernock RD, et al. p16 positive oropharyngeal squamous cell carcinoma:an entity with a favorable prognosis regardless of tumor HPV status. Am J Surg Pathol 2010;34: 1088–96.

30. Stevens TM, Bishop JA. HPV-related carcinomas of the head and neck: morphologic features, variants, and practical considerations for the surgical pathologist. Virchows Arch 2017;471(2):295–307.

31. Bishop JA, Guo TW, Smith DF, et al. Human papillomavirus-related carcinomas of the sinonasal tract. Am J Surg Pathol 2013;37:185–92.

32. Massand RP, El-Mofty SK, Ma XJ, et al. Adenosquamous carcinoma of the head and neck: relationship to human papillomavirus and review of the literature. Head Neck Pathol 2011;5:108–16.

33. Bishop JA, Cowan ML, Shum CH, et al. MAML2 rearrangements in variant forms of mucoepidermoid carcinoma: ancillary diagnostic testing for the ciliated and warthin-like variants. Am J Surg Pathol 2018;42:130–6.

34. Radkay-Gonzalez L, Faquin W, McHugh JB, et al. Ciliated adenosquamous carcinoma: expanding the phenotypic diversity of human papillomavirus-associated tumors. Head Neck Pathol 2016;10: 167–75.

35. Bishop JA, Westra WH. Human papillomavirus-related small cell carcinoma of the oropharynx. Am J Surg Pathol 2011;35:1679–84.

36. Bishop JA, Andreasen S, Hang JF, et al. HPV-related multiphenotypic sinonasal carcinoma: an expanded series of 49 cases of the tumor formerly known as HPV-related carcinoma with adenoid cystic carcinoma-like features. Am J Surg Pathol 2017;41: 1690–701.

37. Lewis JS Jr. Sinonasal squamous cell carcinoma: a review with emphasis on emerging histologic subtypes and the role of human papillomavirus. Head Neck Pathol 2016;10:60–7.

38. Maniakas A, Moubayed SP, Ayad T, et al. North-American survey on HPV-DNA and p16 testing for head and neck squamous cell carcinoma. Oral Oncol 2014;50:942–6.

39. Shoushtari AN, Rahimi NP, Schlesinger DJ, et al. Survey on human papillomavirus/p16 screening use in oropharyngeal carcinoma patients in the United States. Cancer 2010;116:514–9.

40. Witt BL, Albertson DJ, Coppin MG, et al. Use of in situ hybridization for HPV in head and neck tumors: experience from a national reference laboratory. Head Neck Pathol 2015;9:60–4.

41. Lewis JS Jr, Beadle B, Bishop JA, et al. Human papillomavirus testing in head and neck carcinomas: guideline from the College of American Pathologists. Arch Pathol Lab Med 2018;142(5):559–97.

42. Bishop JA, Ma XJ, Wang H, et al. Detection of transcriptionally active high-risk HPV in patients with head and neck squamous cell carcinoma as visualized by a novel E6/E7 mRNA in situ hybridization method. Am J Surg Pathol 2012;36:1874–82.

43. Chernock RD, Wang X, Gao G, et al. Detection and significance of human papillomavirus, CDKN2A(p16) and CDKN1A(p21) expression in squamous cell carcinoma of the larynx. Mod Pathol 2013;26:223–31.

44. Poling JS, Ma XJ, Bui S, et al. Human papillomavirus (HPV) status of non-tobacco related squamous cell carcinomas of the lateral tongue. Oral Oncol 2014;50:306–10.

45. Routine HPV testing in head and neck squamous cell carcinoma. U.S. Department of Health and Human Services, 2013. Available at: https://goo.gl/i5KZNi. Accessed January 5, 2018.

46. Dataset for histopathology reporting of mucosal malignancies of the pharynx. The Royal College of Pathologists, 2013. Available at: https://goo.gl/D4dsHt. Accessed January 5, 2018.

47. Jordan RC, Lingen MW, Perez-Ordonez B, et al. Validation of methods for oropharyngeal cancer HPV status determination in US cooperative group trials. Am J Surg Pathol 2012;36:945–54.

48. Munger K, Baldwin A, Edwards KM, et al. Mechanisms of human papillomavirus-induced oncogenesis. J Virol 2004;78:11451–60.

49. Schache AG, Liloglou T, Risk JM, et al. Evaluation of human papilloma virus diagnostic testing in oropharyngeal squamous cell carcinoma: sensitivity, specificity, and prognostic discrimination. Clin Cancer Res 2011;17:6262–71.

50. Smeets SJ, Hesselink AT, Speel EJ, et al. A novel algorithm for reliable detection of human papillomavirus in paraffin embedded head and neck cancer specimen. Int J Cancer 2007;121:2465–72.

51. Rooper LM, Gandhi M, Bishop JA, et al. RNA in-situ hybridization is a practical and effective method for determining HPV status of oropharyngeal squamous cell carcinoma including discordant cases that are p16 positive by immunohistochemistry but HPV negative by DNA in-situ hybridization. Oral Oncol 2016;55:11–6.

52. Chaudhary AK, Pandya S, Mehrotra R, et al. Comparative study between the Hybrid Capture II test and PCR based assay for the detection of human papillomavirus DNA in oral submucous fibrosis and oral squamous cell carcinoma. Virol J 2010;7:253.

53. Gao Y, Chen X, Wang J, et al. A novel approach for copy number variation analysis by combining multiplex PCR with matrix-assisted laser desorption ionization time-of-flight mass spectrometry. J Biotechnol 2013;166:6–11.

54. Ukpo OC, Flanagan JJ, Ma XJ, et al. High-risk human papillomavirus E6/E7 mRNA detection by a novel in situ hybridization assay strongly correlates with p16 expression and patient outcomes in oropharyngeal squamous cell carcinoma. Am J Surg Pathol 2011;35:1343–50.

55. Kerr DA, Arora KS, Mahadevan KK, et al. Performance of a branch chain RNA in situ hybridization assay for the detection of high-risk human papillomavirus in head and neck squamous cell carcinoma. Am J Surg Pathol 2015;39:1643–52.

56. Lingen MW, Xiao W, Schmitt A, et al. Low etiologic fraction for high-risk human papillomavirus in oral cavity squamous cell carcinomas. Oral Oncol 2013;49:1–8.

57. Begum S, Gillison ML, Nicol TL, et al. Detection of human papillomavirus-16 in fine-needle aspirates to determine tumor origin in patients with metastatic squamous cell carcinoma of the head and neck. Clin Cancer Res 2007;13:1186–91.

58. Weinberger PM, Yu Z, Haffty BG, et al. Molecular classification identifies a subset of human papillomavirus–associated oropharyngeal cancers with favorable prognosis. J Clin Oncol 2006;24:736–47.

59. Leemans CR, Braakhuis BJ, Brakenhoff RH. The molecular biology of head and neck cancer. Nat Rev Cancer 2011;11:9–22.

60. van Houten VM, Snijders PJ, van den Brekel MW, et al. Biological evidence that human papillomaviruses are etiologically involved in a subgroup of head and neck squamous cell carcinomas. Int J Cancer 2001;93:232–5.

61. Schache AG, Liloglou T, Risk JM, et al. Validation of a novel diagnostic standard in HPV-positive

oropharyngeal squamous cell carcinoma. Br J Cancer 2013;108:1332–9.

62. Singhi AD, Westra WH. Comparison of human papillomavirus in situ hybridization and p16 immunohistochemistry in the detection of human papillomavirus-associated head and neck cancer

based on a prospective clinical experience. Cancer 2010;116:2166–73.

63. Begum S, Cao D, Gillison M, et al. Tissue distribution of human papillomavirus 16 DNA integration in patients with tonsillar carcinoma. Clin Cancer Res 2005;11:5694–9.

Updates in Lung Cancer Cytopathology

Paul A. VanderLaan, MD, PhD

KEYWORDS

- Non–small cell lung cancer (NSCLC) • Adenocarcinoma • Cytology • Ancillary testing
- Minimally invasive • PD-L1 • Biomarker

Key points

- The diagnosis, staging, and selection of therapy for patients with lung cancer are increasingly reliant on cytology and small biopsy specimens obtained via minimally invasive means.
- Combining cytomorphologic features with immunohistochemical testing can provide the accurate and specific lung cancer diagnosis required for clinical decision making.
- Molecular testing for a growing number of targetable genomic alterations is standard of care for patients diagnosed with advanced stage non–small cell lung cancer.
- PD-L1 is an evolving biomarker for the selection of patients for immune checkpoint inhibitor therapy.

ABSTRACT

Lung cancer diagnosis and ancillary testing are increasingly relying on cytology and small biopsy specimens obtained via minimally invasive means. Paired with traditional immunohistochemical characterization of tumors, biomarker testing and comprehensive genomic profiling are becoming essential steps in the workup of lung cancer to identify targetable alterations and guide optimal therapy selection. Recent advances in immune checkpoint inhibitor therapy have led to an increasingly complex and unresolved landscape for tumor PD-L1 testing. The prevalence and importance of lung cancer cytology specimens are growing, with more required by the cytopathologist in directing the care of patients with lung cancer.

OVERVIEW

Despite the advances in targeted therapeutic options over the past decade, lung cancer remains by far the leading cause of cancer-related death in the United States. Most patients with lung cancer present at an advanced stage and as such are not surgical candidates.[1] For these patients, the only diagnostic materials obtained are generally small biopsy and increasingly cytology specimens, due in part to technological advances in minimally invasive sampling techniques used by interventional pulmonology and interventional radiology. Furthermore, refinements in immunohistochemistry (IHC) and ancillary molecular testing have improved the diagnostic accuracy as well as prognostic/predictive information that can be gleaned from these pulmonary cytology specimens. In this regard, the cytopathologist is becoming an increasingly important member of the clinical team in directing the care of patients with lung cancer.

Pulmonary cytopathology is both a broad and a constantly evolving field. Much has been written on the subject, including a previous *Surgical Pathology Clinics* article only a few years ago.[2] In this brief review, the author focuses on recent updates in the field, including specimen acquisition, diagnostic workup, and molecular/ancillary testing. In truth,

---

Disclosure Statement: The author reports no relevant conflict of interest with respect to the content of this article.

Department of Pathology, Beth Israel Deaconess Medical Center, Harvard Medical School, 330 Brookline Avenue, Boston, MA 02215, USA

E-mail address: PVANDERL@bidmc.harvard.edu

Surgical Pathology 11 (2018) 515–522
https://doi.org/10.1016/j.path.2018.04.004

not much has changed with respect to the cytomorphologic features of lung cancer cytology, but what has evolved is how these samples are obtained and the ancillary testing now required for most lung carcinoma specimens.

MINIMALLY INVASIVE TISSUE SAMPLING TECHNIQUES

In patients with suspected lung cancer based on clinical risk factors (such as smoking history) and radiologic imaging findings (computed tomographic [CT] or PET-CT scans), a tissue sample is necessary for confirmation. As stated in the most recent lung cancer guidelines from the American College of Chest Physicians, "it is recommended that the diagnosis of lung cancer be established by the least invasive and safest method."[3] This diagnostic process has increasingly relied on either bronchoscopic or transthoracic CT-guided sampling modalities, generating cytology aspirates and/or small tissue biopsy specimens. The sampling modality in part depends on the size and location of the tumor, the presence of mediastinal or distant disease, patient comorbidities, and the local expertise and equipment availability in a given practice.[4] Especially for disease limited to the thorax, bronchoscopic sampling techniques (such as endobronchial ultrasound–transbronchial needle aspiration [EBUS-TBNA]) are generally recommended as the preferred choice for mediastinal staging and sampling of central lesions as well as for more peripheral lesions when coupled with radial EBUS or navigational guidance.[3–5] Alternatively, CT-guided transthoracic needle biopsies can be used for peripheral lung lesions, although they harbor a higher risk of pneumothorax. Regardless of the minimally invasive sampling technique used, the acquisition of sufficient cellular tumor material is critically important, with rapid on-site specimen evaluation potentially helpful in ensuring adequate material is obtained and appropriately triaged in such situations.[6] As shall be discussed, in this era of personalized medicine, the definition of "adequate" has evolved to cover not only material for diagnosis but frequently also tumor subtyping by IHC and ancillary/molecular testing for therapy selection.[7]

DIAGNOSTIC WORKUP OF LUNG CARCINOMA

All diagnoses of lung cancer should be made according to the most recent 2015 World Health Organization (WHO) classification system, which incorporates the most recent International Association for the Study of Lung Cancer (IASLC),

American Thoracic Society, European Respiratory Society (ERS) pathologic classification of lung cancer with particular attention given to cytology and small biopsy specimens.[5,8,9] In practice, these pathologic entities can pose diagnostic challenges when evaluated on limited cytologic samples or ones with suboptimal cellular preservation or visualization. Thus, a risk-based categorization schema that is used in many areas of cytology has been recently proposed by the Papanicolaou Society of Cytopathology.[10] These standardized terminology and nomenclature guidelines for respiratory cytology are much in line with the WHO classification and follow the familiar "Nondiagnostic–Negative (for malignancy)–Atypical–Neoplastic–Suspicious for malignancy–Malignant" framework already codified by the cytopathology community.

Most lung cancers encountered on a daily basis include lung adenocarcinoma, squamous cell carcinoma, and the neuroendocrine tumors, both carcinoid tumors and the high-grade neuroendocrine carcinomas: small cell carcinoma and large cell neuroendocrine carcinoma (LCNEC). Admittedly, these tumors can display a broad spectrum of cytomorphologic features depending on the degree of differentiation, preceding treatment effects, or to a lesser extent the cytologic preparation method used, but classic cytologic exemplars of these tumors are illustrated in **Fig. 1**. In the modern-day workup of lung cancer, the cytology community is well aware that a diagnosis of "non–small cell lung carcinoma (NSCLC)" is no longer sufficient, given the divergent pattern of driver mutations and therapeutic strategies for lung adenocarcinoma as compared with squamous cell carcinoma or other tumors falling under the umbrella of NSCLC. Further subclassification is needed. For NSCLC, if the cytomorphologic features are not clear, a limited IHC panel of generally mutually exclusive markers is recommended, composed of thyroid transcription factor 1 (TTF-1) or novel aspartic proteinase A (Napsin-A) for adenocarcinoma versus p40 or cytokeratin 5/6 (CK5/6) for squamous cell carcinoma.[8] For squamous cell carcinoma, p40 (N-terminal truncation isoform of p63) has been shown to be more specific with similar sensitivity as compared with p63, and as such, is a preferred first-line squamous marker.[11,12] If neuroendocrine features are present or there are suggestive clinical or radiologic findings, only then is it recommended to perform neuroendocrine markers (synaptophysin and chromogranin, and if needed the more sensitive but less specific CD56). If the cytomorphology and immunohistochemical staining profile remains ambiguous, then a cytologic diagnosis of NSCLC-

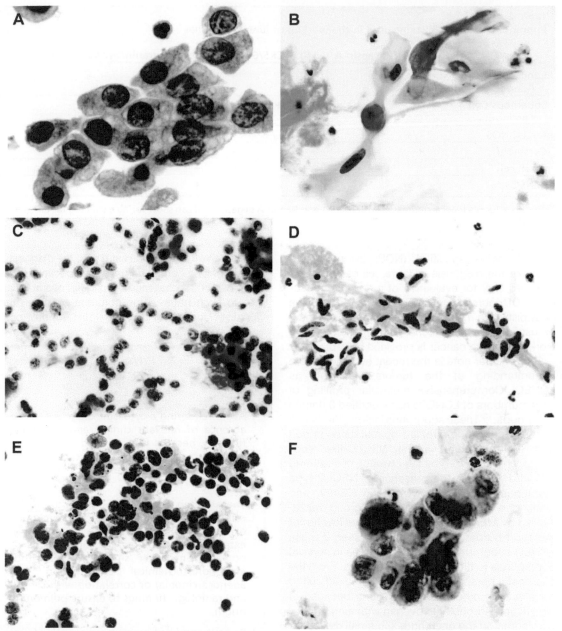

Fig. 1. Cytomorphologic examples of lung cancer. (*A*) Lung adenocarcinoma with eccentrically placed nuclei, prominent nucleoli, finely vacuolated cytoplasm, and 3-dimensional cell clusters. (*B*) Keratinizing squamous cell carcinoma with dense orangeophilic cytoplasm with sharp irregular borders, dark hyperchromatic elongated nuclei with coarse chromatin, present in a background of necrotic debris. (*C*) Carcinoid tumor typified by a hypercellular specimen composed of relatively monotonous cells with round to oval nuclei, characteristic "salt and pepper" chromatin, only rare mitoses, and a clean background. (*D*) Carcinoid tumor demonstrating more spindled morphology but with similar speckled chromatin pattern and rare mitoses. (*E*) Small cell carcinoma is characterized by cells with high nuclear to cytoplasmic ratio, some nuclear molding, finely granular chromatin without prominent nucleoli, and frequent mitotic figures, present in a background of necrotic debris. (*F*) LCNEC can closely resemble lung adenocarcinoma with round to oval nuclei with prominent nucleoli and moderate amounts of finely vacuolated cytoplasm; however, the presence of background necrosis, frequent mitotic figures, and an aggressive clinical presentation might prompt immunohistochemical stain selection to differentiate lung adenocarcinoma from LCNEC. All images are alcohol-fixed Papanicolaou stained smears taken under ×100 oil objective magnification.

Table 1
Immunohistochemical stains used in the workup of lung carcinomas

	TTF-1	Napsin-A	p40	CK5/6	CK7	Chromogranin/Synaptophysin/CD56
Lung Adenocarcinoma[a]	+	+	−	−	+	−
Squamous Cell Carcinoma	−	−	+	+	−/+	−
NSCLC-NOS	−/+	−/+	−/+	−/+	+/−	−
Carcinoid	+	−	−	−	+	+
Small cell	+	−	−	−	+	+
LCNEC	+	−/+	−	−	+	+

[a] Mucinous lung adenocarcinomas are often TTF-1 and Napsin-A negative and can show variable staining for CK7, CK20, and CDX-2.

not otherwise specified (NOS) is warranted, because the diagnosis of large cell carcinoma is reserved only for evaluation of a resection specimen. Of course, one must always consider the possibility of a metastasis to the lung. A summary of useful immunohistochemical markers in the work-up of lung cancer is provided in **Table 1**.

Of particular note is the recent evolution in the understanding of the tumors classified as LCNEC. Comprehensive molecular profiling of large numbers of LCNECs has identified 3 unique subgroups.[13] These subgroups include the "small cell-like" subgroup, typified by mutations in *p53* and *RB1* mutation/loss; the "NSCLC-like" subgroup, characterized by the absence of coaltered *p53* and *RB1* but the presence of NSCLC-type mutations like *STK11*, *KRAS*, and *KEAP1*; and finally, the rare "carcinoid-like" subgroup, represented by *MEN1* mutations and overall low tumor mutation burden. It remains to be seen if these LCNEC subgroups portent differences in survival or response to different therapy options. From the diagnostic perspective, LCNEC can be difficult to diagnose on cytologic preparations because of significant morphologic overlap with lung adenocarcinoma on the one hand, and small cell carcinoma on the other. For the latter, prominent nucleoli and moderate amounts of cytoplasm are signs supporting LCNEC over small cell carcinoma. In differentiating LCNEC from lung adenocarcinoma, Napsin-A IHC can be a useful tool, because in general lung neuroendocrine carcinomas are Napsin-A negative.[14,15] However, weak, focal Napsin-A positivity has been recently reported in 15% of LCNECs, regardless of Napsin-A antibody clone used.[16] As such, one should consider the possibility of LCNEC when confronted with NSCLC that is TTF-1 positive but Napsin-A negative, especially in a clinical context of widespread metastatic disease.

Although straightforward at times, the diagnostic workup of lung cancer on cytology specimens can pose particular challenges. To help avoid falling prey to such traps, some common pitfalls in the workup of lung cancer are outlined in the *Pitfalls* box.

Pitfalls
CYTOLOGIC WORKUP
OF LUNG CANCER

! Avoid rendering a cytologic diagnosis in the absence of relevant clinical and radiologic findings, because this can lead to overdiagnosis of malignancy in reactive conditions, or misdiagnosis of metastatic disease as lung primary.

! There are no cytomorphologic features that can reliably predict primary adenocarcinoma or squamous cell carcinoma of the lung; extensive morphologic overlap with carcinomas from other sites warrants either immunohistochemical confirmation (for adenocarcinoma) or correlation with clinical and radiologic findings to ensure pulmonary origin.

! Be cautious when making a diagnosis of malignancy based on a hypocellular specimen or one with few atypical cells, because this could represent a benign reactive process.

! Crushed small biopsy or poorly prepared smears of carcinoid tumors can be confused with small cell carcinoma; use of MIB-1/Ki-67 staining (high proliferative index in small cell carcinoma), RB1 loss by IHC, and *RB1/p53* mutations by molecular testing would all support small cell carcinoma.

! When encountering a TTF-1-positive but Napsin-A-negative tumor, consider the possibility of a neuroendocrine tumor.

ANCILLARY TESTING

The advances in precision oncology for lung cancer have significantly changed what is both needed and expected from cytology and small biopsy specimens. In the past, the cytopathologist's role in managing patients with lung cancer ended with the diagnosis. Now additional ancillary testing and interpretation, such as IHC for anaplastic lymphoma kinase (ALK), ROS proto-oncogene 1 (ROS1), or programmed death-ligand 1 (PD-L1), are often performed by the cytology laboratory as well as close coordination with molecular laboratories (either in-house or send-out) for mutational analysis. Testing success in large part depends on several preanalytic factors that the cytopathology laboratory should focus on to minimize tissue loss during processing and diagnostic workup, while maximizing materials for downstream ancillary testing.[17] Broadly speaking, attention to the steps of specimen acquisition, processing, and selection for ancillary testing can maximize testing success in the molecular laboratory, as comprehensively discussed elsewhere.[18,19]

Biomarker testing of lung cancer specimens is critically important for the optimal selection of patients to receive targeted therapies, because it has been widely shown that patients with an actionable driver mutation identified by molecular testing (increasingly via multiplexed assays or comprehensive genomic profiling) and given a targeted therapy have increased survival as compared with patients who either do not have a driver mutation or did not receive targeted therapy.[20] As the number of US Food and Drug Administration (FDA)-approved targeted therapies in NSCLC grows, so does the number of potentially actionable genomic alterations that should be tested for.[21] Thus, much information needs to be gleaned from the diagnostic cytology specimens to direct oncologic care for patients with advanced stage lung cancer. Of interest for cytopathologists, the most recent College of American Pathologists, IASLC, and Association for Molecular Pathology (CAP/IASLC/AMP) guidelines have updated the recommendation on which cytology specimens are preferred substrates, now acknowledging that either cell blocks or other cytologic preparations (such as direct smears) are suitable specimens for lung cancer biomarker molecular testing.[22]

A comprehensive discussion of each actionable genomic alteration in NSCLC and how they are tested (via IHC, fluorescent in situ hybridization, or polymerase chain reaction-based molecular methods) is beyond the scope of this article. For this information, the reader is directed to several excellent recent reviews on the subject.[23–25]

Evidence-based guideline recommendations and their recent update put forth by the CAP/IASLC/AMP and endorsed by American Society of Clinical Oncology outline the minimum number of molecular targets that must be tested for in advanced stage NSCLC (predominantly adenocarcinoma): EGFR (epidermal growth factor receptor), ALK, and ROS1.[22,26] In addition to these 3 targets, the most recent National Comprehensive Cancer Network guidelines currently also recommend mandatory testing for BRAF (proto-oncogene B-Raf) as well as PD-L1 (discussed later) based on effective FDA-approved therapies for tumors that harbor these genomic alterations.[4] Moving beyond these more established biomarkers, there are a growing number of "emerging" targets that both guidelines indicate should be tested for, especially if part of a comprehensive next-generation sequencing assay. These genomic targets include MET (hepatocyte growth factor receptor), RET (rearranged during transfection protooncogene), ERBB2 (HER2), and KRAS.[4,22] The prevalence of these driver mutations in NSCLC varies depending on clinical variables, such as age, gender, ethnicity, and smoking status.[27,28] However, based on data compiled from 6 large studies with a cumulative total of more than 25,000 NSCLCs sequenced, the average percentages for each of the major aforementioned genomic alterations are presented in **Fig. 2**.[29–34]

PROGRAMMED DEATH-LIGAND 1 BIOMARKER TESTING

With the recent promising developments in the field of immunotherapy for NSCLC, there has been increased demand for biomarker testing to best select those patients most likely to respond to immune checkpoint inhibitor therapy. Following initial FDA approvals beginning in 2015, there have been a growing number of immune checkpoint inhibitor drugs available to oncologists for the treatment of NSCLC. These drugs primarily target the PD-L1-receptor axis and in general have been shown to have superior response rates, survival, and toxicity profiles as compared with conventional chemotherapy in patients with high PD-L1 tumor expression.[35] This expression is evaluated via IHC with a semiquantitative readout of tumor proportion score (TPS): the percentage of tumor cells showing partial or complete membranous staining of any intensity for PD-L1, with varying clinical cutoffs depending on treatment setting (first vs second/third line) and drug-assay choice.

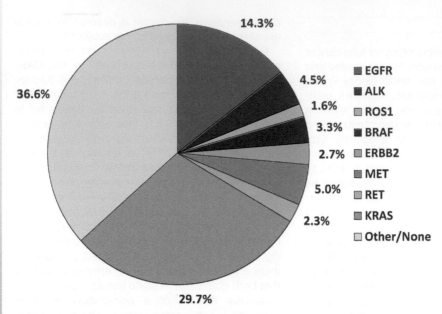

14.3%

36.6%

4.5%

1.6%

3.3%

2.7%

5.0%

2.3%

29.7%

- ■ EGFR
- ■ ALK
- ▤ ROS1
- ■ BRAF
- ▤ ERBB2
- ■ MET
- ■ RET
- ■ KRAS
- ☐ Other/None

Fig. 2. Frequency of major genomic alterations in NSCLC. Based on reported mutation or gene rearrangement frequencies compiled from 6 large-scale studies, the average percentages of each genomic alterations is shown. (*Data from* Refs.[29–34])

With respect to the latter, there are currently 5 different drugs that are either approved or in late-stage clinical trials for treatment of NSCLC (pembrolizumab, nivolumab, atezolizumab, durvalumab, and avelumab), and each drug has a paired assay consisting of a different antibody clone (22C3, 28-8, SP142, SP263, and 73-10, respectively), run on different staining platforms (Dako Autostainer Link 48 vs Ventana BenchMark UL-TRA), with different clinical cutoff definitions of positivity (≥50%, ≥1%, ≥25%), and with one (atezolizumab) even requiring evaluation of PD-L1 expression on both tumor cells and tumor infiltrating immune cells.[36] Unfortunately, this has led to uncertainty regarding the comparability of results across different testing platforms, with ongoing studies attempting to decipher this complexity for testing laboratories.[37,38]

Of particular interest to cytopathology, to date, all of the large-scale clinical trials leading to the approval of immune checkpoint inhibitors have used formalin-fixed, paraffin-embedded (FFPE) surgical pathology tissue specimens as PD-L1 IHC testing substrates. Given that a large proportion of diagnostic specimens for advanced stage lung cancer are cytology specimens (EBUS-TBNA, fine-needle aspirate, or effusion specimens) and may be the only clinically available specimen for testing, it is important to determine if cytology specimens, namely FFPE cell block specimens, can be reliably used as PD-L1 testing substrates. At this point, only a handful of studies on the topic have been published, but early results are promising. By using the 22C3 pharmDx assay, 2 groups have shown overall similar PD-L1 tumor expression patterns in cytology cell block–tested specimens compared with surgical pathology–tested specimens.[36,39] Furthermore, a cohort of patients with lung cancer with paired cytology cell block and surgical pathology specimens showed strong correlation of PD-L1 tumor positivity scores between their 2 specimens.[40] As such, it appears as if cytology cell blocks may be a viable option for PD-L1 biomarker testing, although more validation type studies are needed. Although PD-L1 IHC remains the best biomarker for selection of patients for immune checkpoint inhibitor therapy, it remains to be seen whether tumor mutation burden, used either in conjunction with or in place of PD-L1 TPS, may actually be a better tool for the selection of patients who may respond to immune checkpoint inhibitory therapy.[41]

SUMMARY

This is an exciting time for pulmonary cytopathology, given the concurrent advances in interventional pulmonology and thoracic oncology. The cytopathologist has become a key player in guiding the care of patients with lung cancer, both by providing accurate diagnoses on small cytology specimens obtained via minimally invasive means and by ensuring the processing and handling of cytology specimens are done in ways to maximize the likelihood of ancillary testing success.[42] Treatment of advanced stage lung cancer has become a more dynamic process, with optimal therapy selection increasingly being reassessed by the treating oncologist via repeat tumor biopsy (or more recently liquid biopsy) testing to identify potential resistance mechanisms in the setting of targeted therapies.[43,44] Coupling the need for longitudinal tumor sampling during the course of treatment with the global trend in medicine toward less invasive diagnostic procedures, the reliance on both the cytopathologist and the cytopathology laboratory should only increase in the years ahead. By leveraging the tried-and-true diagnostic cytomorphologic expertise of our specialty with the ever growing field of molecular pathology, the cytopathologist is positioned both now and in the future to be a leader in the multidisciplinary approach to providing optimal care to patients with cancer.

REFERENCES

1. National Cancer Institute (NCI) Surveillance, Epidemiology, and End Results (SEER) program. Cancer stat facts: lung and bronchus cancer. Available at: https://seer.cancer.gov/statfacts/html/lungb.html. Accessed February 22, 2018.
2. Schmitt F, Machado JC. Ancillary studies, including immunohistochemistry and molecular studies, in lung cytology. Surg Pathol Clin 2014;7:35–46.
3. Detterbeck FC, Lewis SZ, Diekemper R, et al. Executive summary: diagnosis and management of lung cancer, 3rd ed: American College of Chest Physicians evidence-based clinical practice guidelines. Chest 2013;143:7S–37S.
4. National Comprehensive Cancer Network. Non-Small Cell Lung Cancer (Version 2.2018). Available at: https://www.nccn.org/professionals/physician_gls/pdf/nscl.pdf. Accessed February 13, 2018.
5. Postmus PE, Kerr KM, Oudkerk M, et al. Early and locally advanced non-small-cell lung cancer (NSCLC): ESMO clinical practice guidelines for diagnosis, treatment and follow-up. Ann Oncol 2017;28:iv1–21.
6. Kraft AO. Specimen acquisition: ROSEs, gardeners, and gatekeepers. Cancer 2017;125:449–54.
7. Sung S, Crapanzano JP, DiBardino D, et al. Molecular testing on endobronchial ultrasound (EBUS) fine needle aspirates (FNA): impact of triage. Diagn Cytopathol 2018;46:122–30.
8. Travis WD, Brambilla E, Burke AP, et al, editors. WHO classification of tumours of the lung, pleura, thymus and heart. 4th edition. Lyon (France): World Health Organization; 2015.
9. Travis WD, Brambilla E, Noguchi M, et al. Diagnosis of lung cancer in small biopsies and cytology: implications of the 2011 International Association for the Study of Lung Cancer/American Thoracic Society/European Respiratory Society classification. Arch Pathol Lab Med 2013;137:668–84.
10. Layfield LJ, Baloch Z, Elsheikh T, et al. Standardized terminology and nomenclature for respiratory cytology: the Papanicolaou Society of Cytopathology guidelines. Diagn Cytopathol 2016;44:399–409.
11. Bishop JA, Teruya-Feldstein J, Westra WH, et al. p40 (ΔNp63) is superior to p63 for the diagnosis of pulmonary squamous cell carcinoma. Mod Pathol 2012;25:405–15.
12. Tatsumori T, Tsuta K, Masai K, et al. p40 is the best marker for diagnosing pulmonary squamous cell carcinoma: comparison with p63, cytokeratin 5/6, desmocollin-3, and sox2. Appl Immunohistochem Mol Morphol 2014;22:377–82.
13. Rekhtman N, Pietanza MC, Hellmann MD, et al. Next-generation sequencing of pulmonary large cell neuroendocrine carcinoma reveals small cell carcinoma-like and non-small cell carcinoma-like subsets. Clin Cancer Res 2016;22:3618–29.
14. Masai K, Tsuta K, Kawago M, et al. Expression of squamous cell carcinoma markers and adenocarcinoma markers in primary pulmonary neuroendocrine carcinomas. Appl Immunohistochem Mol Morphol 2013;21:292–7.
15. Zhang C, Schmidt LA, Hatanaka K, et al. Evaluation of napsin A, TTF-1, p63, p40, and CK5/6 immunohistochemical stains in pulmonary neuroendocrine tumors. Am J Clin Pathol 2014;142:320–4.
16. Rekhtman N, Pietanza CM, Sabari J, et al. Pulmonary large cell neuroendocrine carcinoma with adenocarcinoma-like features: napsin A expression and genomic alterations. Mod Pathol 2018;31:111–21.
17. Roy-Chowdhuri S, Stewart J. Preanalytic variables in cytology: lessons learned from next-generation sequencing-the MD Anderson Experience. Arch Pathol Lab Med 2016;140:1191–9.
18. Roy-Chowdhuri S, Aisner DL, Allen TC, et al. Biomarker testing in lung carcinoma cytology specimens: a perspective from members of the pulmonary pathology society. Arch Pathol Lab Med 2016;40:1267–72.
19. da Cunha Santos G, Saieg MA. Preanalytic specimen triage: smears, cell blocks, cytospin preparations, transport media, and cytobanking. Cancer Cytopathol 2017;125:455–64.
20. Kris MG, Johnson BE, Berry LD, et al. Using multiplexed assays of oncogenic drivers in lung cancers to select targeted drugs. JAMA 2014;311:1998–2006.
21. Reck M, Rabe KF. Precision diagnosis and treatment for advanced non-small-cell lung cancer. N Engl J Med 2017;377:849–61.
22. Lindeman NI, Cagle PT, Aisner DL, et al. Updated molecular testing guideline for the selection of lung cancer patients for treatment with targeted tyrosine kinase inhibitors: guideline from the College of American Pathologists, the International Association for the Study of Lung Cancer, and the Association for Molecular Pathology. Arch Pathol Lab Med 2018;142(3):321–46.
23. Sholl LM. The molecular pathology of lung cancer. Surg Pathol Clin 2016;9:353–78.

24. Calvayrac O, Pradines A, Pons E, et al. Molecular biomarkers for lung adenocarcinoma. Eur Respir J 2017;49(4), [pii:1601734].

25. Bernicker EH, Miller RA, Cagle PT. Biomarkers for selection of therapy for adenocarcinoma of the lung. J Oncol Pract 2017;13:221–7.

26. Lindeman NI, Cagle PT, Beasley MB, et al. Molecular testing guideline for selection of lung cancer patients for EGFR and ALK tyrosine kinase inhibitors: guideline from the College of American Pathologists, International Association for the Study of Lung Cancer, and Association for Molecular Pathology. Arch Pathol Lab Med 2013;137:828–60.

27. Yamaguchi N, Vanderlaan PA, Folch E, et al. Smoking status and self-reported race affect the frequency of clinically relevant oncogenic alterations in non-small-cell lung cancers at a United States-based academic medical practice. Lung Cancer 2013;82:31–7.

28. VanderLaan PA, Rangachari D, Majid A, et al. Tumor biomarker testing in non-small-cell lung cancer: a decade of change. Lung Cancer 2018;116:90–5.

29. Suh JH, Johnson A, Albacker L, et al. Comprehensive genomic profiling facilitates implementation of the national comprehensive cancer network guidelines for lung cancer biomarker testing and identifies patients who may benefit from enrollment in mechanism-driven clinical trials. Oncologist 2016;21:684–91.

30. Jordan EJ, Kim HR, Arcila ME, et al. Prospective comprehensive molecular characterization of lung adenocarcinomas for efficient patient matching to approved and emerging therapies. Cancer Discov 2017;7:596–609.

31. Collisson EA, Campbell JD, Brooks AN, et al. Cancer genome atlas research network. Comprehensive molecular profiling of lung adenocarcinoma. Nature 2014;511:543–50.

32. Sholl LM, Aisner DL, Varella-Garcia M, et al. Multi-institutional Oncogenic driver mutation analysis in lung adenocarcinoma: the lung cancer mutation consortium experience. J Thorac Oncol 2015;10: 768–77.

33. Illei PB, Belchis D, Tseng LH, et al. Clinical mutational profiling of 1006 lung cancers by next generation sequencing. Oncotarget 2017;8:96684–96.

34. Barlesi F, Mazieres J, Merlio JP, et al. Routine molecular profiling of patients with advanced non-small-cell lung cancer: results of a 1-year nationwide programme of the French Cooperative Thoracic Intergroup (IFCT). Lancet 2016;387:1415–26.

35. Reck M, Rodríguez-Abreu D, Robinson AG, et al. Pembrolizumab versus chemotherapy for PD-L1-positive non-small-cell lung cancer. N Engl J Med 2016;375:1823–33.

36. Torous VF, Rangachari D, Gallant B, et al. PD-L1 testing using the clone 22C3 pharmDx kit for selection of patients with non-small cell lung cancer to receive immune checkpoint inhibitor therapy: are cytology cell blocks a viable option? J Am Soc Cytopathol 2018;7(3):133–41.

37. Hirsch FR, McElhinny A, Stanforth D, et al. PD-L1 immunohistochemistry assays for lung cancer: results from phase 1 of the blueprint PD-L1 IHC assay comparison project. J Thorac Oncol 2017;12: 208–22.

38. Hendry S, Byrne DJ, Wright GM, et al. Comparison of four PD-L1 immunohistochemical assays in lung cancer. J Thorac Oncol 2018;13:367–76.

39. Heymann JJ, Bulman WA, Swinarski D, et al. PD-L1 expression in non-small cell lung carcinoma: comparison among cytology, small biopsy, and surgical resection specimens. Cancer 2017;125: 896–907.

40. Russell-Goldman E, Kravets S, Dahlberg SE, et al. Cytologic-histologic correlation of programmed death-ligand 1 immunohistochemistry in lung carcinomas. Cancer Cytopathol 2018;126(4):253–63.

41. Carbone DP, Reck M, Paz-Ares L, et al. First-line nivolumab in stage IV or recurrent non-small-cell lung cancer. N Engl J Med 2017;376:2415–26.

42. Zakowski MF. Analytic inquiry: molecular testing in lung cancer. Cancer Cytopathol 2017;125:470–6.

43. Sholl LM, Aisner DL, Allen TC, et al. Liquid biopsy in lung cancer: a perspective from members of the pulmonary pathology society. Arch Pathol Lab Med 2016;140:825–9.

44. Hiley CT, Le Quesne J, Santis G, et al. Challenges in molecular testing in non-small-cell lung cancer patients with advanced disease. Lancet 2016;388: 1002–11.

Updates in Effusion Cytology

Christin M. Lepus, MD, PhD, Marina Vivero, MD*

KEYWORDS

• Effusion • Cytology • Molecular • Immunohistochemistry • Mesothelioma

Key points

- Serous effusions are most commonly benign and, with the exception of connective tissue disease, usually present nonspecific cytologic findings.
- Effusion cytology yields an overall sensitivity and specificity of up to 80% and 98%, respectively, for malignant disease. These both improve with ancillary diagnostic testing.
- Immunohistochemistry, cytogenetic, and molecular analysis can all be done on cell blocks, smears, and liquid-based preparations of effusion fluids for diagnostic and predictive purposes.
- Immunohistochemical loss of BAP1 protein expression, seen in 57% to 67% of mesotheliomas, can be useful to distinguish between benign and malignant mesothelial proliferations.
- Immunohistochemical staining of effusion samples is helpful in the diagnosis of rare mimics of more common epithelial malignancies.

ABSTRACT

Effusion cytology plays multiple roles in the management of benign and malignant disease, from primary diagnosis to tissue allocation for ancillary diagnostic studies and biomarker testing of therapeutic targets. This article summarizes recent advances in pleural effusion cytology, with a focus on the practical application of immunohistochemical markers, cytogenetic techniques, flow cytometry, and molecular techniques for the diagnosis and management of primary and secondary neoplasms of the pleura.

OVERVIEW

Cytologic examination of serous effusions provides a unique opportunity to obtain clinically impactful information with minimal discomfort and risk to patients. Reported rates of malignancy in effusions range from 15% to 50%,[1,2] of which 15% to 42% may represent the first manifestation of disease.[1-3] Interobserver concordance and sensitivity varies based on experience, fluid type, diagnosis (benign vs malignant), number of specimens examined, and preparation type.[2,4,5] Overall, sensitivity and specificity of effusion cytology for the detection of malignancy in effusions varies from 40% to 80% and 89% to 98%, respectively.[2,5] Significant cytomorphologic overlap exists in effusion specimens between benign and malignant mesothelial cells and adenocarcinomas, as well as between carcinomas of different primary origins.[4,6,7] Ancillary techniques are frequently used to resolve these diagnostic challenges and avoid diagnostic pitfalls, as well as to increase the sensitivity and specificity of effusion cytology to 94% and 100%, respectively.[2,5]

ANCILLARY TESTING OF EFFUSIONS

IMMUNOHISTOCHEMISTRY

Immunohistochemistry is widely adopted in cytologic diagnosis of effusions and allows for

Disclosure Statement: Neither author has financial disclosures.
Department of Pathology, Brigham and Women's Hospital, 75 Francis Street, Boston, MA 02115, USA
* Corresponding author.
E-mail address: mvivero@bwh.harvard.edu

Surgical Pathology 11 (2018) 523–544
https://doi.org/10.1016/j.path.2018.05.003

accurate classification of most tumors. Cell block preparations are most commonly used owing to the ease of morphologic interpretation, existing validation of immunohistochemical stains on formalin-fixed paraffin-embedded material, minimal background staining, and the ability to evaluate numerous antigens on a single preparation.[8] Immunohistochemical stains also provide a cost-effective way to evaluate predictive biomarkers, such as quantification of hormone receptors in metastatic breast carcinoma and anaplastic lymphoma kinase (ALK), ROS proto oncogene 1 (ROS1), and programmed cell death-ligand 1 (PD-L1) staining in lung cancer.[9–11] Although inherent intratumor heterogeneity may limit interpretation of immunohistochemistry on targeted needle and excisional biopsies owing to sampling bias,[12] intertumor heterogeneity may be a more significant factor in effusions because metastatic disease and treated tumor may show differing immunophenotypes compared with the primary source.[9,13,14]

FLOW CYTOMETRY

Flow cytometric immunophenotyping of effusion specimens has emerged as another sensitive, reproducible, and low-cost quantitative ancillary diagnostic technique with a quick turnaround time, particularly for the detection and classification of hematolymphoid neoplasms.[15] Lymphocyte-rich effusions often present a diagnostic challenge for cytopathologists. Low-grade lymphomas can look deceptively bland, whereas reactive lymphocytes can show marked atypia, requiring flow cytometry to differentiate between them. Although not routine practice, protein expression can also be assessed by flow cytometry in nonhematologic malignant effusions to detect metastatic disease or monitor treatment response, and is highly sensitive and specific.[16]

CYTOGENETIC ANALYSIS

Because mechanical and enzymatic tissue disaggregation is unnecessary, cytology specimens are appealing substrates for cytogenetic studies. Both karyotype and fluorescence in situ hybridization (FISH) studies can be performed, and a variety of preparations, including fresh cell suspensions, cytocentrifugation preparations, thin-layer slides, and cell blocks, can be used.[17] Cytogenetic analysis can be used for diagnostic purposes, particularly for mesothelioma, lymphomas, and sarcomas.[18–21] Or it can be used for predictive purposes, such as assessment of ALK and ROS1 gene rearrangements in non-small cell lung carcinoma.[22,23]

MOLECULAR TESTING

In some patients, effusions may be the only available specimen for molecular profiling of genetic alterations that are increasingly important in diagnosis and prediction of drug responsiveness, metastatic potential, and likelihood of recurrence.[24] The development of improved DNA extraction protocols and next-generation sequencing (NGS) platforms requiring less DNA input has enabled use of cytologic specimens for high-throughput mutational analysis,[25,26] allowing multiple target genes to be analyzed in a single assay. A variety of routine cytologic preparations, including cell blocks, smears, and liquid-based preparations, all of which can be prepared from effusion fluid, can be used for molecular testing.[27–44] A subset of studies evaluating molecular analysis of cytology specimens have focused on effusion fluids using different methods, with occasional comparison to surgical specimens (**Table 1**).

Among other preanalytic factors, including preparation type, tumor fraction, and tumor quantity,[26–29] the success of gene sequencing, particularly NGS techniques that show superiority compared with traditional Sanger sequencing,[29,35] is strongly affected by DNA yield as opposed to tumor cell content alone.[27] In 1 study, EGFR mutations matching those detected in surgical samples were seen in 42% of cytologic specimens containing no tumor cells,[35] raising the possibility that NGS may be sufficiently sensitive to detect cell-free DNA in effusion specimens. Moreover, some studies have reported the detection of mutations in cytology specimens that were not detected in corresponding surgical biopsies despite adequate sequence coverage, possibly reflecting the potential of cytologic specimens to more accurately sample tumor heterogeneity during tumor progression and metastasis.[42]

DIAGNOSIS OF BENIGN SEROUS EFFUSIONS

Benign effusions, defined as effusions lacking microscopic evidence of malignant cells, account for up to 74% of all effusions and are typically associated with nonspecific cytologic findngs.[45] Benign effusions occur due to several causes, including inflammatory conditions, hemodynamic disturbances, malignancy (as a secondary result of lymphatic obstruction), obstructive pneumonia, or other mechanical issues.

INFECTION

Infection, either via direct involvement or parapneumonic involvement, is the most common

Table 1
Performance of molecular testing of effusion cytology specimens

Publication	Malignancy	Effusion Type	Preparation	Mean DNA Yield (ng/µL)	Methods or Platform	Number of Successfully Sequenced Specimens (%)	Concordance with Surgical Samples (%)
Allegrini et al,[37] 2012	Lung adenocarcinoma	Pleural, peritoneal	Smears, cell blocks	—	7500 Fast Real-Time PCR System (Applied Biosystems)	12/13 (92)	—
Buttitta et al,[35] 2013	Lung adenocarcinoma	Pleural	Papanicolaou stained smears	—	Sanger, NGS (Roche 454 Junior)	15/15 (100)	—
Liu et al,[38] 2013	Lung adenocarcinoma or adenosquamous carcinoma	Pleural	Cell blocks	—	ARMS (ADx-ARMS)	21/21 (100)	17/21 (81)
Sun et al,[34] 2013	NSCLC	Pleural	Smears, cell blocks	180, 49.5[a]	Pyrosequencing	17/17 (100)	14/17 (82)
Shah et al,[42] 2015	HGSC	Pleural, peritoneal	Cytospins	47.46	NGS (Illumina HiSeq 2000)	5/5 (100)	5/5 (100)
Dibardino et al,[43] 2016	NSCLC	Pleural, pericardial	Unknown	—	NGS (Illumina HiSeq 2500)	6/6 (100)	5/6 (83)[b]
Wei et al,[32] 2016	Lung adenocarcinoma	Pleural, pericardial	Fresh or PreservCyt	191	NGS (Illumina MiSeq)	4/4 (100)	—
Velizheva et al,[36] 2017	Lung adenocarcinoma	Pleural	Smears, cell blocks	131	NGS (Roche 454 Junior)	3/3 (100)	1/1 (100)
Leichsenring et al,[40] 2018	Various carcinomas	Pleural, peritoneal	Cell blocks	20.44	NGS (ThermoFisher Ion Torrent PGM)	20/20 (100)	14/20 (70)

Abbreviations: HGSC, high-grade serous carcinoma; NSCLC, non-small cell lung carcinoma.
[a] Smears in this study yielded a mean of 180 ng/µL, cell blocks yielded a mean yield of 49.5 ng/µL.
[b] One patient was subsequently found to harbor an EGFR mutation on a surgical pleural biopsy.

nonmalignant cause of serous effusions.[45] More than 40% of patients with bacterial pneumonia develop parapneumonic effusions,[46,47] whereas fungal infections only cause 1% to 5% of pleural effusions, even in at-risk populations.[47,48] Cytologically, bacterial and fungal parapneumonic effusions are neutrophil-rich, with potentially significant eosinophilia in fungal infections.[49,50] Microbiological culture is the current gold standard for identification of organisms in cytology, although sensitivity for the identification of fungi can be as low as 58%.[47,51] Sensitive and rapid molecular methods for the detection and identification of microorganisms in clinical samples are undergoing active investigation[52]; however, this may not be feasible in small laboratories. As such, neutrophilic effusions should prompt Gram and fungal staining if clinical suspicion for infection is high and cultures are unavailable. Although highly specific, Gram stain has a low sensitivity (48%) for the detection of bacteria[47] and is not appropriate for speciation. *Aspergillus*, *Coccidioides*, *Cryptococcus*, *Nocardia*, *Pneumocystis*, and other fungi are potential causes of effusions in immunocompromised hosts, with significant morbidity or mortality.[49,53] Many of these may be recognized morphologically; however, diagnostic accuracy of fungal stains for speciation is variable (78%–95%).[54,55]

Tuberculous and viral effusions are both characterized by polymorphous lymphocytosis.[56,57] Up to 59% of pleural effusions are Epstein-Barr virus (EBV)-positive by polymerase chain reaction (PCR),[58] although the significance thereof is uncertain because more than 90% of the adult population has been exposed to the virus.[57] The sensitivity of acid-fast bacilli stains depends on bacterial burden and culture is generally more sensitive.[59] Lymphocytic effusions are also associated with malignancy and heart failure, thus routine evaluation of lymphocytic effusions for microorganisms or the presence of viral antigens is not recommended.

CONNECTIVE TISSUE DISEASE

Effusions are a common manifestation of connective tissue disease, occurring in about 30% to 40% of systemic lupus erythematosus (SLE) patients and 3% to 4% of patients with rheumatoid arthritis.[60,61] Pleuritis and effusion development may occasionally precede other manifestations of disease[61] and are, therefore, important to recognize.

Lupus erythematosus (LE) cells, consisting of neutrophils or macrophages with glassy cytoplasmic inclusions (hematoxylin bodies) that are thought to represent phagocytosed apoptotic nuclei, are pathognomonic for SLE and present in 27% of cases (**Fig. 1A, B**).[60] Care must be taken to distinguish LE cells from the morphologically similar tart cells, macrophages containing ingested nuclear material with a more recognizable chromatin structure, which are nonspecific and of uncertain clinical significance.[60] Serous fluids from patients with rheumatoid arthritis characteristically show histiocytes and giant cells among amorphous granular and necrotic debris that mirrors the findings in rheumatoid nodules (**Fig. 1C, D**).[62]

EOSINOPHILIC EFFUSIONS

Eosinophilic effusions, defined as effusions that contain at least 10% eosinophils, represent as many as 16% of exudative pleural effusions.[50] They are usually associated with conditions that introduce blood or air into the pleural space, including pneumothorax, hemothorax, chest trauma, and thoracentesis.[50,63,64] Other etiologic factors include malignancy, drug reactions, infection (particularly parasitic and fungal), pulmonary emboli, and immune disorders, including Churg-Straus and hypereosinophilia syndrome.[50] These are less common and should only be considered if supporting clinical and laboratory findings are present.

DIAGNOSIS OF MALIGNANT SEROUS EFFUSIONS

Ninety-five percent of malignant serous effusions represent metastatic disease, consisting primarily of adenocarcinomas (70%–77%).[1–3,6,65,66] The most common primary sites of malignancy in pleural and peritoneal fluids are summarized in **Table 2**.[1–3,6,65–67] As many as 8% of patients have multiple prior malignancies, and 5% to 6% present with occult malignancies.[68] Therefore, differential diagnostic considerations depend on patient history and clinical features, although lung cancer is more common in pleural effusions; for example, breast cancer is more prevalent in women with a history of breast carcinoma.[68] Additionally, both benign and malignant mesothelial proliferations are significant sources of interpretive error.[4,6] Therefore, carefully selected immunohistochemical panels are often necessary to distinguish between carcinomas and exclude the possibility of mesothelioma. Claudin-4 (**Fig. 2**), which is absent in mesothelioma, melanoma, and most sarcomas,[69] has recently emerged as the most sensitive and specific epithelial marker, although it may occasionally show nonspecific

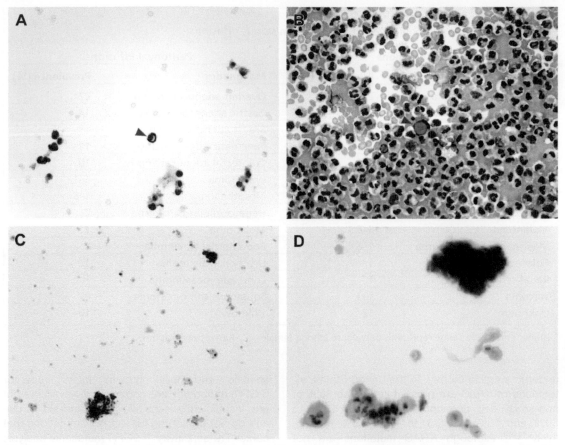

Fig. 1. Cytomorphologic findings in connective tissue disease–associated effusions. LE cells are characterized by large, homogeneous inclusions (*arrowheads*) within macrophages and neutrophils that are thought to represent ingested cell nuclei and are exclusively seen in SLE (*A, B*). Effusions in patients with rheumatoid pleuritis are characterized by a cellular background comprised of elongated macrophages and giant cells, with occasional clusters of amorphous necrotic debris (*C, D*).

cytoplasmic staining in histiocytes[70] and should be combined with other epithelial markers in difficult cases. Mesothelial markers and tumor-specific markers may be added to a panel as clinical context dictates. Cytologic, immunohistochemical, and genetic features of malignancies most commonly seen in serous effusions are summarized in **Table 3**.

LUNG ADENOCARCINOMA

Malignant pleural effusion, seen at presentation in approximately 8% to 15% of lung adenocarcinoma patients,[71] confers poor survival, and is currently considered metastatic disease for treatment purposes. As treatment becomes increasingly focused on tumor-specific genetic alterations, timely diagnosis of lung adenocarcinoma in effusion specimens will become integral to patient management.

Lung adenocarcinoma demonstrates heterogeneous microarchitecture in pleural fluids, with large rounded clusters, papillae, micropapillary clusters, or single cells (**Fig. 3**A, B). Nuclei may be uniform or pleomorphic, round or irregular, and may have 1 or multiple variably prominent nucleoli. Fine cytoplasmic vacuolization, large intracytoplasmic vacuoles, and granular cytoplasm may all be seen. Tumors are typically cytokeratin (CK)7-positive or CK20-negative, although CK20 and CDX2 positivity may be seen in a subset of adenocarcinomas, mimicking an enteric phenotype.[72] Thyroid transcription factor (TTF)-1 (**Fig. 3**C) is highly specific for lung adenocarcinoma but demonstrates variable sensitivity, whereas napsin A (**Fig. 3**D) is slightly more sensitive but less specific and can also be seen in renal, ovarian, and breast neoplasms (see **Table 3**).[73–77]

Molecular testing of lung adenocarcinomas in effusions is appropriate in patients who cannot

Table 2
Prevalence of secondary malignant involvement in serous effusions

Pleural Effusions		Peritoneal Effusions	
Malignancy	**Prevalence (%)**	**Malignancy**	**Prevalence (%)**
Lung adenocarcinoma	29–37	Ovarian adenocarcinoma	27
Breast adenocarcinoma	8–40[a]	Gastric adenocarcinoma	14
Ovarian adenocarcinoma	18–20	Breast adenocarcinoma	13
Gastric adenocarcinoma	2	Pancreatic adenocarcinoma	11
Pancreatic adenocarcinoma	3	Colorectal adenocarcinoma	10
Squamous cell carcinoma	3–8	Lymphoma	5–12
Lymphoma	3–16	Mesothelioma	1–8
Small cell carcinoma (lung)	6–9	Hepatocellular carcinoma	2
Melanoma	5–6	Melanoma	2
Malignant mesothelioma	1–6	Endometrial carcinoma	1
Colorectal	1	Urothelial carcinoma	1
Renal cell carcinoma	1	Lung adenocarcinoma	1
Sarcoma	1–3	Squamous cell carcinoma	0.1–1
Unknown	12	Unknown	10

[a] Higher end of the range represents prevalence among female-only patient populations.

undergo surgical biopsy. In the United States, alterations of *KRAS* are present in 30% to 35% of non-small cell carcinomas, *EGFR* in 16% to 30%, and *ALK* and *ROS1* in 7% and 5%, respectively.[78–80] Although *KRAS* mutations are not currently treated with targeted therapy, *EGFR*, *ALK*, and *ROS1* alterations confer sensitivity to general or alteration-specific tyrosine kinase inhibitors (TKIs). Molecular testing of all lung adenocarcinoma specimens is inefficient and cost-prohibitive; therefore, algorithms that incorporate screening immunohistochemistry or sequential molecular testing are routinely used. Mutation-specific endothelial growth factor receptor (EGFR) antibodies are commercially available but are insufficiently sensitive for stand-alone use and do not detect the full range of mutations that confer TKI-sensitivity.[44] *EGFR* mutational analysis can be performed using a variety of PCR-based gene-sequencing techniques, with a sensitivity of 82% and specificity of 80% in effusion specimens.[30,35,37,38] The sensitivity and specificity of ALK immunohistochemistry are 100% and 86.3% to 100% in effusion specimens, respectively.[11,23] ROS1 immunohistochemical staining is also highly sensitive for gene rearrangement but shows lower

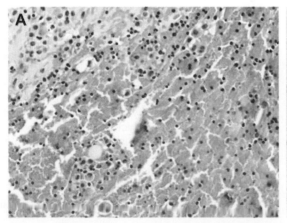
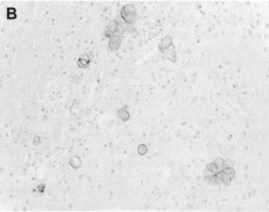

Fig. 2. Scattered clusters of lung adenocarcinoma (*A*) are highlighted by a claudin-4 immunohistochemical stain (*B*), which demonstrates membranous positivity in lesional cells.

Table 3
Morphologic, immunophenotypic, and genetic features of common malignant serous effusions

Diagnosis	Cytomorphology	Morphologic Differential Diagnosis	Immunohistochemical Profile	Associated Genes or Syndromes
Lung Adenocarcinoma	+/− nuclear pleomorphism, +/− nucleoli, rounded clusters, micropapillae, papillary structures, single cells	Breast, esophagogastric, colon, mesothelioma	CK7+, CK20−, TTF-1+ (54%–80%), napsin A+ (65%–83%)	*KRAS* (31%), *EGFR* (16%–31%) *ALK* (7%), *BRAF* (5%–7%) *MET* (7%), *ROS1* (5%), *ERBB2* (5%), *RET* (4%)
Breast Carcinoma, Ductal	+/− nuclear pleomorphism, +/− nucleoli, rounded clusters, branched clusters	Lung, mesothelioma	CK7+, GCDFP-15 (5%–47%), mammaglobin (22%–87%), GATA3+ (94%–100%), ER (86%), PR (80%), HER2 (13%–15%)	• *PIK3CA* (21%–40%), *PTEN* (6%–7%) • *BRCA1/BRCA2* germline mutations
Breast Carcinoma, Lobular	Low to moderate N/C ratio, single cells, intracytoplasmic vacuoles	Mesothelial cells, histiocytes, mesothelioma, melanoma	CK7+, GATA3 (100%), ER/PR (>95%), HER2 (<5%)	*CDH1* (12%–83%)
Ovarian carcinoma, high-grade serous	Papillary or scalloped clusters, high N/C ratio, prominent nucleoli	Mesothelioma, Müllerian clear cell carcinoma, endometrioid adenocarcinoma	CK7+, CK20−, Pax8+(>95%), WT-1+ (80%–97%), ER+ (97%–100%), napsin A− (0)	• *TP53* (63%–95%) • *BRCA1/BRCA2* germline mutations
Ovarian carcinoma, clear cell	Clusters with scalloped borders, finely vacuolated or granular cytoplasm, moderate to high N/C ratio, amorphous hyalinized amorphous matrix with or without surrounding neoplastic cells	Serous carcinoma, endometrioid adenocarcinoma, pancreatic ductal adenocarcinoma, renal cell carcinoma, adrenal cortical carcinoma	CK7+, CK20−, Pax8+ (>95%), napsin A+ (>95%), HNF1β (89%), WT-1− (3%), ER− (0%–28%)	• *ARID1A* (50%), KRAS, BRAF, PTEN, PIK3CA, HER2 • Lynch syndrome

(continued on next page)

Table 3
(continued)

Diagnosis	Cytomorphology	Morphologic Differential Diagnosis	Immunohistochemical Profile	Associated Genes or Syndromes
Ovarian carcinoma, endometrioid	Rounded clusters, moderate to abundant cytoplasm, +/− nucleoli, +/− intracytoplasmic neutrophils	Ovarian serous carcinoma, ovarian clear cell carcinoma, lung, colon	CK7+, CK20−, Pax8+ (>95%), ER+ (>95%), napsin A− (10%)	• PTEN (67%), ARID1A (34%)
Gastric adenocarcinoma	Single cells or clusters, signet ring cell or intestinal morphology	Lobular carcinoma of breast, lung, mesothelioma	CK7+, CK20+/− (53%), CDX −2+/− (61%), HER2+ (20%)	HER2 (20%)
Pancreatic ductal adenocarcinoma	Rounded clusters, single cells, nuclear size variation (4x or more)	Lung, breast, stomach, colon, ovarian	CK7+, CK20+/− (20%−22%), CDX-2+/− (16%), SMAD4− (loss, 54%)	KRAS (90%−92%), CDKN2A (90%), TP53 (75%), SMAD4 (55%)
Lymphoma	Single cells, high N/C ratio, clumped chromatin, variable nucleoli (depends on subtype), lymphoglandular bodies in background	Small cell carcinoma, melanoma, poorly differentiated non-small cell carcinoma	• Depends on subtype • General: LCA, CD3, CD20, kappa light chain, lambda light chain, Ki-67 • CD5, CD10, CD23, BCL-2, BCL-6, CD30, CD138, CyclinD1 (mantle cell), HHV8 (PEL), EBER (DLBCL, PEL, PBL), MYC (DLBCL, Burkitt), ALK (ALCL)	Follicular: BCL-2, t (14,18) Mantle Cell: CCND1, t (11;14) Burkitt: MYC, t (8;14) DLBCL: C-MYC, BCL-2
Mesothelioma	Scalloped clusters, +windows, single cells, −pleomorphism, + central nuclei and nucleoli	Adenocarcinoma	CK7+, CK20−, CK5/6+, WT-1+, calretinin+, D2-40+, mesothelin+, BerEP4−−, B72.3−, CEA−, MOC31−, claudin-4−, BAP1 (loss, 55%−80%)	CDKN2A (60%), NF2 (50%−60%), BAP1 (60%−80%)

Abbreviations: ALCL, anaplastic large cell lymphoma; DLBCL, diffuse large B-cell lymphoma, including double hit and triple hit; HER2, human epidermal growth factor receptor 2; HHV, human herpesvirus; N/C, nuclear-to-cytoplasmic; PBL, plasmablastic lymphoma; PEL, primary effusion lymphoma; TTF, thyroid transcription factor.

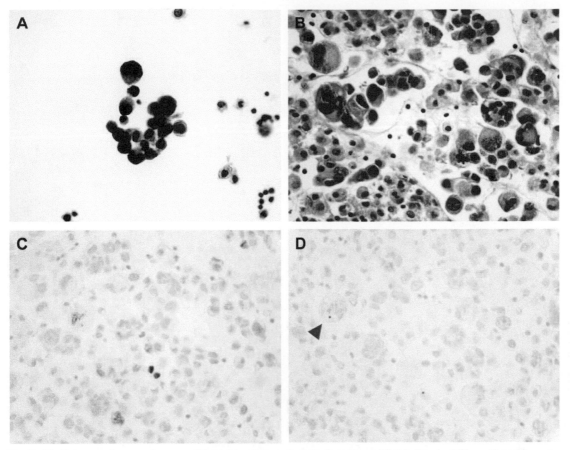

Fig. 3. (*A, B*) Lung adenocarcinoma with giant cell morphology in a pleural fluid. Poorly differentiated lung tumors may be difficult to identify in effusions, and may demonstrate absent or only weak and focal (*C*) thyroid transcription factor (TTF)-1 and (*D*) napsin A (*arrowhead*) staining.

specificity in surgical biopsies,[10] and has not yet been evaluated in effusions. As such, a positive ALK or ROS1 immunohistochemical result should be confirmed using FISH, reverse transcription (RT)-PCR, or NGS techniques, all of which are highly specific for gene rearrangements.[10,11,22,23,36]

Recently, the US Food and Drug Administration has also approved immune checkpoint inhibitors for first-line and second-line treatment of patients with advanced non-small cell carcinoma.[81,82] Approved use of immune checkpoint therapy is currently contingent on immunohistochemical screening of PD-L1 expression in surgical biopsies. PD-L1 immunohistochemistry performed on cytology specimens, including effusions, does seem to correlate with staining in surgical specimens,[83] although additional studies are needed to establish diagnostic thresholds and clinical significance of staining in these specimens because sampling technique may affect results.[12]

BREAST CARCINOMA

Ductal carcinoma of the breast in serous effusions typically consists of clusters of cells and single cells with irregular nuclear borders and variable nuclear to cytoplasmic ratio (**Fig. 4**A). Lobular carcinoma of the breast most frequently presents as singly-dispersed cells with a moderate to low nuclear-to-cytoplasmic ratio, low-grade nuclei, and cytoplasmic vacuoles (**Fig. 4**C, D). A low threshold for immunohistochemical staining of effusion specimens should be used in patients with a history of lobular carcinoma because the tumor cells may mimic histiocytes or mesothelial cells.

Gross cystic disease fluid protein 15 (GCDFP-15), mammaglobin, and GATA3 (**Fig. 4**E) immunohistochemical stains may be used to determine breast origin in effusions (see **Table 3**).[84–87] GATA3 has shown the highest sensitivity and stains up to 85% of triple-negative breast cancers but must be interpreted in clinical context because it may also

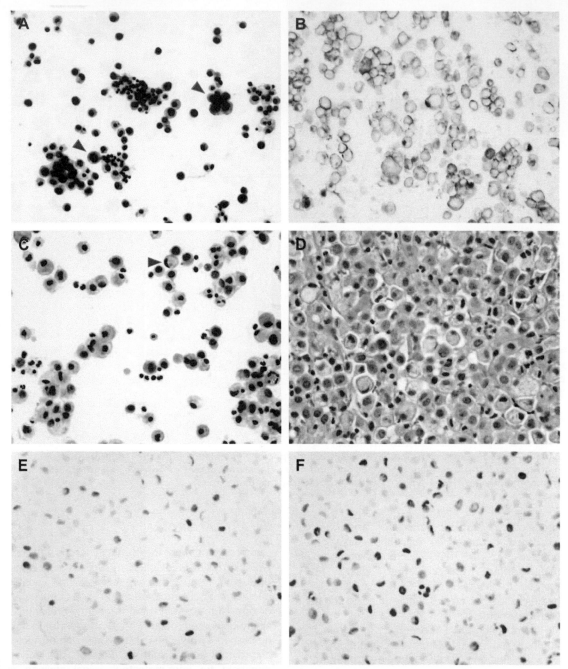

Fig. 4. Pleural fluid in a patient with ductal adenocarcinoma, demonstrating small, scalloped clusters and single cells (*A, arrowheads*) that show strong (3+) HER2 positivity (*B*), which predicts therapeutic response to trastuzumab. Lobular carcinoma typically demonstrates a single cell (*arrowhead*) pattern (*C, D*) and may mimic histiocytes or mesothelial cells but can be distinguished with GATA3 (*E*) and estrogen receptor (ER) (*F*) immunohistochemical stains.

be seen in benign mesothelial cells, urothelial carcinomas, and other solid tumor types.[85,87] SOX10 has also shown a sensitivity of 38% for metastatic triple negative carcinoma in surgical biopsies[88] but has not been evaluated in effusions.

Current management of breast carcinoma depends on tumor hormone and human epidermal growth factor receptor 2 (HER2) expression status (**Fig.** 4B–F). The specificity of estrogen and progesterone receptor immunohistochemistry approaches

100% in effusions; however, sensitivity compared with surgical biopsies is lower, particularly for progesterone receptor (see **Table 3**).[9] Studies of HER2 status in effusions have shown considerable variability in both sensitivity and specificity,[9,13] possibly due to frequent differences in receptor status between primary and locoregional or distant metastatic disease and posttreatment disease.[14]

OVARIAN CARCINOMA

Serous tumors are the most common ovarian carcinomas seen in effusion specimens, accounting for 81% of cases.[84] Although clear cell and endometrioid tumors each represent less than 10% of malignant serous effusions,[84] they are managed differently and a subset are associated with Lynch syndrome.[89,90] High-grade serous carcinomas typically show papillary clusters and singly dispersed cells with scant to moderate amounts of cytoplasm, increased nucleocytoplasmic ratio, irregular hyperchromatic nuclei, prominent central nucleoli, and frequent psammoma bodies.[91] Clear cell carcinomas often display abundant, finely vacuolated or granular cytoplasm, inconspicuous nucleoli, hobnail morphology, and are associated with an amorphous, hyalinized matrix that may either be surrounded by or intermixed with tumor cells.[91,92] There may be significant morphologic overlap between high-grade and low-grade serous tumors, clear cell carcinomas, and endometrioid carcinomas. A panel including PAX8, WT-1, estrogen receptor (ER), and napsin A can be helpful in establishing Müllerian origin and distinguishing between ovarian neoplasms (see **Table 3**).[93,94] PAX8 is highly sensitive for Müllerian carcinomas in effusions[84,94]; however, inclusion of general epithelial markers in a diagnostic panel is recommended because reactive and malignant mesothelial cells may show significant PAX8 expression.[95] Within context, napsin A is nearly 100% sensitive and specific for clear cell carcinoma,[93,94] which tends to be WT-1 and ER negative, whereas serous and endometrioid tumors are mostly WT-1/ER positive and napsin A negative.[93,94] Napsin A should be interpreted carefully if renal cell carcinoma is in the differential because 70% of papillary and 24% of clear cell renal cell tumors show positivity.[77] Mucinous adenocarcinomas of the ovary typically do not mimic serous, clear cell, or endometrioid carcinomas but can demonstrate focal CK20 and CDX-2 positivity and harbor KRAS mutations[96–98]; distinguishing these from pancreaticobiliary and gastric neoplasms depends on clinical and radiologic findings.

Ovarian carcinomas frequently demonstrate TP53, KRAS, PTEN, and ARID1A mutations.[78–80] Although this information may ultimately predict treatment response to conventional or targeted chemotherapy, it is of limited diagnostic value because sequencing or immunohistochemical evidence of alterations in these genes may be seen in several other tumor types.[78–80]

GASTRIC AND PANCREATIC ADENOCARCINOMA

Diagnosis of stomach and pancreatic tumors may be challenging owing to nonspecific immunohistochemical profiles. Stomach and pancreatic tumors demonstrate CK7 positivity, and a subset, particularly gastric adenocarcinomas, are CK20 and CDX-2 positive (**Fig. 5**).[96,99] Inactivation of the DPC4(SMAD4) tumor suppressor gene with concomitant loss of protein expression is seen in approximately half of pancreatic adenocarcinomas (**Fig. 6**).[100] KRAS mutations are also common in pancreatic adenocarcinomas; however, similar mutations are also present at significant rates in lung and mucinous ovarian adenocarcinomas and, therefore, of limited diagnostic utility.[78–80,98] Of esophagogastric tumors, 15% to 20% demonstrate overexpression of HER2, which may be used to select patients for trastuzumab therapy.[101]

Diffuse Malignant Mesothelioma

Malignant mesothelioma presents with effusion in 54% to 89% of patients[102,103] but causes fewer than 5% of serous effusions, most frequently in the pleura, followed by the peritoneal cavity, pericardium, and other sites.[104] Mesothelioma occurs primarily in men (male/female ratio 4:1 in pleura, 1.3:1 in peritoneum). It is usually associated with occupational asbestos exposure (80% cases), with fewer cases attributable to other fibers or therapeutic radiation.[104–106] Current diagnostic guidelines require demonstration of invasive or nodular growth, and distinction from carcinoma using a panel of at least 2 mesothelial markers and 2 adenocarcinoma or general epithelial markers (**Table 4**).[107] Because tissue invasion cannot be assessed in cytologic preparations, mesotheliomatous effusions pose unique challenges; therefore, the reported sensitivity of effusion cytology for mesothelioma is low compared with other malignancies, at 32% to 53%.[108,109]

Mesothelioma demonstrates a clustered or discohesive pattern with features of mesothelial lineage, such as clear spaces between cells or 2-toned cytoplasm, and varying degrees of nuclear atypia (**Fig. 7**).[107] Because of the significant morphologic overlap between malignant and reactive mesothelial proliferations, several studies have evaluated immunohistochemical stains to

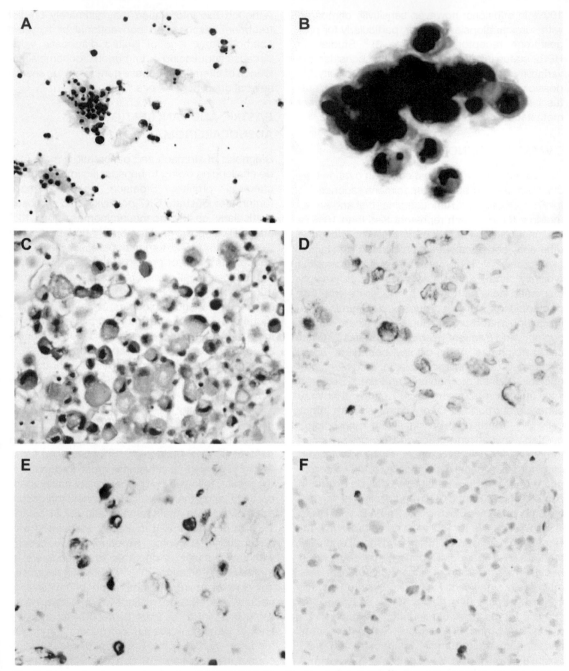

Fig. 5. Stomach adenocarcinoma frequently presents with signet ring cell features and a dispersed pattern in effusions (*A–C*). Cells may mimic histiocytes or intermingle with inflammatory elements within the effusion but may be distinguished using immunohistochemistry for CK7 (*D*), CK20 (*E*), and/or CDX-2 (*F*) in most cases.

distinguish between the 2, most of which have not shown sufficient sensitivity or specificity for diagnostic use (**Table 5**).[110–114]

Mesothelioma carcinogenesis is primarily driven by loss of tumor suppressor function. *CDKN2A*, *NF2*, and *BAP1* are altered in 67% to 95%, 50% to 65%, and 42% to 80% of mesotheliomas,

respectively.[19,115–118] Although cytogenetic analysis increases the sensitivity and specificity of effusion cytology for mesothelioma,[20] expense and time constraints can limit the practical use thereof. Loss of p16 protein expression by immunohistochemistry, however, does not reliably indicate *CDKN2A* deletion, whereas *NF2* alterations

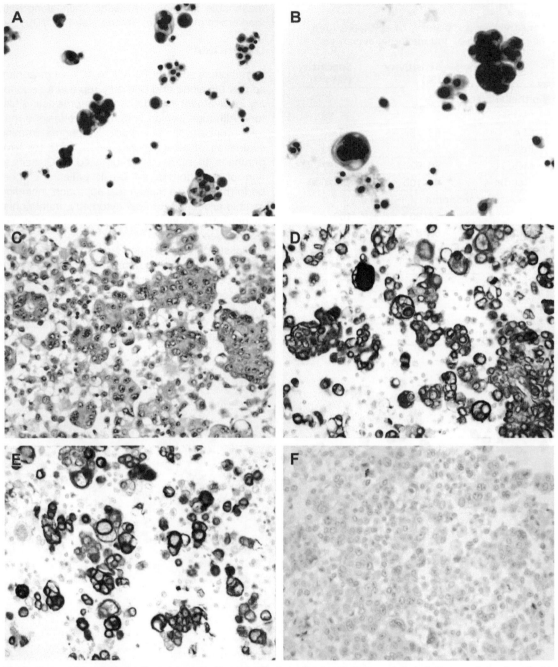

Fig. 6. Pancreatic adenocarcinoma in a peritoneal effusion, demonstrating rounded clusters and single cells (*A–C*). Approximately 20% of pancreatic adenocarcinomas demonstrate a CK7+ (*D*) and CK20+ (*E*) phenotype. Loss of SMAD4 expression (*F*) is seen in about 50% of pancreatic ductal carcinomas, and contrasts with background staining of inflammatory cells.

are frequently homozygous and mutations in the gene do not correlate with protein expression.[119] Methylthioadenosine phosphorylase (*MTAP*) is frequently codeleted with *CDKN2A*,[19] and MTAP immunohistochemistry is potentially a highly specific surrogate for *CDKN2A* deletion but has low sensitivity for mesothelioma on its own.[120] Loss of BAP1 protein expression is rarely seen in carcinomas and has shown the most promise as an immunohistochemical marker of mesothelioma, with a sensitivity of up to 67%, and specificity of 100% across studies,[118,121] making it a

Table 4
Sensitivity and specificity of epithelial, lung adenocarcinoma, and mesothelial markers

	Sensitivity (%)	Specificity (%)
Epithelial markers		
CD15	51–70	95–98
CEA	63–78	98
BerEP4	74–89	95–98
MOC31	86–92	87–97
Claudin-4	91–100	99–100
Lung Adenocarcinoma		
TTF-1	54–80	100
Napsin-A	65–87	98–100
Mesothelial markers		
CK5/6	46–76	89–100
Calretinin	85–96	87–100
WT-1	78	62
D2-40	79	100
Mesothelin	75	71

reasonable first-line diagnostic stain along with markers of mesothelial lineage (see **Fig. 7**D).

LYMPHOMAS

Lymphomas account for 3% to 15% of malignant serous effusions and primarily represent secondary involvement in patients with a preexisting history. Although benign lymphocytic effusions may raise concern for low-grade lymphoma, routine evaluation of all lymphocyte-rich fluids for lymphoma is, therefore, not suggested.[122] Classification of lymphomas in at-risk patients is best performed using a multimodal approach, including sample allocation for flow cytometry, immunohistochemistry, in situ hybridization, and molecular testing (see **Table 3**).[123,124]

Classic primary effusion lymphomas (PELs) are rare, accounting for less than 0.5% of effusions,[125] and occur predominantly in male patients with a history of human immunodeficiency virus (HIV).[125–128] Occasional cases have also been reported in the setting of solid organ transplant, chronic infection, and in HIV-negative individuals

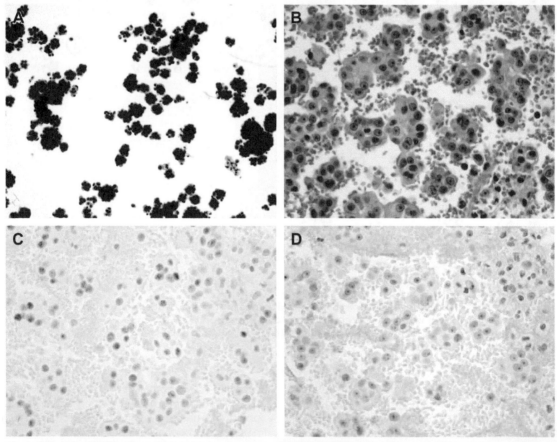

Fig. 7. Effusions affected by malignant mesothelioma are often cellular (A), demonstrating numerous scalloped clusters of mesothelial cells with low-grade nuclei and central nucleoli (B). WT-1 positive tumor cells (C) demonstrate a diagnostic loss of BAP1 protein expression (D), which is seen in approximately 60% of cases.

Table 5
Performance of immunohistochemical and fluorescence in situ hybridization markers in the distinction between reactive and malignant mesothelial proliferations

	Reactive Mesothelium (% Cases)	Mesothelioma (% Cases)	Sensitivity for Mesothelioma (%)	Specificity for Mesothelioma (%)
IHC Marker				
Desmin	84–86	0–10	48	97
EMA	4–6	71–100	68–99	74–97
GLUT-1	0–37	40–100	40–99	80–100
P53	0–14	16–86	41–61	91
IMP3	0–27	36–91	36–77	73–100
CD146	3	71	71–94	98
BAP1	0	57–80	57–67	100
MTAP	0	45	45	100
NF2	0	4	4	100
LATS2	27	20	27	80
YAP	92	80	92	20
FISH Assay				
CDKN2A (p16)	0	29–100	29–100	100
NF2	0	35–65	35–65	100
BAP1	0	30–61	42–80	100

from human herpesvirus (HHV)8-endemic areas.[125,128] Pleural and peritoneal involvement are equally common, and peripheral white blood cell counts and bone marrow biopsies are frequently normal.[126,127] Overall survival is approximately 3 to 6 months, and approximately one-third of patients are resistant to chemotherapy.[125–127]

PEL is characterized by large cells with moderate to abundant cytoplasm, irregular nuclei, coarse chromatin, and single or multiple prominent nucleoli.[125,128] Immunoblastic or plasmablastic features and lymphoglandular bodies may also be present.[128] PEL are typically CD20-negative; however, nearly all cases are positive for CD45, CD30 and CD38.[125–127] Most cases are also positive for HHV8 by PCR or immunohistochemistry, and approximately 50% show EBV coinfection.[126–129] Molecular studies may show clonal IgH gene rearrangement, although polyclonal patterns have also been described, and diagnosis can usually be achieved by cytologic and immunohistochemical evaluation alone.[127]

MESENCHYMAL TUMORS

Sarcomas involve approximately 3% of serous effusions, usually as metastatic disease.[130] A cellular fluid with numerous keratin-negative cells should prompt exclusion of sarcomatoid carcinoma, melanoma, and lymphoma, as well as evaluation for epithelioid mesenchymal neoplasms. In particular, epithelioid hemangioendothelioma (EHE) and angiosarcoma have been described as potential clinical and pathologic mimics of epithelial tumors, presenting with pleural thickening and adenocarcinoma-like cytology.[131] EHE in fluids is seen as single cells and small clusters of cells, with 1 or multiple low-grade to intermediate-grade nuclei, moderate amounts of cytoplasm, and occasional cytoplasmic vacuoles that may contain red blood cells (**Fig. 8C**).[130,132] Angiosarcomas may demonstrate similar features but typically have a higher nucleocytoplasmic ratio, greater nuclear atypia, and lack the cytoplasmic vacuoles of EHE (**Fig. 8A**).[131,133] Both tumors stain with the endothelial markers CD31, CD34, and ERG (**Fig. 8B**), and may show some keratin positivity.[130–133] Translocations involving the *CAMTA-1* (and, rarely, *TFE3*) genes have recently been described in EHE, resulting in a nuclear pattern of immunohistochemical protein expression (**Fig. 8D**).[21]

NUT CARCINOMA

NUT carcinoma is a rare, poorly differentiated variant of squamous cell carcinoma associated

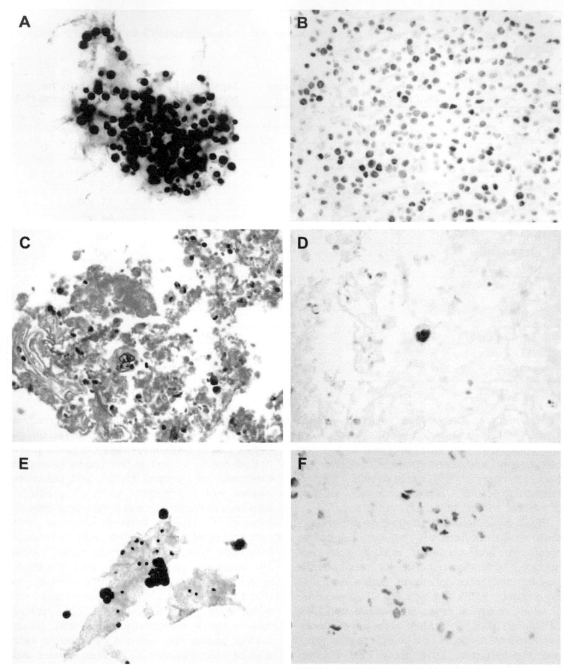

Fig. 8. Rare malignant morphologic pitfalls for adenocarcinoma, small cell carcinoma, and lymphoma in pleural effusions. Angiosarcoma (*A*) and EHE (*C*) usually demonstrate a single cell dispersion pattern with epithelioid morphology, and are positive for ERG (*B*). Of EHEs, 86% demonstrate nuclear positivity for CAMTA1 (*D*). NUT carcinoma (*E*) is rare in serous effusions but rapidly fatal and may be distinguished by a granular pattern of nuclear NUT expression (*F*).

with translocations of the *NUT* gene, with a predilection for the head and neck and thorax.[134,135] Although NUT carcinoma is rare, it may demonstrate focal aberrant expression of multiple nuclear transcription factors (including TTF-1), and may mimic lymphoma, small cell carcinoma, or poorly differentiated adenocarcinoma in effusions (Fig. 8E). It is p63, p40, and NUT positive (Fig. 8F), although typically negative for neuroendocrine markers.[134,135]

REFERENCES

1. Rossi ED, Bizzarro T, Schitt F, et al. The role of liquid-based cytology and ancillary techniques in pleural and pericardic effusions: an institutional experience. Cancer Cytopathol 2015;123(4): 258–66.
2. Motherby H, Nadjari B, Friegel P, et al. Diagnostic accuracy of effusion cytology. Diagn Cytopathol 1999;20(6):350–7.
3. Irani DR, Underwood RD, Johnson EH, et al. Malignant pleural effusions. A clinical cytopathologic study. Arch Intern Med 1987;147(6):1133–6.
4. Tabatabai ZL, Nayar R, Souers RJ, et al. Performance characteristics of body fluid cytology: analysis of 344, 380 responses from the College of American Pathologists interlaboratory comparison program in nongynecologic cytopathology. Arch Pathol Lab Med 2017. https://doi.org/10.5858/arpa.2016-0509-CP.
5. Metzgeroth G, Kuhn C, Schultheis B, et al. Diagnostic accuracy of cytology and immunocytology in carcinomatous effusions. Cytopathology 2008; 19:205–11.
6. Kalogeraki A, Tamiolakis D, Datseri G, et al. Pleural effusion cytology due to malignancy. A combined cytomorphological-immunocytochemical study of 500 cases. Rev Port Pneumol (2006) 2016;22(5): 290–1.
7. Idowu MO, Powers CN. Lung cancer cytology: potential pitfalls and mimics - a review. Int J Clin Exp Pathol 2010;3(4):367–85.
8. Fetsch PA, Abati A. Immunocytochemistry in effusion cytology: a contemporary review. Cancer 2001;93:293–308.
9. Shabaik A, Lin G, Peterson M, et al. Immunohistochemistry on cell block of FNA and serous effusions from patients with primary and metastatic breast carcinoma. Diagn Cytopathol 2011;39(5):328–32.
10. Sholl LM, Sun H, Butaney M, et al. ROS1 immunohistochemistry for detection of ROS1-rearranged lung adenocarcinomas. Am J Surg Pathol 2013; 37(9):1441–9.
11. Zhou J, Yao H, Zhao J, et al. Cell block samples from malignant pleural effusion might be valid alternative samples for anaplastic lymphoma kinase detection in patients with advanced non-small-cell lung cancer. Histopathology 2015;66(7):949–54.
12. Ilie M, Long-Mira E, Bence C, et al. Comparative study of the PD-L1 status between surgically resected specimens and matched biopsies of NSCLC patients reveal major discordances: a potential issue for anti-PD-L1 therapeutic strategies. Ann Oncol 2016;27:147–53.
13. Francis IM, Alath P, George SS, et al. Metastatic breast carcinoma in pleural fluid: correlation of receptor and HER2 status with the primary carcinoma – a pilot study. Diagn Cytopathol 2016; 44(12):980–6.
14. Rossi S, Basso M, Strippoli A, et al. Hormone receptor status and HER2 expression in primary breast cancer compared with synchronous axillary metastases or recurrent metastatic disease. Clin Breast Cancer 2015;15(5):307–12.
15. Bode-Lesniewska B. Flow cytometry and effusions in lymphoproliferative processes and other hematologic neoplasias. Acta Cytol 2016;60(4):354–64.
16. Risberg B, Davidson B, Dong HP, et al. Flow cytometric immunophenotyping of serous effusions and peritoneal washings: comparison with immunocytochemistry and morphological findings. J Clin Pathol 2000;53(7):513–7.
17. Dal Cin P, Qian X, Cibas ES. The marriage of cytology and cytogenetics. Cancer Cytopathol 2013;121(6):279–90.
18. Factor RE, Dal Cin P, Fletcher JA, et al. Cytogenetics and fluorescence in situ hybridization as adjuncts to cytology in the diagnosis of malignant mesothelioma. Cancer 2009;117(4):247–53.
19. Illei PB, Rusch VW, Zakowski MF, et al. Homozygous deletion of CDKN2A and codeletion of the methylthioadenosine phosphorylase gene in the majority of pleural mesotheliomas. Clin Cancer Res 2003;9:2108–13.
20. Illei PB, Ladanyi M, Rusch VW, et al. The use of CDKN2A deletion as a diagnostic marker for malignant mesothelioma in body cavity effusions. Cancer 2003;99(1):51–6.
21. Doyle LA, Fletcher CD, Hornick JL. Nuclear expression of CAMTA1 distinguishes epithelioid hemangioendothelioma from histologic mimics. Am J Surg Pathol 2016;40(1):94–102.
22. Bozzetti C, Nizzoli R, Tiseo M, et al. ALK and ROS1 rearrangements tested by fluorescence in situ hybridization in cytological smears from advanced non-small cell lung cancer patients. Diagn Cytopathol 2015;43(11):941–6.
23. Liu L, Zhan P, Zhou X, et al. Detection of EML4-ALK in lung adenocarcinoma using pleural effusion with FISH, IHC, and RT-PCR methods. PLoS One 2015; 10(3):e0117032.
24. Cross D, Burmester JK. The promise of molecular profiling for cancer identification and treatment. Clin Med Res 2004;2(3):147–50.
25. Tian SK, Killian JK, Rekhtman N, et al. Optimizing workflows and processing of cytologic samples for comprehensive analysis by next-generation sequencing: Memorial Sloan Kettering Cancer Center experience. Arch Pathol Lab Med 2016. https://doi.org/10.5858/arpa.2016-0108-RA.
26. Roy-Chowdhuri S, Chow C-W, Kane MK, et al. Optimizing the DNA yield for molecular analysis from

cytologic preparations. Cancer Cytopathol 2016; 124(4):254–60.

27. Roy-Chowdhuri S, Goswami RS, Chen H, et al. Factors affecting the success of next-generation sequencing cytology specimens. Cancer Cytopathol 2015;123(11):659–68.

28. Dejmek A, Zendehrokh N, Tomaszewska M, et al. Preparation of DNA from cytological material: effects of fixation, staining, and mounting medium on DNA yield and quality. Cancer Cytopathol 2013;121(7):344–53.

29. Kanagal-Shamanna R, Portier BP, Singh RR, et al. Next-generation sequencing-based multi-gene mutation profiling of solid tumors using fine needle aspiration samples: promises and challenges for routine clinical diagnostics. Mod Pathol 2014; 27(2):314–27.

30. Scarpa A, Sikora K, Fassan M, et al. Molecular typing of lung adenocarcinoma on cytological samples using a multigene next generation sequencing panel. PLoS One 2013;8(11):e80478.

31. de Biase D, Visani M, Baccarini P, et al. Next generation sequencing improves the accuracy of KRAS mutation analysis in endoscopic ultrasound fine needle aspiration pancreatic lesions. PLoS One 2014;9(2):e87651.

32. Wei S, Lieberman D, Morrissette JJD, et al. Using "residual" FNA rinse and body fluid specimens for next-generation sequencing: an institutional experience. Cancer Cytopathol 2016;124(5):324–9.

33. Valero V, Saunders TJ, He J, et al. Reliable detection of somatic mutations in fine needle aspirates of pancreatic cancer with next-generation sequencing: implications for surgical management. Ann Surg 2016;263(1):153–61.

34. Sun PL, Jin Y, Kim H, et al. High concordance of EGFR mutation status between histologic and corresponding cytologic specimens of lung adenocarcinomas. Cancer Cytopathol 2013;121(6):311–9.

35. Buttitta F, Felicioni L, Del Grammastro M, et al. Effective assessment of EGFR mutation status in bronchoalveolar lavage and pleural fluids by next-generation sequencing. Clin Cancer Res 2013; 19(3):691–8.

36. Velizheva NP, Rechsteiner MP, Wong CE, et al. Cytology smears as excellent starting material for next-generation sequencing-based molecular testing of patient with adenocarcinoma of the lung. Cancer 2017;125(1):30–40.

37. Allegrini S, Antona J, Mezzapelle R, et al. Epidermal growth factor receptor gene analysis with a highly sensitive molecular assay in routine cytologic specimens of lung adenocarcinoma. Am J Clin Pathol 2012;138(3):377–81.

38. Liu X, Lu Y, Zhu G, et al. The diagnostic accuracy of pleural effusion and plasma samples versus tumour tissue for detection of EGFR mutation in patients with advanced non-small cell lung cancer: comparison of methodologies. J Clin Pathol 2013; 66(12):1065–9.

39. Liu X, Mody K, de Abreu FB, et al. Molecular profiling of appendiceal epithelial tumors using massively parallel sequencing to identify somatic mutations. Clin Chem 2014;60(7):1004–11.

40. Leichsenring J, Volckmar A-L, Kirchner M, et al. Targeted deep sequencing of effusion cytology samples is feasible, informs spatiotemporal tumor evolution, and has clinical and diagnostic utility. Genes Chromosomes Cancer 2018;57(2): 70–9.

41. Hwang DH, Garcia EP, Ducar MD, et al. Next-generation sequencing of cytologic preparations: an analysis of quality metrics. Cancer 2017;125(10): 786–94.

42. Shah RH, Scott SN, Brannon AR, et al. Comprehensive mutation profiling by next-generation sequencing of effusion fluids from patients with high-grade serous ovarian carcinoma. Cancer Cytopathol 2015;123(5):289–97.

43. DiBardino DM, Saqi A, Elvin JA, et al. Yield and Clinical Utility of Next-Generation Sequencing in Selected Patients With Lung Adenocarcinoma. Clin Lung Cancer 2016;17(6):517–522.e3.

44. Lindeman NI, Cagle PT, Beasley MB, et al. Molecular testing guideline for selection of lung cancer patients for EGFR and ALK tyrosine kinase inhibitors: guideline from the College of American Pathologists, International Association for the Study of Lung Cancer, and Association for Molecular Pathology. J Thorac Oncol 2013;8(7): 823–59.

45. Dragoescu EA, Liu L. Pericardial fluid cytology: an analysis of 128 specimens over a 6-year period. Cancer Cytopathol 2013;121(5):242–51.

46. Light RW. Parapneumonic effusions and empyema. Proc Am Thorac Soc 2006;3(1):75–80.

47. Ferrer A, Osset J, Alegre J, et al. Prospective clinical and microbiological study of pleural effusions. Eur J Clin Microbiol Infect Dis 1999;18(4): 237–41.

48. Chen Y, Brennesel D, Walters J, et al. Human immunodeficiency virus-associated pericardial effusion: report of 40 cases and review of the literature. Am Heart J 1999;137(3):516–21.

49. Merchant M, Romero AO, Libke RD, et al. Pleural effusion in hospitalized patients with Coccidioidomycosis. Respir Med 2008;102(4):537–40.

50. Kalomenidis I, Light RW. Eosinophilic pleural effusions. Curr Opin Pulm Med 2003;9(4):254–60.

51. Tarrand JJ, Lichterfeld M, Warraich I, et al. Diagnosis of invasive septate mold infections. A correlation of microbiological culture and histologic or cytologic examination. Am J Clin Pathol 2003; 119(6):854–8.

52. Denning DW, Park S, Lass-Florl C, et al. High-frequency triazole resistance found in nonculturable Aspergillus fumigatus from lungs of patients with chronic fungal disease. Clin Infect Dis 2011;52: 1123–9.

53. Joseph J, Strange C, Sahn SA. Pleural effusions in hospitalized patients with AIDS. Ann Intern Med 1993;118(11):856–9.

54. Sangoi AR, Rogers WM, Longacre TA, et al. Challenges and pitfalls of morphologic identification of fungal infections in histologic and cytologic specimens: a ten-year retrospective review at a single institution. Am J Clin Pathol 2009;131(3):364–75.

55. Kung VL, Chernock RD, Burnham CD. Diagnostic accuracy of fungal identification in histopathology and cytopathology specimens. Eur J Clin Microbiol Infect Dis 2017. https://doi.org/10.1007/s10096-017-3116-3.

56. Choi H, Chon HR, Kim K, et al. Clinical and laboratory differences between lymphocyte- and neutrophil-predominant pleural tuberculosis. PLoS One 2016;11(10):e0165428.

57. Takei H, Mody D. Epstein-Barr virus-positive pleural effusion: clinical features, cytomorphologic characteristics, and flow cytometric immunophenotyping. Am J Clin Pathol 2014;142(6):788–94.

58. Thijsen SFT, Luderer R, van Gorp JMH, et al. A possible role for Epstein-Barr virus in the pathogenesis of pleural effusion. Eur Respir J 2005; 26(4):662–6.

59. Caulfield AJ, Wengenack NL. Diagnosis of active tuberculosis disease: from microscopy to molecular techniques. J Clin Tuberc Other Mycobact Dis 2016;4:33–43.

60. Naylor B. Cytological aspects of pleural, peritoneal and pericardial fluids from patients with systemic lupus erythematosus. Cytopathology 1992;3(1): 1–8.

61. Walker WC, Wright V. Rheumatoid pleuritis. Ann Rheum Dis 1967;26(6):467–74.

62. Naylor B. The pathognomonic cytologic picture of rheumatoid pleuritis. The 1989 Maurice Goldblatt Cytology award lecture. Acta Cytol 1990;34(4): 465–73.

63. Smit HJ, van den Heuvel MM, Barbierato SB, et al. Analysis of pleural fluid in idiopathic spontaneous pneumothorax; correlation of eosinophil percentage with the duration of air in the pleural space. Respir Med 1999;93(4):262–7.

64. Heidecker J, Kaplan A, Sahn SA. Pleural fluid and peripheral eosinophilia from hemothorax: hypothesis of the pathogenesis of EPE in hemothorax and pneumothorax. Am J Med Sci 2006;332(3):148–52.

65. Ebata T, Okuma Y, Nakahara Y, et al. Retrospective analysis of unknown primary cancers with malignant pleural effusion at initial diagnosis. Thorac Cancer 2016;7(1):39–43.

66. Dey S, Nag D, Nandi A, et al. Utility of cell block, to detect malignancy in fluid cytology: adjunct or necessity? J Cancer Res Ther 2017;13(3):425–9.

67. Nasser H, Kuntzman TJ. Pleural effusion in women with a known adenocarcinoma: the role of immunostains in uncovering another hidden primary tumor. Acta Cytol 2011;55(5):438–44.

68. Saab J, Hoda RS, Narula N, et al. Diagnostic yield of cytopathology in evaluating pericardial effusions: clinicopathologic analysis of 419 specimens. Cancer 2017;125(2):128–37.

69. Ordonez NG. Value of claudin-4 immunostaining in the diagnosis of mesothelioma. Am J Clin Pathol 2013;139(5):611–9.

70. Jo VY, Cibas ES, Pinkus GS. Claudin-4 immunohistochemistry is highly effective in distinguishing adenocarcinoma from malignant mesothelioma in effusion cytology. Cancer Cytopathol 2014;122(4): 299–306.

71. Morgensztern D, Waqar S, Subramanian J, et al. Prognostic impact of malignant pleural effusion at presentation in patients with metastatic non-small cell lung cancer. J Thorac Oncol 2012;7(10):1485–9.

72. Yatabe Y, Koga T, Mitsudomi T, et al. CK20 expression, CDX2 expression, K-ras mutation, and goblet cell morphology in a subset of lung adenocarcinomas. J Pathol 2004;203(2):645–52.

73. Kim JH, Kim YS, Choi YD, et al. Utility of napsin A and thyroid transcription factor 1 in differentiating metastatic pulmonary from on-pulmonary adenocarcinoma in pleural effusion. Acta Cytol 2011; 55(3):266–70.

74. El Hag M, Schmidt L, Roh M, et al. Utility of TTF-1 and Napsin-A in the work-up of malignant effusions. Diagn Cytopathol 2016;44(4):299–304.

75. Ng WK, Chow JC, Ng PK. Thyroid transcription factor-1 is highly sensitive and specific in differentiating metastatic pulmonary from extrapulmonary adenocarcinoma in effusion fluid cytology specimens. Cancer 2002;96(1):43–8.

76. Dejmek A, Naucler P, Smedieback A, et al. (TA02) is a useful alternative to thyroid transcription factor-1 (TTF-1) for the identification of pulmonary adenocarcinoma cells in pleural effusions. Diagn Cytopathol 2007;35(8):493–7.

77. Ordonez NG. Value of PAX8, PAX2, napsin A, carbonic anhydrase IX, and claudin-4 immunostaining in distinguishing pleural epithelioid mesothelioma from metastatic renal cell carcinoma. Mod Pathol 2013;26(8):1132–43.

78. The cBioPortal for Cancer Genomics. Available at: http://www.cbioportal.org/index.do. Accessed December 14, 2017.

79. Gao J, Aksov BA, Dogrusoz U, et al. Integrative analysis of complex cancer genomics and clinical profiles using the cBioPortal. Sci Signal 2013; 6(269):pl1.

80. Cerami E, Gao J, Dogrusoz U, et al. The cBio cancer genomics portal: an open platform for exploring multidimensional cancer genomics data. Cancer Discov 2012;2(5):401–4.

81. Weinstock C, Khozin S, Suzman D, et al. U.S. Food and Drug Administration approval summary: atezolizumab for metastatic non-small cell lung cancer. Clin Cancer Res 2017;23(16):4534–9.

82. Langer CJ, Gadgeel SM, Borghaei H, et al. Carboplatin and pemetrexed with or without pembrolizumab for advanced, non-squamous non-small cell lung cancer: a randomised, phase 2 cohort of the open-label KEYNOTE-021 study. Lancet Oncol 2016;17:1497–508.

83. Heymann JJ, Bulman WA, Swinarski D, et al. Programmed death-ligand 1 expression in non-small cell lung carcinoma: comparison among cytology, small biopsy, and surgical resection specimens. Cancer Cytopathol 2017;125(12):896–907.

84. Yan Z, Gidley J, Horton D, et al. Diagnostic utility of mammaglobin and GCDFP-15 in the identification of metastatic breast carcinoma in fluid specimens. Diagn Cytopathol 2009;37(7):475–8.

85. Lew M, Pang JC, Jing X, et al. Young investigator challenge: the utility of GATA3 immunohistochemistry in the evaluation of metastatic breast carcinomas in malignant effusions. Cancer Cytopathol 2015;123(10):576–81.

86. Braxton DR, Cohen C, Siddiqui MT. Utility of GATA3 immunohistochemistry for diagnosis of metastatic breast carcinoma in cytology specimens. Diagn Cytopathol 2015;43(4):271–7.

87. Shield PW, Papadimos DJ, Walsh MD. GATA3: a promising marker for metastatic breast carcinoma in serous effusion specimens. Cancer Cytopathol 2014;122(4):307–12.

88. Nelson ER, Sharma R, Argani P, et al. Utility of Sox10 labeling in metastatic breast carcinomas. Hum Pathol 2017;67:205–10.

89. Wiseman W, Michael CW, Roh MH. Diagnostic utility of PAX8 and PAX2 immunohistochemistry in the identification of metastatic Müllerian carcinoma in effusions. Diagn Cytopathol 2011;39(9):651–6.

90. Vierkoetter KR, Ayabe AR, VanDrunen M, et al. Lynch syndrome in patients with clear cell and endometrioid cancers of the ovary. Gynecol Oncol 2014;135(1):81–4.

91. Chui MH, Ryan P, Radigan J, et al. The histomorphology of Lynch syndrome-associated ovarian carcinomas: toward a subtype-specific screening strategy. Am J Surg Pathol 2014;38(9):1173–81.

92. Shield P. Peritoneal washing cytology. Cytopathology 2004;15(3):131–41.

93. Damiani D, Suciu V, Genestie C, et al. Cytomorphology of ovarian clear cell carcinomas in peritoneal effusions. Cytopathology 2016;27(6):427–32.

94. Kandalaft PL, Gown AM, Isacson C. The lung-restricted marker napsin A is highly expressed in clear cell carcinomas of the ovary. Am J Clin Pathol 2014;142(6):830–6.

95. Kobel M, Kalloger SE, Carrick J, et al. A limited panel of immunomarkers can reliably distinguish between clear cell and high grade serous carcinoma of the ovary. Am J Surg Pathol 2009;33(1):14–21.

96. Chapel DB, Husain AN, Krausz T, et al. PAX8 expression in a subset of malignant peritoneal mesotheliomas and benign mesothelium has diagnostic implications in the differential diagnosis of ovarian serous carcinoma. Am J Surg Pathol 2017;41(12):1675–82.

97. Vang R, Gown AM, Barry TS, et al. Cytokeratins 7 and 20 in primary and secondary mucinous tumors of the ovary: analysis of coordinate immunohistochemical expression profiles and staining distribution in 179 cases. Am J Surg Pathol 2006;30(9):1130–9.

98. Tomillo L, Moch H, Diener PA, et al. CDX-2 immunostaining in primary and secondary ovarian carcinomas. J Clin Pathol 2004;57(6):641–3.

99. Nodin B, Zendehrokh N, Sundstrom M, et al. Clinicopathologic correlates and prognostic significance of KRAS mutation status in a pooled prospective cohort of epithelial ovarian cancer. Diagn Pathol 2013;8:106.

100. Bayrak R, Haltas H, Yenidunya S. The value of CDX2 and cytokeratins 7 and 20 expression in differentiating colorectal adenocarcinomas from extraintestinal gastrointestinal adenocarcinomas: CK7-/20+ phenotype is more specific than CDX2 antibody. Diagn Pathol 2012;7:9.

101. Wilentz RE, Su GH, Dai JL, et al. Immunohistochemical labeling for dpc4 mirrors genetic status in pancreatic adenocarcinomas: a new marker of DPC4 inactivation. Am J Pathol 2000;156(1):37–43.

102. Kim WH, Gomez-Izquierdo L, Vilardell F, et al. HER2 status in gastric and gastroesophageal junction cancer: results of the large, multinational HER-EAGLE study. Appl Immunohistochem Mol Morphol 2016. https://doi.org/10.1097/PAI.0000000000000423.

103. Senyigit A, Bayram H, Babayigit C, et al. Malignant pleural mesothelioma caused by environmental exposure to asbestos in the Southeast of Turkey: CT findings in 117 patients. Respiration 2000;67(6):615–22.

104. Ribak J, Lilis R, Suzuki Y, et al. Malignant mesothelioma in a cohort of asbestos insulation workers: clinical presentation, diagnosis, and causes of death. Br J Ind Med 1988;45(3):182–7.

105. Delgermaa V, Takahashi K, Park EK, et al. Global mesothelioma deaths reported to the World Health Organization between 1994 and 2008.

Bull World Health Organ 2011;89(10):716–24, 724A–C.

106. Hodgson JT, Darnton A. The quantitative risks of mesothelioma and lung cancer in relation to asbestos exposure. Ann Occup Hyg 2000;44(8): 565–601.

107. Metintas M, Hillerdal G, Metintas S, et al. Endemic malignant mesothelioma: exposure to erionite is more important than genetic factors. Arch Environ Occup Health 2010;65(2):86–93.

108. Hjerpe A, Ascoli V, Bedrossian C, et al. Guidelines for cytopathologic diagnosis of epithelioid and mixed type malignant mesothelioma. Complementary statement from the International Mesothelioma Interest Group, also endorsed by the International Academy of Cytology and the Papanicolaou Society of Cytopathology. Cytojournal 2015;12:26.

109. Renshaw AA, Dean BR, Cibas ES, et al. The role of cytologic evaluation of pleural fluid in the diagnosis of malignant mesothelioma. Chest 1997;111: 106–9.

110. Rakha EA, Patil S, Abdulla K, et al. The sensitivity of cytologic evaluation of pleural fluid in the diagnosis of malignant mesothelioma. Diagn Cytopathol 2010;38(12):874–9.

111. Ikeda K, Tate G, Suzuki T, et al. Diagnostic usefulness of EMA, IMP3, and GLUT-1 for the immunocytochemical distinction of malignant cells from reactive mesothelial cells in effusion cytology using cytospin preparations. Diagn Cytopathol 2011; 39(6):395–401.

112. Hasteh F, Lin GY, Weidner N, et al. The use of immunohistochemistry to distinguish reactive mesothelial cells from malignant mesothelioma in cytologic effusions. Cancer Cytopathol 2010; 118(2):90–6.

113. Shen J, Pinkus GS, Deshpande V, et al. Usefulness of EMA, GLUT-1, and XIAP for the cytologic diagnosis of malignant mesothelioma in body cavity fluids. Am J Clin Pathol 2009;131(4): 516–23.

114. Attanoos RL, Griffin A, Gibbs AR. The use of immunohistochemistry in distinguishing reactive from neoplastic mesothelium. A novel use for desmin and comparative evaluation with epithelial membrane antigen, p53, platelet-derived growth factor receptor, P-glycoprotein, and Bcl-2. Histopathology 2003;43(3):231–8.

115. Minato H, Kurose N, Fukushima M, et al. Comparative immunohistochemical analysis of IMP3, GLUT1, EMA, CD146, and desmin for distinguishing malignant mesothelioma from reactive mesothelial cells. Am J Clin Pathol 2014;141(1): 85–93.

116. Chiosea S, Krasinskas A, Cagle PT, et al. Diagnostic importance of 9p21 homozygous deletion in malignant mesotheliomas. Mod Pathol 2008;21: 742–7.

117. Bott M, Brevet M, Taylor BS, et al. The nuclear deubiquitinase BAP1 is commonly inactivated by somatic mutations and 3p21 losses in malignant pleural mesothelioma. Nat Genet 2011;43(7): 668–72.

118. Yoshikawa Y, Sato A, Tsujimura T, et al. Frequent inactivation of the BAP1 gene in epithelioid-type malignant mesothelioma. Cancer Sci 2012;103: 868–74.

119. Cigognetti M, Lonardi S, Fisogni S, et al. BAP1 (BRCA1-associated protein 1) is a highly specific marker for differentiating mesothelioma from reactive mesothelial proliferations. Mod Pathol 2015; 28(8):1043–57.

120. Sheffield BS, Lorette J, Shen Y, et al. Immunohistochemistry for NF2, LATS1/2, and TAP/TAZ fails to separate benign from malignant mesothelial proliferations. Arch Pathol Lab Med 2016;140(5):391.

121. Hida T, Hamasaki M, Mastumoto S, et al. Immunohistochemical detection of MTAP and BAP1 protein loss for mesothelioma diagnosis: comparison with 9p21 FISH and BAP1 immunohistochemistry. Lung Cancer 2017;104:98–105.

122. Cozzi I, Oprescu FA, Rullo E, et al. Loss of BRCA1-associated protein 1 (BAP1) expression is useful in diagnostic cytopathology of malignant mesothelioma in effusions. Diagn Cytopathol 2017. https://doi.org/10.1002/dc23837.

123. Walts AE, Marchevsky AM. Low cost-effectiveness of CD3/CD20 immunostains for initial triage of lymphoid-rich effusions: an evidence-based review of the utility of these stains in selecting cases for full hematopathologic workup. Diagn Cytopathol 2012; 40(7):565–9.

124. Tong LC, Ko HM, Saleg MA, et al. Subclassification of lymphoproliferative disorders in serous effusions: a 10-year experience. Cancer Cytopathol 2013;121(5):261–70.

125. Chen L, Zhang JS, Liu DG, et al. An algorithmic approach to diagnose haematolymphoid neoplasms in effusion by combining morphology, immunohistochemistry, and molecular cytogenetics. Cytopathology 2017. https://doi.org/10.1111/cyt.12449.

126. Jones D, Weiberg DS, Pinkus GS, et al. Cytologic diagnosis of primary serous lymphoma. Am J Clin Pathol 1996;106(3):359–64.

127. Komanduri KY, Luce JA, McGrath MS, et al. The natural history and molecular heterogeneity of HIV-associated primary malignant lymphomatous effusions. J Acquir Immune Defic Syndr Hum Retrovirol 1996;13(3):215–26.

128. Boulanger E, Agbalika F, Maarek O, et al. A clinical, molecular, and cytogenetic study of 12 cases of

human herpesvirus 8 associated primary effusion lymphoma in HIV-infected patients. Hematol J 2001;2(3):172–9.

129. Wakely PE Jr, Menezes G, Nuovo GJ. Primary effusion lymphoma: cytopathologic diagnosis using in situ molecular genetic analysis for human herpesvirus 8. Mod Pathol 2002;15(9):944–50.

130. Abadi MA, Zakowski MF. Cytologic features of sarcomas in fluids. Cancer Cytopathol 1998;84(2):71–6.

131. Zhang PJ, Livolsi VA, Brooks JJ. Malignant epithelioid vascular tumors of the pleura: report of a series and literature review. Hum Pathol 2000;31(1):29–34.

132. Enbom ET, Abasolo PA, Dixon JR, et al. Cytomorphological features of epithelioid hemangioendothelioma in ascitic fluid with radiological, clinical, and histopathological correlations. Acta Cytol 2014;58(2):211–6.

133. Boucher LD, Swanson PE, Stanley MW, et al. Cytology of angiosarcoma. Findings in fourteen fine-needle aspiration biopsy specimens and one pleural fluid specimen. Am J Clin Pathol 2000;114(2):210–9.

134. Sholl LM, Nishino M, Pokharel S, et al. Primary pulmonary NUT midline carcinoma: clinical, radiographic, and pathologic characterizations. J Thorac Oncol 2015;10(6):951–9.

135. Bishop JA, French CA, Ali SZ. Cytopathologic features of NUT midline carcinoma: a series of 26 specimens from 13 patients. Cancer Cytopathol 2016;124(12):901–8.

Evaluation of Carcinoma of Unknown Primary on Cytologic Specimens

Erika E. Doxtader, MD*, Deborah J. Chute, MD

KEYWORDS

• Carcinoma • Unknown primary • Cytology • Immunohistochemistry • Molecular profiling

---

Key points

- Carcinoma of unknown primary is a distinct entity defined as metastatic carcinoma without a clinically obvious primary tumor.

- Determining the tissue of origin in patients diagnosed with carcinoma of unknown primary is important so site-directed therapy can be given, which may improve patient outcomes.

- Immunohistochemistry is the most widely used tool for the work-up of metastases, but molecular profiling assays are now also available for this purpose.

- This review provides an overview of helpful immunohistochemical stains used in the work-up of metastatic carcinoma, with a focus on newer site-specific markers, and discusses the role of gene expression profiling assays for determining tissue of origin.

- The utility of cytopathology specimens in the evaluation of carcinoma of unknown primary also is highlighted.

ABSTRACT

Carcinoma of unknown primary is defined as metastatic carcinoma without a clinically obvious primary tumor. Determining the tissue of origin in carcinoma of unknown primary is important for site-directed therapy. Immunohistochemistry is the most widely used tool for the work-up of metastases, but molecular profiling assays are also available. This review provides an overview of immunohistochemical stains in the work-up of metastatic carcinoma, with a focus on newer site-specific markers, and discusses the role of gene expression profiling assays for determining tissue of origin. The utility of cytopathology specimens in the evaluation of carcinoma of unknown primary also is highlighted.

OVERVIEW

Carcinoma of unknown primary (CUP) is defined as metastatic carcinoma without a clinically obvious primary tumor and is diagnosed only after a thorough clinical history and physical examination, imaging studies, and serum tumor marker analysis fail to elucidate a primary site.[1,2] CUP accounts for approximately 3% to 5% of all carcinomas,[1,3,4] and comprises a heterogeneous collection of tumors, including poorly differentiated carcinoma, adenocarcinoma, squamous cell carcinoma, and neuroendocrine carcinoma. Although a majority of patients with CUP have unfavorable outcomes and an aggressive clinical course, some clinically recognized subgroups of patients have more favorable outcomes, including women with isolated metastases to the axillary

---

Disclosures: The authors have no conflicts of interest or funding to disclose.
Department of Pathology, Cleveland Clinic, 9500 Euclid Avenue, Cleveland, OH 44195, USA
* Corresponding author.
E-mail address: doxtade@ccf.org

Surgical Pathology 11 (2018) 545–562
https://doi.org/10.1016/j.path.2018.04.006

surgpath.theclinics.com

lymph nodes, patients with metastatic squamous cell carcinoma to neck lymph nodes, and men with bone metastasis and elevated prostate-specific antigen (PSA); these patients may be given locoregional treatment based on the most likely primary site.[1,4] Patients with unfavorable outcomes tend to have widely metastatic disease and adenocarcinoma histology[1,4,5] and are often treated with platinum-based combination chemotherapy.[6] In autopsy-based studies, a small, clinically undetectable primary is found in up to 73% of patients with CUP, mostly from the lung and pancreas.[7]

survival than patients given empiric CUP regimens.

IHC is the most widely used tool by pathologists to identify a likely primary site based on tumor expression of site-specific markers. In recent years, the utility of IHC has been bolstered by new lineage-specific transcription factors that have greater sensitivity and specificity than traditional cytoplasmic markers for identifying likely primary sites.[9] In addition, new gene expression profiling assays have been developed for identifying tissue of origin in patients with CUP; these assays have gained popularity with clinicians, although they are less familiar to the average practicing pathologist, despite their reportedly superior accuracy over IHC in identifying a primary site.[10,11]

From a pathologist's point of view, tumors that fall into the category of CUP are not always easy to recognize, and whether or not a tumor needs to be worked up extensively by IHC is not always clear. Pathologists may not be privy to all of the available clinical information; furthermore, the clinical work-up may be incomplete at the time of the initial biopsy. In many cases, limited IHC panels are used to confirm clinically suspected primary sites. It is not uncommon, however, for a pathologist to need to perform an extensive work-up; common scenarios include patients with widely metastatic disease and no obvious dominant mass, patients who have a history of more than 1 primary carcinoma, or patients in whom there is a remote history of carcinoma. Even after a thorough IHC work-up, a primary site is unable to be identified in up to a third of metastatic carcinomas.[12]

This review provides an overview and update of useful immunohistochemical stains for the work-up of CUP and discusses the current molecular approaches that are commercially available for identifying tissue of origin. The term CUP is used broadly to include situations where at least initially there is no clinically known primary, and the pathologist is asked to try to identify a primary site by morphology and IHC, while recognizing that "true" CUPs are often morphologically and immunohistochemically ambiguous. In addition, issues specific to cytopathology specimens are discussed, because these specimens are increasingly used in the work-up of these patients.

Key Points
CARCINOMA OF UNKNOWN PRIMARY

- CUP is a clinical entity defined as metastatic carcinoma without a clinically apparent primary site.

- Because therapeutic strategies are based primarily on site of origin and histologic features, pathologists have an important role in assigning a primary site in cases of CUP.

- Immunohistochemistry (IHC) is the most widely used and cost-effective method to evaluate CUP, but molecular profiling assays are also commercially available for determining site of origin.

- Even after IHC and/or molecular analysis, a primary site is not identified in a significant proportion of CUP cases.

Management of patients with carcinoma is dependent on the anatomic site and histologic classification of the tumor. Attempts by a pathologist to identify the site of origin in patients with CUP are made with the hopes that tumor site-specific therapy will be the best treatment of the patient; furthermore, on identifying a primary site, tumor-specific molecular testing can be performed to guide therapy (ie, personalized or targeted therapy). The clinical utility of assigning a primary site is based on the assumption that the CUP would behave as the assigned primary tumor, but it is not known if CUP has distinct biology from tumors of known primary origin or if outcomes in patients with CUP will improve from receiving site-specific therapy.[6] In a study by Hainsworth and colleagues,[8] patients with CUP who received anatomic site-directed therapy had longer median

IMMUNOHISTOCHEMISTRY

Most of the data on the use of IHC are from the surgical pathology literature. Over the past few decades, the number of clinically useful immuno-histochemical stains has increased, and as more and more cases are tested, the utility of each of these stains has become clearer. Although cyto-keratins, especially CK7 and CK20, have tradition-ally been used to identify the general location of a primary site, their role is now supplemented by newer, site-specific nuclear transcription factors. Because the use of differential cytokeratins is well established, this review focuses on these newer IHC stains.

ADENOCARCINOMA

Adenocarcinomas are by far the largest sub-group of CUPs.[1] Although morphologic features can sometimes suggest a given primary site, there is significant overlap, especially when tu-mors become less differentiated. IHC, therefore, becomes necessary to attempt to establish site of origin. In a review of autopsy studies in pa-tients with CUP, the most common primary sites identified were lung and pancreas.[7] The most useful markers to distinguish between adenocar-cinomas of various primary sites are discussed; a summary of these immunostains is presented in **Table 1**.

LUNG

Thyroid transcription factor-1 (TTF-1) is a nuclear transcription factor involved in the embryogenesis of lung and thyroid epithelium. TTF-1 is expressed in normal lung and thyroid tissue as well as most carcinomas that arise in these organs. Nuclear TTF-1 positivity is seen in approximately 75% to 80% of lung adenocarcinomas and is negative in a majority of nonpulmonary (and nonthyroid) adenocarcinomas, making it a useful marker in the work-up of CUP.[13,14] The sensitivity of TTF-1 for lung adenocarcinoma can decrease with loss of differentiation as well as in mucinous ade-nocarcinomas, which are positive in only approx-imately one-third of cases.[13-15] The specificity of TTF-1 for lung adenocarcinomas also depends on the clone used. The most commonly used commercially available clones are 8G7G3/1 and SPT24; the former has slightly lower sensitivity but higher specificity for lung adenocarcinoma than the latter.[13] TTF-1 can be expressed in up to 15% of carcinomas of the gynecologic (GYN) tract and can occasionally be positive in adeno-carcinomas of the gastrointestinal (GI) tract, breast, and genitourinary tract.[13,16-20] Positive staining with TTF-1 is more common in nonpul-monary adenocarcinomas with the less specific clone SPT24 as well as the newer clone SP141, which seems to have higher sensitivity for pulmo-nary adenocarcinoma but lower specificity.[20] Specifically, sarcomatoid mesothelioma and squamous cell carcinomas of the lung can stain with SP141, with potential for misclassification.[21] Given its imperfect specificity for lung adenocar-cinoma, TTF-1 should be used in combination with other site-specific markers in the assessment of CUP.

Napsin A is a cytoplasmic marker expressed in a majority of lung adenocarcinomas; the combination of napsin A and TTF-1 is more sen-sitive for lung adenocarcinoma than either marker alone[14] and is especially useful to identify the occasional lung adenocarcinomas that are negative or weakly and/or focally positive for TTF-1 but positive for napsin A.[22] Napsin A, how-ever, can also be expressed in carcinomas of the endometrium, ovary (especially clear cell carci-nomas), thyroid, kidney, and liver.[14,22-24] In a study by Mukhopadhyay and Katzenstein,[22] in which the expression of polyclonal and mono-clonal napsin A antibodies were compared be-tween metastatic pulmonary and nonpulmonary carcinomas, the specificity of the monoclonal napsin A antibody for pulmonary adenocarci-nomas was higher than the polyclonal antibody, the latter staining 30% of nonpulmonary carci-nomas. A well-described pitfall associated with polyclonal napsin A is apical cytoplasmic stain-ing in adenocarcinomas of the GI tract.[22,25] This staining pattern is not seen with the mono-clonal antibody.

Table 1
Immunohistochemical markers commonly used in the work-up of carcinoma of unknown primary

Marker	Site of Origin	Sensitivity (%)
TTF-1	Lung (adenocarcinoma)	70–90
	Thyroid	90–100
Napsin A	Lung (adenocarcinoma)	70–90
CDX2	Colorectal	70–100
SATB2	Colorectal	80–97
GATA3	Breast	80–100
	Urothelial	75–100
PAX8	Kidney	80–100
	GYN tract	90–100
	Thyroid	30–100
NKX3.1	Prostate	90–100

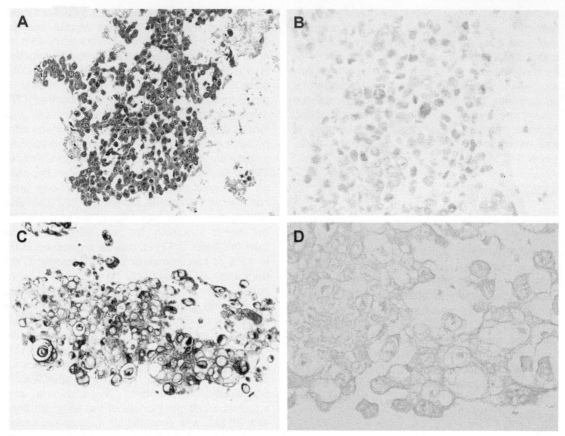

Fig. 1. Immunohistochemical staining profile of lung adenocarcinoma. A poorly differentiated carcinoma diagnosed in a station 7 lymph node by endobronchial ultrasound-guided transbronchial needle aspiration (*A*) (hematoxylin-eosin, cell block, ×200) is positive for TTF-1 (*B*) (×400) and for napsin A (*C*) (×400) and is negative for PAX8 (*D*) (×400), consistent with a lung primary.

In the context of a TTF-1/napsin A–positive metastatic carcinoma, PAX8 can be useful in distinguishing between thyroid and lung primaries; PAX8 is positive in a majority of thyroid carcinomas[26] but is invariably negative in lung adenocarcinomas.[27,28] Thus, a carcinoma that is TTF-1-positive, napsin A–positive, and PAX8-negative is highly likely to be a lung primary (**Fig. 1**), whereas a carcinoma that is positive for TTF-1 or napsin A but also strongly and diffusely positive for PAX8 is extremely unlikely to be metastasis from the lung (**Fig. 2**).

Because approximately 20% of lung adenocarcinomas are negative for TTF-1 and/or napsin A, the absence of staining for these markers does not exclude the lung as a possible primary site.[14,22] As discussed previously, this is especially true for most (70%) mucinous adenocarcinomas. The utility of TTF-1 and napsin A has also been validated in the cytology literature.[15,29,30]

Key Points
PAX8 IMMUNOHISTOCHEMISTRY

- PAX8 is a nuclear marker that is highly expressed in carcinomas of the thyroid, müllerian system, kidney, and thymus.

- PAX8 is helpful in the setting of a TTF-1 and/ or napsin A–positive CUP, because PAX8 is usually positive in thyroid carcinomas but negative in lung adenocarcinoma.

- PAX8 may be positive in occasional cholangiocarcinomas and pancreatic adenocarcinomas, which may be a potential pitfall.

- Expression of PAX8 has been described in pancreatic neuroendocrine tumors, although its utility in establishing site of origin of neuroendocrine tumors is not clear.

- PAX8 is negative in mesothelial cells and, therefore, is useful in the setting of a malignant effusion

Pitfalls
Thyroid Transcription Factor-1

! Approximately 20% of lung adenocarcinomas are negative for TTF-1.

! Mucinous adenocarcinomas of the lung may be TTF-1–negative in up to two-thirds of cases.

! TTF-1 can occasionally be positive in adenocarcinomas of the GYN tract, GI tract, breast, and genitourinary tract, especially when the less specific clone SPT24 is used.

! Extrapulmonary small cell carcinomas may express TTF-1; therefore, TTF-1 has a limited role in the evaluation of metastatic small cell CUP.

! In cytopathology material, TTF-1 staining may be weak and difficult to interpret.

GASTROINTESTINAL TRACT

One of the most common markers used in the work-up of CUP is CDX2, a nuclear transcription factor that is a marker of GI epithelial differentiation. CDX2 shows strong and diffuse positivity in a majority of colorectal and duodenal adenocarcinomas and shows heterogeneous expression in adenocarcinomas of the stomach, esophagus, and pancreatobiliary tract.[31] CDX2 reactivity is retained in colorectal metastases, although its expression can decrease in poorly differentiated tumors.[32] It has been shown to have superior sensitivity over villin, a cytoplasmic marker of GI differentiation that also stains adenocarcinomas of the GI tract.[31] Although CDX2 has excellent sensitivity for colorectal tumors, it can also be expressed in non–GI tract adenocarcinomas, with high levels of expression reported in up to 60% of mucinous ovarian carcinomas and 30% to 50% of adenocarcinomas of the bladder.[9,31,33] It can occasionally be positive in adenocarcinomas of the

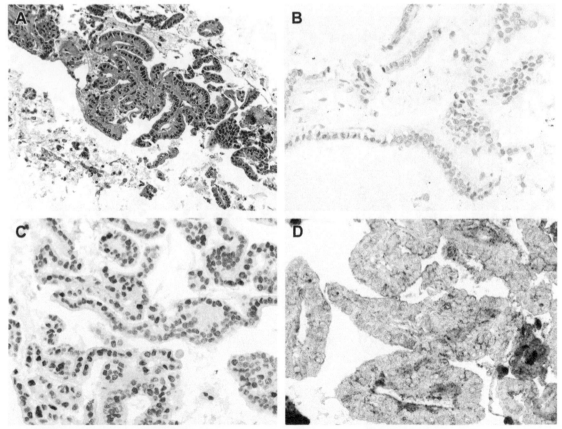

Fig. 2. TTF-1 positivity is not limited to lung adenocarcinoma. In this metastatic carcinoma in a 4R lymph node sampled by endobronchial ultrasound-guided transbronchial needle aspiration (*A*) (hematoxylin-eosin, cell block, ×200), positivity for TTF-1 (*B*) (×400), PAX8 (*C*) (×400), and thyroglobulin (*D*) (×400) is consistent with thyroid origin.

lung,[34] especially mucinous adenocarcinomas; as discussed previously, two-thirds of pulmonary mucinous adenocarcinomas may be TTF-1 and napsin A–negative and may be misclassified if CDX2 is positive. CDX2 reactivity has also been described in occasional endometrial carcinomas and hepatocellular carcinomas.[32,35,36] Despite its limited specificity, CDX2 remains a useful marker in evaluating metastases diagnosed on cytologic specimens (Fig. 3). In a study of CDX2 expression in cell block material, Saad and colleagues[37] showed that CDX2 was positive in 86% of metastases from the GI tract and was negative in all non–GI tract adenocarcinomas tested.

SATB2 is a relatively new, sensitive nuclear marker of GI differentiation and stains 85% to 97% of all colorectal adenocarcinomas.[38,39] It can be a useful adjunct in the assessment of CUP, owing to its increased specificity over CDX2 for tumors of colorectal origin.[40] SATB2 can be helpful in distinguishing colorectal metastases from gastric or pancreatic metastases, which may be CDX2-positive but are seldom positive for SATB2.[39] Another diagnostic setting in which SATB2 may be of use is in the evaluation of metastases involving the ovary. In a study by Yang and colleagues,[41] SATB2 was a highly sensitive and specific marker for distinguishing metastatic adenocarcinoma ex–goblet cell carcinoid tumor involving the ovary from metastases to the ovary from other primary sites, which showed only focal and weak staining. Because SATB2 is negative in most primary ovarian tumors, it can also help distinguish metastatic colorectal or appendiceal adenocarcinomas involving the ovary from primary mucinous ovarian tumors, which may be CDX2 positive.[42] Matsushima and colleagues[43] assessed SATB2 staining in pulmonary enteric–type adenocarcinomas and colorectal metastases involving the lung and concluded that SATB2 is a useful marker in differentiating the two, because SATB2 was positive in only 13% of pulmonary enteric adenocarcinomas but was positive in 100% of metastatic colorectal adenocarcinomas. The utility of SATB2 staining in mucinous adenocarcinomas of the lung has not yet been widely

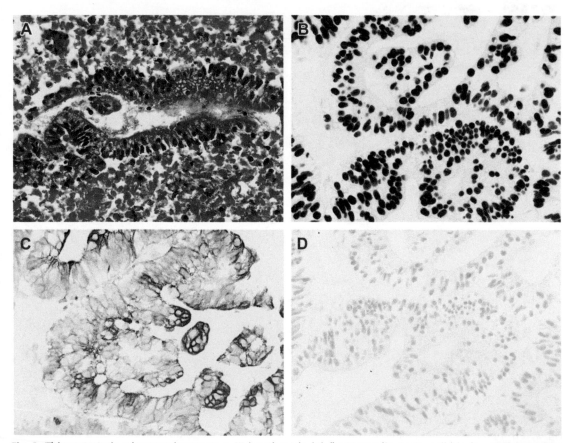

Fig. 3. This metastatic adenocarcinoma to a 4R lymph node (A) (hematoxylin-eosin, cell block, ×400) is positive for CDX2 (B) (×400) and CK20 (C) (×400), consistent with a colorectal primary. TTF-1 (D) (×400) and napsin A were negative.

studied. Primary bladder adenocarcinomas, which are frequently CDX2 positive, also stain for SATB2 in 49% of cases; thus, CDX2 and SATB2 are not helpful in distinguishing primary bladder adenocarcinoma from colorectal metastasis.[44]

BREAST

Metastasis from the breast should routinely be considered in the work-up of CUP, especially in women. GATA-binding protein 3 (GATA3) is a transcription factor that has become increasingly used in the work-up of CUP as a marker of breast and urothelial origin. It is exquisitely sensitive for breast carcinomas, with expression in more than 90% of cases, regardless of histologic subtype or grade.[45,46] Reactivity may decrease with increasing tumor grade,[47] and tumors that are triple negative for estrogen receptor (ER), progesterone receptor (PR), and human epidermal growth factor receptor-2, may show reduced GATA3 reactivity or may be negative.[45,47] GATA3 has been shown to have higher sensitivity for breast origin than the cytoplasmic breast markers gross cystic disease fluid protein-15 (GCDFP-15) and

mammaglobin.[45,48] In a large study of GATA3 expression in 2500 epithelial and nonepithelial tumors, Miettinen and colleagues[45] showed that GATA3 was expressed in more than 90% of primary and metastatic ductal and lobular carcinomas of the breast, whereas GCDFP-15 expression was present in 78%. Furthermore, GATA3 expression was identified in all histologic subtypes of breast carcinoma tested, including tumors with ductal, lobular, papillary, and mucinous differentiation. Although GATA3 is reported to have high specificity for breast and urothelial origin,[47] caution should be used in the interpretation because GATA3 expression has also been demonstrated in pancreatic ductal adenocarcinomas, squamous cell carcinomas, mesotheliomas, salivary gland tumors, parathyroid tumors, and some mesenchymal tumors.[45] Nonetheless, GATA3 is a useful marker in the cytologic evaluation of breast metastases; in a study including 53 fine-needle aspirates of breast lesions, GATA3 was positive in 82% of metastases.[47] An example of a metastatic breast carcinoma diagnosed on a cytology specimen is illustrated in **Fig. 4**.

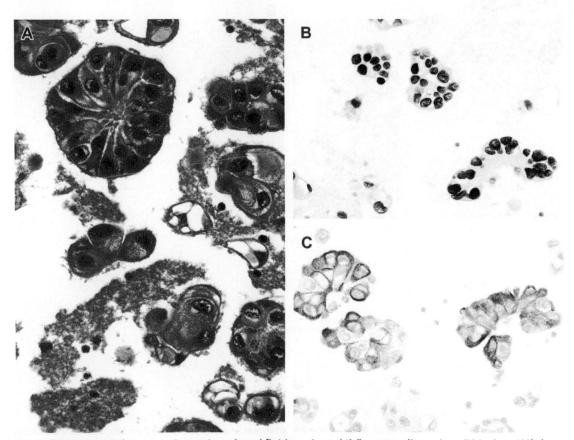

Fig. 4. This metastatic breast carcinoma in a pleural fluid specimen (*A*) (hematoxylin-eosin, cell block, ×400) shows strong and diffuse nuclear positivity for GATA3 (*B*) (×400) and cytoplasmic positivity for mammaglobin (*C*) (×400).

As discussed previously, triple-negative breast carcinomas may be negative for site-specific breast markers, such as GATA3, and thus can be difficult to classify. In cases of metastatic triple-negative breast carcinoma, Sox10 may be a useful marker of breast origin, because a subset of these cases has been recently shown to be Sox10-positive.[49]

GENITOURINARY TRACT

Prostate origin should be considered in any metastatic carcinoma presenting in a man, especially if there is metastasis to the bone. Metastatic prostate carcinomas are typically pan-keratin–positive but CK7-negative and CK20-negative.[50] The prostate-specific cytoplasmic markers PSA and prostate-specific acid phosphatase (PSAP) have been widely used as markers of prostate origin. A newer nuclear marker, NKX3.1, however, has been shown to have high sensitivity and specificity for identifying metastases from the prostate.[51] In a tissue microarray study, Gurel and colleagues[51]

showed that NKX3.1 has higher sensitivity than PSA (98.6% vs 94%) and equivalent sensitivity to PSAP; NKX3.1 specificity was 99.7%, staining only 1 of 349 nonprostatic tumors. NKX3.1 has been shown to be a useful marker for identifying prostate metastases in cytology cell block material.[52] Because it is a nuclear marker, NKX3.1 may be easier to interpret than PSA and PSAP, especially in small biopsy or cytology specimens (**Fig. 5**).

The morphology of metastatic urothelial carcinoma often overlaps with that of carcinomas of other primary sites, as does its expression of nonspecific markers, such as CK7 and p63. The cytoplasmic markers uroplakin III and thrombomodulin, although specific for urothelial origin, lack sensitivity.[53,54] As discussed previously, GATA3 is a sensitive marker of urothelial origin, identifying 86% of urothelial carcinomas in 1 study.[47] In a microarray study of paired regional metastases and bladder primaries, GATA3 staining was present in the metastases in 79% of cases and in the primary tumor in 75%.[55] Reactivity is generally

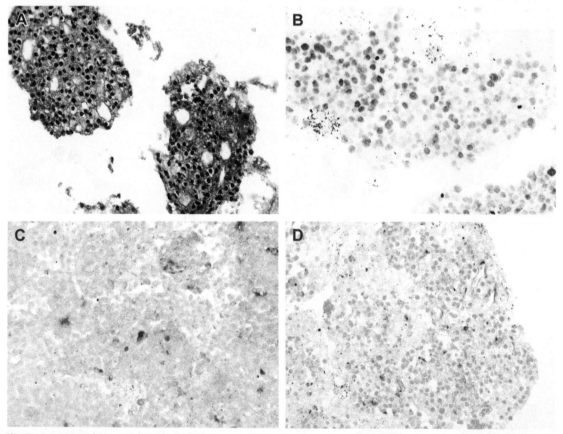

Fig. 5. A metastasis to a 4L lymph node from a prostatic adenocarcinoma, sampled by endobronchial ultrasound-guided transbronchial needle aspiration (*A*) (hematoxylin-eosin, cell block, ×400), is positive for the nuclear marker NKX3.1 (*B*) (×400) as well as PSAP (*C*) (×400) and PSA (*D*) (×400).

strong and diffuse and is present across subtypes of urothelial carcinoma,[48,55] with the exception of sarcomatoid and small cell variants.[56] GATA3 should be included in a panel of IHC stains in the evaluation of CUP when urothelial carcinoma enters the differential diagnosis.

PAX-8, a transcription factor involved in the development of the thyroid gland, kidney, and müllerian system, has emerged as a reliable marker of metastatic renal cell carcinoma (RCC), owing to its positivity in most RCCs in both primary and metastatic sites.[57,58] In a study by Tong and colleagues,[58] PAX8 was expressed in 98% of clear cell RCC, 90% of papillary RCC, and 71% of sarcomatoid RCC, and was detected in 85% of metastatic renal tumors. PAX8 is more sensitive for RCC than the classic renal markers, including CD10 and RCC.[59] PAX8 has limited sensitivity for renal tumors, however, due to its expression in carcinomas of the thyroid and GYN tract[57]; in addition, it can occasionally be positive in thymic neoplasms, cholangiocarcinoma, and pancreatic adenocarcinoma.[9] Use of the monoclonal antibody BC12 reportedly shows less cross-reactivity than the polyclonal antibody in B lymphocytes and pancreatic adenocarcinomas.[28] PAX8 positivity in a metastatic carcinoma should be interpreted in the context of a panel of markers, especially when a GYN or thyroid primary is also in the differential diagnosis. Other sites, including breast, prostate, stomach, colon/rectum and adrenal gland, are generally PAX8-negative.[28] An example of a PAX8-positive metastatic clear cell RCC diagnosed on a cytology specimen is shown in **Fig. 6**.

GYNECOLOGIC TRACT

The identification of GYN tract origin in metastatic CUP, which was previously dependent on expression of ER and PR, has greatly benefited from the introduction of the PAX8 antibody. PAX8 is expressed in a majority of carcinomas of müllerian origin, with positivity in up to 98% of serous, 94% of endometrioid, and 100% of clear cell tumors from the uterus, ovary, omentum, and fallopian tube.[57,60] Its expression is retained in a majority of metastases from the ovary and endometrium,

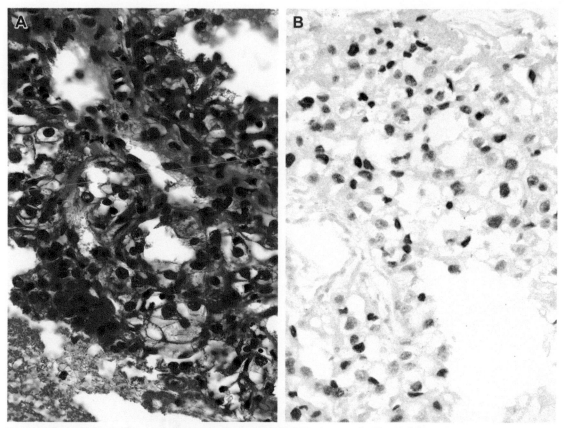

Fig. 6. In this metastatic clear cell carcinoma to an 11L lymph node, sampled by endobronchial ultrasound-guided transbronchial needle aspiration (*A*) (hematoxylin-eosin, cell block, ×400), PAX8 is positive (*B*) (×400), confirming renal origin.

making it a useful marker of GYN tract origin in the metastatic setting. As discussed previously, PAX8 is not entirely specific, because it is also positive in carcinomas of the thyroid and kidney as well as in thymic tumors.[61]

Ovarian carcinomas commonly involve the peritoneal fluid. PAX8 is a useful marker in the evaluation of malignant serous effusions in women, because it is positive in up to 70% of metastatic ovarian and endometrial carcinomas in serous effusion specimens.[62] WT1, another sensitive nuclear marker of ovarian serous carcinoma,[9] is also positive in mesothelial cells; because PAX8 is not expressed in mesothelial cells, it is a superior marker over WT1 in the setting of a malignant effusion.[63,64] An example of a metastatic high-grade serous carcinoma diagnosed on a fluid cytology specimen is illustrated in **Fig. 7**.

SQUAMOUS CELL CARCINOMA

Recognition of squamous differentiation can be challenging on surgical and cytologic material. Particularly given the better prognosis for patients with squamous cell CUP, it is important to exclude this tumor subtype on evaluation.[1] Markers, such as p63 and p40, are helpful in recognition of squamous differentiation but are not specific for site of origin.[65] p63 is positive in urothelial cell carcinomas and rarely in other neoplasms (such as basal cell–phenotype breast cancer and lung adenocarcinoma), so evaluation with a panel of stains is helpful in excluding other neoplasms. p40, an antibody that recognizes the p63 isoform ΔNp63, has higher specificity for squamous differentiation than p63 and, therefore, may be superior to p63 in the metastatic setting.[66]

Unfortunately, there is no immunohistochemical marker that is specific for site of origin of a metastatic squamous cell carcinoma, with 2 exceptions.[67] When high-risk human papillomavirus (HPV) is demonstrated in the tumor cells, possible primary sites can be narrowed down to the oropharynx, uterine cervix, and rarely vulva or anus. p16, a surrogate marker of high-risk HPV infection, does not have high specificity outside of the oropharynx or cervix, because other primary sites can show strong and diffuse positivity, including squamous cell carcinomas of the lung,

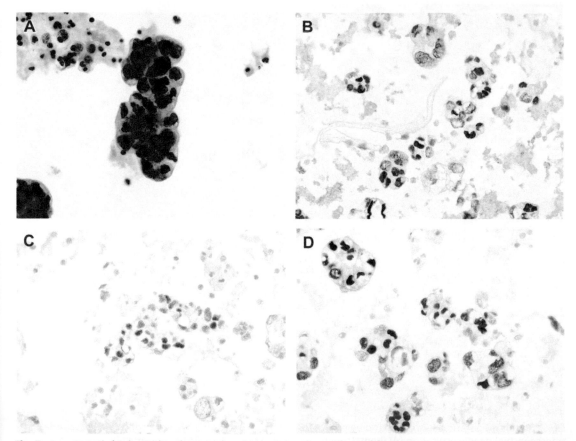

Fig. 7. A metastatic high-grade adenocarcinoma involving the peritoneal fluid (*A*) (hematoxylin-eosin, cell block, ×400) is positive for PAX8 (*B*) (×400), WT1 (*C*) (×400), and p53 (*D*) (×400), consistent with endometrial origin.

skin, and nonoropharyngeal head and neck sites.[68] Thus, confirmation of high-risk HPV infection using in situ hybridization or molecular testing may be helpful. p16 IHC is frequently unreliable in cytology cell blocks and may be falsely negative[67]; thus, HPV-specific testing is often more helpful on cytologic samples. The second useful exception is Epstein-Barr virus (EBV), which when positive suggests origin in the nasopharynx. EBV testing should be considered when HPV testing is negative, especially if a head and neck primary is suspected. The most commonly used marker is chromogenic in situ hybridization for EBV, which is highly specific for EBV infection, including in cytology samples.[69] Both HPV-associated and EBV-associated squamous cell carcinomas frequently present as small primary tumors that may go unrecognized on imaging studies.[67]

NEUROENDOCRINE CARCINOMA

Determination of primary site in neuroendocrine carcinomas can be difficult, and high-grade lesions are an especially vexing problem. In low-grade metastatic neuroendocrine carcinomas, expression of TTF-1 is suggestive of either lung or thyroid origin, because TTF-1 is expressed in a majority of pulmonary carcinoid tumors[70] (although staining can be patchy and weak) and in most medullary thyroid carcinomas[71] but is generally negative in other low-grade neuroendocrine carcinomas.[72] Absence of TTF-1 staining, however, does not exclude lung origin, because up to a quarter of lung carcinoids can be negative.[70] Furthermore, PAX8 is not especially helpful in distinguishing between lung and thyroid origin in this setting; although most pulmonary carcinoid tumors are PAX8-negative, with a reported range of positivity between 0% and 8%,[26,27,46,70] more than half of medullary thyroid carcinomas are also PAX8 negative.[26] PAX8 expression alone has limited value in the setting of metastatic neuroendocrine carcinomas of unknown primary, because PAX8 can be positive in well-differentiated neuroendocrine tumors of the pancreas (due to cross-reactivity of the polyclonal antibody with PAX6),[73] tumors originating from the duodenum, rectum, stomach, and a subset of medullary thyroid carcinoma.[26] A panel of immunostains, including CDX2 and calcitonin, may help in the differential diagnosis of a PAX8-positive, TTF-1–negative low-grade neuroendocrine carcinoma, because CDX2 is specific for neuroendocrine tumors of GI origin[72] and calcitonin positivity supports metastatic medullary thyroid carcinoma.

Unlike low-grade neuroendocrine carcinomas, in which TTF-1 expression is restricted to subsets of lung and medullary thyroid carcinoma, high-grade neuroendocrine carcinomas can express TTF-1 regardless of primary site. TTF-1 expression has been demonstrated in 44% of nonpulmonary small cell carcinomas, including those from the prostate, bladder, and uterine cervix.[71] Determining site of origin in a metastatic, high-grade neuroendocrine carcinoma remains a challenge.

> ### *Key Points*
> #### IMMUNOHISTOCHEMISTRY IN NEUROENDOCRINE TUMORS OF UNKNOWN PRIMARY
>
> - Establishing site of origin in metastatic neuroendocrine tumors is difficult, especially in higher-grade carcinomas.
>
> - In low-grade neuroendocrine tumors, TTF-1 expression suggests either lung or thyroid primary.
>
> - CDX2 expression is specific for GI origin in metastatic neuroendocrine tumors.
>
> - PAX8 can be expressed in neuroendocrine tumors of the thyroid, pancreas, duodenum, rectum, and stomach and, therefore, has limited value in the setting of a metastatic low grade neuroendocrine tumor of unknown primary.
>
> - TTF-1 positivity in small cell carcinomas is not specific for site of origin, because nonpulmonary small cell carcinomas may be positive.

IMMUNOHISTOCHEMISTRY IN CYTOPATHOLOGY SPECIMENS

Suspected metastases are often sampled by fine-needle aspiration, which is an effective, minimally invasive technique for evaluating superficial or deep-seated lesions. Metastases may also be diagnosed on pleural, pericardial, and peritoneal fluid samples; these types of specimens are common in patients with CUP, who often present with a malignant effusion.[74] In cytopathology specimens, IHC is typically performed on cell block material. There are several issues with cell block preparation, however, that may have an impact on the extent of the work-up for a given sample. It may be difficult to obtain an adequately cellular cell block for an exhaustive IHC work-up. Cell block preparation methods vary widely between laboratories,[75] and preparation of a sufficient cell block is often operator-dependent. In cases in which a cytopathologist is present for rapid-onsite evaluation, the cytopathologist can request extra passes dedicated for cell block preparation to try to ensure adequate cellularity. In many cases, however, rapid-onsite evaluation is not practical, and specimens lacking adequate cellularity for IHC remain a common problem. In situations in which the cell block is paucicellular, IHC can be performed on destained smears that contain tumor, although only a limited number of stains are possible. The cell transfer technique has been developed to remove tumor cells from a smear and transfer them to another slide for IHC; multiple immunohistochemical stains can potentially be performed depending on the amount of tumor present.[76,77] These methods are likely not applicable, however, in cases in which multiple stains are necessary and may result in destruction of slides and loss of material that may potentially be needed for molecular testing.

Key Points
IMMUNOHISTOCHEMISTRY ON CYTOPATHOLOGY SPECIMENS FOR CARCINOMA OF UNKNOWN PRIMARY

- Cell block specimens may suffer from low cellularity; assessment of tumor cells on IHC can be difficult.

- Most IHC assays are validated on formalin-fixed paraffin-embedded (FFPE) tissue; separate validation of each IHC stain is warranted in laboratories that use alcohol-based fixatives.

- Quality of IHC stains may differ between FFPE samples and alcohol-fixed cytology samples.

- Contaminating normal cells may be difficult to evaluate on cell blocks and can be overinterpreted as neoplastic on IHC (eg, napsin A in alveolar macrophages or TTF-1 in normal bronchial cells).

Another issue affecting IHC performance on cytopathology specimens is the lack of standardization across laboratories regarding specimen collection methods and fixatives. In general, specimens can either be collected in alcohol-based fixatives or formalin. In laboratories that use a liquid-based cytology platform, the use of an automated system, such as the Cellient Automated Cell Block System (Hologic, Bedford, Massachusetts), is a faster and less labor-intensive method of generating cell blocks than creating FFPE cell blocks. Because most laboratories validate immunohistochemical stains on FFPE tissue, however, cytopathology laboratories that use alcohol-based fixatives should separately validate each immunohistochemical stain to ensure that the assay achieves consistent results.[78,79] In a study by Sauter and colleagues[79] in which they compared the results of IHC on formalin-fixed and alcohol-fixed cell blocks, almost half of antibodies tested failed initial validation on alcohol-fixed material using conditions optimized for FFPE tissue, highlighting the challenges of IHC on alcohol-fixed material. Despite the technical difficulties sometimes encountered, cytology specimens remain a robust source of diagnostic material that can be used for both IHC and molecular testing.

MOLECULAR PROFILING ASSAYS

In the past decade, molecular profiling assays have been developed to complement standard pathologic examination of CUP[80–85]; these assays may be most helpful when an IHC work-up fails to identify a possible primary site.[4] The premise behind the use of gene expression profiling for CUP is that different tissue types have specific gene expression profiles, and metastatic tumors retain some of the same molecular characteristics as the tissue of origin.[86] Gene expression profiling assays use either an oligonucleotide-microarray approach or real-time polymerase chain reaction (RT-PCR) to evaluate expression of multiple genes in a given sample; the sample is then compared with a database containing gene expression profiles for known tumor types. In general, for microarray analysis, messenger RNA (mRNA) or microRNA is isolated from the tumor sample, amplified, labeled with a fluorescent probe, and hybridized to a microarray containing probes complementary to known gene sequences. Detection of fluorescent signals in specific locations on the microarray provides a unique gene expression profile for a tumor sample, which can then be compared with a database of gene expression profiles of known tumor types. With the use of microarray platforms, expression of thousands of genes can be measured in a given sample.[7] RT-PCR assays were also developed because they are more suited for clinical use; however, fewer genes can be tested for using this method.[82] As of this writing, 3 gene expression profiling assays are commercially available: CancerTYPE ID, Rosetta Cancer Origin Test, and miRview mets (**Table 2**). The reported accuracy of gene expression profiling assays for determining the

Table 2
Gene expression profiling assays for determining site of origin in carcinoma of unknown primary

Assay (Manufacturer; Web Site[a])	Assay Type	Reported Accuracy	Tumor Classes Identified (No.)	Specimen Requirements	Commercially Available?	Selected References
CupPrint (Agendia BV; N/A)	1900-gene microarray based	83%	49	FFPE	No	Horlings et al,[80] 2008
Tissue of Origin Test (Cancer Genetics Incorporated; cancergenetics.com)	1550-gene microarray based	88%	15	FFPE	Yes	Monzon et al,[81] 2009
CancerTYPE ID (bioTheranostics, Inc.; cancertypeid.com)	92-gene RT-PCR	87%	31	FFPE	Yes	Ma et al,[82] 2006
CUP Assay (Veridex; N/A)	mRNA	79%	6	FFPE	No	Talantov et al,[83] 2006; Varadhachary et al,[84] 2008
miRview mets (Teva Pharmaceutical Industries; oncotest.co.il)	48-microRNA	86%	25	FFPE	Yes	Lu et al,[85] 2005

[a] Web sites accessed December 3, 2017.

correct tissue of origin ranges from 80% to 90% in patients with a known primary.[81,82,86] Some data suggest, however, that classification performance may decrease in poorly differentiated carcinomas; Ma and colleagues[82] reported 94%, 84%, and 71% accuracy in classifying well differentiated, moderately differentiated, and poorly differentiated tumors, respectively.

Key Points
MOLECULAR PROFILING ASSAYS FOR CARCINOMA OF UNKNOWN PRIMARY

- There are currently 3 commercially available gene expression profiling assays for evaluating CUP.

- These assays report 80% to 90% accuracy in classifying metastatic carcinomas.

- Molecular profiling assays require FFPE tissue; only cytopathology material fixed in formalin is acceptable.

- Molecular profiling may not be a practical application for cytopathology laboratories that primarily use alcohol-based fixatives.

In patients presenting with CUP, the accuracy of molecular profiling assays can be difficult to evaluate, because an obvious primary site is not known.[87] The performance of gene expression profiling assays in this subset of patients has been addressed in a few studies. In a study of the CancerTYPE ID assay in patients with CUP, molecular profiles of 171 metastatic tumors of unknown origin were compared with clinical data, including latent primary tumors found months or years after initial presentation as well as IHC diagnoses. The molecular profiling assay was found to be in agreement with both clinical and IHC diagnoses approximately 75% of the time,[4] suggesting that gene expression profiling has value in the assessment of CUP. In a similar study, Varadhachary and colleagues[84] evaluated the molecular profiles from tumors in 120 patients with CUP and identified a likely tissue of origin in 61%; in these patients, the molecular results were deemed compatible with clinicopathologic features and response to treatment. In a multicenter validation study of the Tissue of Origin test, 547 frozen specimens representing either metastatic tumors or poorly differentiated primary tumors were studied to simulate the types of tumors that commonly present as CUP. The overall sensitivity and specificity of the assay in this subgroup of tumors were 87.8% and 99.4%, respectively, although accurate classification of metastatic tumors was slightly lower than for primary tumors (84.5% vs 90.7%, respectively).[81]

When directly compared with IHC, molecular profiling assays have been reported to have comparable or slightly superior accuracy in assigning a primary site. Weiss and colleagues[11] compared IHC analysis versus the 92-gene classifier Cancer-TYPE ID in 131 high-grade, predominantly metastatic tumors and found that the molecular assay had an accuracy of 79% versus 69%, respectively, for standard morphology and IHC. In a similar study of the Tissue of Origin test, 157 metastatic carcinomas with clinically known primary sites were evaluated by both molecular profiling and IHC; molecular profiling was significantly more accurate significantly more accurate than IHC in identifying the correct primary site (89% vs 83%, respectively) and was especially more superior in the subset of poorly differentiated carcinomas tested.[10]

Although the reported accuracy of molecular profiling assays is on par with or slightly superior to IHC, there are significant drawbacks to its routine use, including cost and prolonged turnaround time, because the specimen must be sent to an outside laboratory for evaluation. In contrast, IHC is in widespread use, is available in most laboratories, and can be performed quickly. Another potential problem of molecular profiling assays is the possibility of misclassification due to contaminating non-neoplastic tissues that may be inadvertently sampled with the tumor. In a study by Monzon and colleagues[81] of 39 inaccurate classifications by the Tissue of Origin test, 11 matched the biopsy site for that sample. Finally, although molecular profiling assays are reported to have high diagnostic accuracy, it is unclear whether or not their use results in clinical benefit to the patient. In a recent update of the National Comprehensive Cancer Network (NCCN) guidelines for occult primary tumors, an expert panel recommended against the routine use of gene expression profiling for identification of the tissue of origin, because a clinical benefit has not been consistently demonstrated.[2]

The role of cytopathology specimens in molecular profiling of CUP is unclear, because there is little published literature on the topic. The commercially available assays have been validated on formalin-fixed tissue only. In a study of the performance of the Tissue of Origin Test in FFPE cell blocks from malignant effusions in patients with known primaries, Stancel and colleagues[88] found a 94% agreement between the results of the molecular profiling assay and the known diagnosis, suggesting that cell block specimens yield adequate diagnostic material for these types of assays. As discussed previously, however, cell block specimens may often be of suboptimal cellularity; furthermore, there is the potential for misclassification by molecular profiling assays due to contaminating benign cells (especially in effusion specimens, in which high numbers of admixed mesothelial cells and lymphocytes are common). More studies are needed to address the potential for cytology specimens to be used in this setting. Currently, it seems that cytology specimens play a limited role in molecular profiling of CUP.

CIRCULATING TUMOR CELLS

The CELLSEARCH circulating tumor cell (CTC) test (Menarini Silicon Biosystems, San Diego, CA), an assay designed to analyze the peripheral blood for the presence of CTCs, has recently been approved by the Food and Drug Administration (FDA) to evaluate prognosis in patients with metastatic breast, colorectal or prostate cancer. The CELLSEARCH CTC assay identifies circulating epithelial tumor cells by assessing immunohistochemical expression of CD45, EpCAM, and cytokeratins 8, 18, and 19 (http://www.cellsearchctc.com, accessed December 31, 2017). If a malignant cell population can be isolated from the peripheral blood, IHC could potentially be used for further characterization. In a recent study by Matthew and colleagues,[89] a post–CELLSEARCH CTC assay was developed to assess the immunohistochemical expression of the CTC population using antibodies to CK7, CK20, TTF-1, ER, and PSA, to attempt to determine site of origin in patients with CUP. The assay was able to detect metastases from patients with known breast and prostate cancer. Although this is a developing area, the use of a minimally invasive blood test in the initial diagnosis of patients with metastatic carcinoma is an intriguing prospect. Prospective clinical testing is needed before further implementation of this new technology.

THE FUTURE OF CARCINOMA OF UNKNOWN PRIMARY

Although current practice is to treat patients with carcinoma based on anatomic site and histologic subtype, in the era of next-generation sequencing and personalized therapy, it is not inconceivable that future treatment strategies for a given tumor could be based on molecular signatures and the presence or absence of actionable mutations. For example, in the past year, the FDA approved pembrolizumab for the treatment of patients with unresectable or metastatic solid tumors that are either microsatellite instability–high or mismatch repair deficient. This is the first FDA-approved cancer treatment based on the genetic signature of a tumor rather than site of origin (https://www.fda.gov/NewsEvents/Newsroom/PressAnnouncements/ucm560167.htm, accessed January 1, 2018). At this time, however, the NCCN clinical guidelines do not recommend blanket genetic testing of all CUPs, citing lack of evidence of clinical benefit.[2] Accordingly, attempting to elucidate the primary site of a CUP remains an important responsibility of the pathologist, and cytopathology remains at the forefront as metastases are increasingly diagnosed using minimally invasive techniques. The ability to accurately assign a primary site will likely increase with the continued addition of sensitive antibodies for site-specific nuclear transcription factors. There is potential in the future for analyzing CTCs with either IHC or mutational analysis, which may obviate invasive procedures to obtain tumor tissue in patients with CUP, but more research is needed in this area.

REFERENCES

1. Pavlidis N, Pentheroudakis G. Cancer of unknown primary site. Lancet 2012;379:1428–35.
2. Ettinger DS, Handorf CR, Agulnik M, et al. NCCN guidelines insights: occult primary, version 3.2014. featured updates to the NCCN guidelines. J Natl Compr Canc Netw 2014;12:969–74.
3. Varadhachary GR, Abbruzzese JL, Lenzi R. Diagnostic strategies for unknown primary cancer. Cancer 2004;100:1776–85.
4. Greco FA. Molecular diagnosis of the tissue of origin in cancer of unknown primary site: useful in patient management. Curr Treat Options Oncol 2013;14: 634–42.
5. Choi J, Nahm JH, Kim SK. Prognostic clinicopathologic factors in carcinoma of unknown primary origin: a study of 106 consecutive cases. Oncotarget 2017;8:62630–40.
6. Pentheroudakis G, Greco FA, Pavlidis N. Molecular assignment of tissue of origin in cancer of unknown primary may not predict response to therapy or outcome: a systematic literature review. Cancer Treat Rev 2009;35:221–7.
7. Pentheroudakis G, Golfinopoulous V, Pavlidis N. Switching benchmarks in cancer of unknown primary: From autopsy to microarray. Eur J Cancer 2007;43:2026–36.
8. Hainsworth JD, Rubin MS, Spigel DR. Molecular gene expression profiling to predict the tissue of origin and direct site-specific therapy in patients with carcinoma of unknown primary site: a prospective trial of the Sarah Cannon Research Institute. J Clin Oncol 2012;31:217–23.
9. Conner JR, Hornick JL. Metastatic carcinoma of unknown primary: diagnostic approach using immunohistochemistry. Adv Anat Pathol 2015;22:149–67.
10. Handorf CR, Kulkarni A, Grenert JP, et al. A multicenter study directly comparing the diagnostic accuracy of gene expression profiling and immunohistochemistry for primary site identification in metastatic tumors. Am J Surg Pathol 2013;37: 1067–75.
11. Weiss LM, Chu P, Schroeder BE, et al. Blinded comparator study of immunohistochemical analysis versus a 92-gene cancer classifier in the diagnosis of the primary site in metastatic tumors. J Mol Diagn 2013;15:263–9.
12. Anderson GG, Weiss LM. Determining tissue of origin for metastatic cancers: meta-analysis and literature review of immunohistochemistry performance. Appl Immunohistochem Mol Morphol 2010; 18:3–8.
13. Ordonez NG. Value of thyroid transcription factor-1 immunostaining in tumor diagnosis: a review and update. Appl Immunohistochem Mol Morphol 2012; 20:429–44.
14. Bishop JA, Sharma R, Illei PB. Napsin A and thyroid transcription factor-1 expression in carcinomas of the lung, breast, pancreas, colon, kidney, thyroid, and malignant mesothelioma. Hum Pathol 2010;41: 20–5.
15. Stoll LM, Johnson MW, Gabrielson E, et al. The utility of napsin-A in the identification of primary and metastatic lung adenocarcinoma among cytologically poorly differentiated carcinomas. Cancer Cytopathol 2010;118:441–9.
16. Fujiwara S, Nawa A, Nakanishi T, et al. Thyroid transcription factor 1 expression in ovarian carcinoma is an independent prognostic factor. Hum Pathol 2010;41:560–5.
17. Zhang PJ, Gao HG, Pasha TL, et al. TTF-1 expression in ovarian and uterine epithelial neoplasia and its potential significance, an immunohistochemical assessment with multiple monoclonal antibodies and different secondary detection systems. Int J Gynecol Pathol 2009;28:10–8.
18. Robens J, Goldstein L, Gown AM, et al. Thyroid transcription factor-1 expression in breast carcinomas. Am J Surg Pathol 2010;34:1881–5.
19. Sakurai A, Sakai Y, Yatabe Y. Thyroid transcription factor-1 expression in rare cases of mammary ductal carcinoma. Histopathology 2011;59:145–8.
20. Bae JM, Kim JH, Park JH, et al. Clinicopathological and molecular implications of aberrant thyroid transcription factor-1 expression in colorectal carcinomas: an immunohistochemical analysis of 1319 cases using three different antibody clones. Histopathol 2018;72(3):423–32.

21. Klebe S, Swalling A, Jonavicius L, et al. An immunohistochemical comparison of two TTF-1 monoclonal antibodies in atypical squamous lesions and sarcomatoid carcinoma of the lung, and pleural malignant mesothelioma. J Clin Pathol 2016;69:136–41.

22. Mukhopadhyay S, Katzenstein A-L. Comparison of monoclonal Napsin A, polyclonal Napsin A, and TTF-1 for determining lung origin in metastatic adenocarcinomas. Am J Clin Pathol 2012;138:703–11.

23. Yamashita Y, Nagasaka T, Naiki-Ito A, et al. Napsin A is a specific marker for ovarian clear cell adenocarcinoma. Mod Pathol 2015;28:111–7.

24. Fadare O, Desouki MM, Gwin K, et al. Frequent expression of napsin A in clear cell carcinoma of the endometrium: potential diagnostic utility. Am J Surg Pathol 2014;38:189–96.

25. Rekhtman N, Kazi S. Nonspecific reactivity of polyclonal napsin A antibody in mucinous adenocarcinomas of various sites: a word of caution. Arch Pathol Lab Med 2015;139:434–6.

26. Ordonez NG. Value of PAX8 immunostaining in tumor diagnosis: a review and update. Adv Anat Pathol 2012;19:140–51.

27. McHugh K, Arrossi AV, Farver CF, et al. Does strong and diffuse PAX-8 positivity occur in primary lung carcinoma? An immunohistochemical study of 418 cases and review of the literature. Appl Immunohistochem Mol Morphol 2017, [Epub ahead of print].

28. Tacha D, Qi W, Zhou D, et al. PAX8 mouse monoclonal antibody [BC12] recognizes a restricted epitope and is highly sensitive in renal cell and ovarian cancers but does not cross-react with B cells and tumors of pancreatic origin. Appl Immunohistochem Mol Morphol 2013;21:59–63.

29. El Hag M, Schmidt L, Roh M, et al. Utility of TTF-1 and Napsin-A in the work-up of malignant effusions. Diagn Cytopathol 2016;44:299–304.

30. Kim J-H, Kim YS, Choi YD, et al. Utility of napsin A and thyroid transcription factor 1 in differentiating metastatic pulmonary from non-pulmonary adenocarcinoma in pleural effusion. Acta Cytol 2011;55:266–70.

31. Werling RW, Yaziji H, Bacchi CE, et al. CDX2, a highly sensitive and specific marker of adenocarcinomas of intestinal origin: an immunohistochemical survey of 476 primary and metastatic carcinomas. Am J Surg Pathol 2003;27:303–10.

32. De Lott LB, Morrison C, Suster S, et al. CDX2 is a useful marker of intestinal-type differentiation: a tissue microarray-based study of 629 tumors from various sites. Arch Pathol Lab Med 2005;129:1100–5.

33. Vang R, Gown AM, Wu L-S-F, et al. Immunohistochemical expression of CDX2 in primary ovarian mucinous tumors and metastatic mucinous carcinomas involving the ovary: comparison with CK20 and correlation with coordinate expression of CK7. Mod Pathol 2006;19:1421–8.

34. Cowan ML, Li QK, Illei PB. CDX-2 expression in primary lung adenocarcinoma. Appl Immunohistochem Mol Morphol 2016;24:16–9.

35. Logani S, Oliva E, Arnell PM, et al. Use of novel immunohistochemical markers expressed in colonic adenocarcinoma to distinguish primary ovarian tumors from metastatic colorectal carcinoma. Mod Pathol 2005;18:19–25.

36. Shah SS, Wu T-T, Tobenson MS, et al. Aberrant CDX2 expression in hepatocellular carcinomas: an important diagnostic pitfall. Hum Pathol 2017;64:13–8.

37. Saad RS, Essig DL, Silverman JF, et al. Diagnostic utility of CDX-2 expression in separating metastatic gastrointestinal adenocarcinoma from other metastatic adenocarcinoma in fine-needle aspiration cytology using cell blocks. Cancer Cytopathol 2004;102:168–73.

38. Magnusson K, de Wit M, Brennan DJ, et al. SATB2 in combination with cytokeratin 20 identifies over 95% of all colorectal carcinomas. Am J Surg Pathol 2011;35:937–48.

39. Lin F, Shi J, Zhu S, et al. Cadherin-17 and SATB2 are sensitive and specific immunomarkers for medullary carcinoma of the large intestine. Arch Pathol Lab Med 2014;138:1015–26.

40. Berg KB, Schaeffer DF. SATB2 as an immunohistochemical marker for colorectal adenocarcinoma. A concise review of benefits and pitfalls. Arch Pathol Lab Med 2017;141:1428–33.

41. Yang C, Sun L, Zhang L, et al. Diagnostic utility of SATB2 in metastatic krukenberg tumors of the ovary. An immunohistochemical study of 70 cases with comparison to CDX2, CK7, CK20, chromogranin and synaptophysin. Am J Surg Pathol 2018;42(2):160–71.

42. Moh M, Krings G, Ates D, et al. SATB2 expression distinguishes ovarian metastases of colorectal and appendiceal origin from primary ovarian tumors of mucinous or endometrioid type. Am J Surg Pathol 2016;40:419–32.

43. Matsushima J, Yazawa T, Suzuki M, et al. Clinicopathological, immunohistochemical, and mutational analysis of pulmonary enteric adenocarcinoma: usefulness of SATB2 and β-catenin immunostaining for differentiation from metastatic colorectal carcinoma. Hum Pathol 2017;64:179–85.

44. Giannico GA, Gown AM, Epstein JI, et al. Role of SATB2 in distinguishing the site of origin in glandular lesions of the bladder/urinary tract. Hum Pathol 2017;67:152–9.

45. Miettinen M, McCue PA, Sarlomo-Rikala M, et al. GATA3: a multispecific but potentially useful marker in surgical pathology. A systematic analysis of 2500

epithelial and nonepithelial tumors. Am J Surg Pathol 2014;38:13–22.

46. Sangoi AR, Shrestha B, Yang G, et al. The novel marker GATA3 is significantly more sensitive than traditional markers mammaglobin and GCDFP15 for identifying breast cancer in surgical and cytology specimens of metastatic and matched primary tumors. Appl Immunohistochem Mol Morphol 2016; 24:229–37.

47. Liu H, Shi J, Wilkerson ML, et al. Immunohistochemical evaluation of GATA3 expression in tumors and normal tissues: a useful biomarker for breast and urothelial carcinomas. Am J Clin Pathol 2012;138: 57–64.

48. Ordoñez NG. Value of GATA3 immunostaining in tumor diagnosis: a review. Adv Anat Pathol 2013;20: 352–60.

49. Nelson ER, Sharma R, Argani P, et al. Utility of Sox10 labeling in metastatic breast carcinomas. Hum Pathol 2017;67:205–10.

50. Chu P, Wu E, Weiss LM. Cytokeratin 7 and cytokeratin 20 expression in epithelial neoplasms: a survey of 435 cases. Mod Pathol 2000;13:962–72.

51. Gurel B, Ali TZ, Montgomery EA. NKX3.1 as a marker of prostatic origin in metastatic tumors. Am J Surg Pathol 2010;34:1097–105.

52. Jia L, Jiang Y, Michael CW. Performance of different prostate specific antibodies in the cytological diagnosis of metastatic prostate adenocarcinoma. Diagn Cytopathol 2017;45:998–1004.

53. Parker DC, Folpe AL, Bell J, et al. Potential utility of uroplakin III, thrombomodulin, high molecular weight cytokeratin, and cytokeratin 20 in noninvavsive, invasive, and metastatic urothelial (transitional cell) carcinomas. Am J Surg Pathol 2003;27:1–10.

54. Kaufmann O, Volmerig J, Dietel M. Uroplakin III is a highly specific and moderately sensitive immunohistochemical marker for primary and metastatic urothelial carcinomas. Am J Clin Pathol 2000;113: 683–7.

55. Zhao L, Antic T, Witten D, et al. Is GATA3 expression maintained in regional metastases? A study of paired primary and metastatic urothelial carcinomas. Am J Surg Pathol 2013;37:1876–81.

56. Liang Y, Heitzman J, Kamat AM, et al. Differential expression of GATA3 in urothelial carcinoma variants. Hum Pathol 2014;45:1466–72.

57. Ozcan A, Shen SS, Hamilton C, et al. PAX 8 expression in non-neoplastic tissues, primary tumors, and metastatic tumors: a comprehensive immunohistochemical study. Mod Pathol 2011;24:751–64.

58. Tong GX, Yu WM, Beaubier NT, et al. Expression of PAX8 in normal and neoplastic renal tissues: an immunohistochemical study. Mod Pathol 2009;22: 1218–27.

59. Mentrikoski MJ, Wendroth SM, Wick MR. Immunohistochemical distinction of renal cell carcinoma from other carcinomas with clear-cell histomorphology: utility of CD10 and CA-125 in addition to PAX-2, PAX-8, RCCma, and adipophilin. Appl Immunohistochem Mol Morphol 2014;22:635–41.

60. Ozcan A, Liles N, Coffey D, et al. PAX2 and PAX8 expression in primary and metastatic müllerian epithelial tumors: a comprehensive comparison. Am J Surg Pathol 2011;35:1837–47.

61. Laury AR, Perets R, Piao H, et al. A comprehensive analysis of PAX8 expression in human epithelial tumors. Am J Surg Pathol 2011;35:816–26.

62. Tong GX, Devaraj K, Hamele-Bena D, et al. PAX8: a marker for carcinoma of Müllerian origin in serous effusions. Diagn Cytopathol 2011;39: 567–74.

63. Zhao L, Guo M, Sneige N, et al. Value of PAX8 and WT1 immunostaining in confirming the ovarian origin of metastatic carcinoma in serous effusion specimens. Am J Clin Pathol 2012;137:304–9.

64. McKnight R, Cohen C, Siddiqui MT. Utility of paired box gene 8 (PAX8) expression in fluid and fine-needle aspiration cytology: an immunohistochemical study of metastatic ovarian serous carcinoma. Cancer Cytopathol 2010;118: 298–302.

65. Mukhopadhyay S, Katzenstein A-L. Subclassification of non-small cell lung carcinomas lacking morphologic differentiation on biopsy specimens: utility of an immunohistochemical panel containing TTF-1, Napsin A, p63, and CK5/6. Am J Surg Pathol 2011;35:15–25.

66. Bishop JA, Teruya-Feldstein J, Westra WH, et al. p40 (ΔNp63) is superior to p63 for the diagnosis of pulmonary squamous cell carcinoma. Mod Pathol 2012;25:405–15.

67. Chernock RD, Lewis JS. Approach to metastatic carcinoma of unknown primary in the head and neck: Squamous cell carcinoma and beyond. Head Neck Pathol 2015;9:6–15.

68. Doxtader EE, Katzenstein AL. The relationship between p16 expression and high-risk human papillomavirus infection in squamous cell carcinomas from sites other than uterine cervix: a study of 137 cases. Hum Pathol 2012;43:327–32.

69. Lee WY, Hsiao JR, Jin YT, et al. Epstein - Barr virus detection in neck metastases by in-situ hybridization in fine needle aspiration cytologic studies: an aid for differentiating the primary site. Head Neck 2000; 22(4):336–40.

70. Weissferdt A, Tang X, Wistuba LL, et al. Comparative immunohistochemical analysis of pulmonary and thymic neuroendocrine carcinomas using PAX8 and TTF-1. Mod Pathol 2013;26: 1554–60.

71. Agoff SN, Lamps LW, Philip AT, et al. Thyroid transcription factor-1 is expressed in extrapulmonary small cell carcinomas but not in other

extrapulmonary neuroendocrine tumors. Mod Pathol 2000;13:238–42.

72. Chan ES, Alexander J, Swanson PE, et al. PDX-1, CDX-2, TTF-1, and CK7: a reliable immunohisto-chemical panel for pancreatic neuroendocrine neo-plasms. Am J Surg Pathol 2012;36:737–43.

73. Lai J-P, Mertens RB, Mirocha J, et al. Comparison of PAX6 and PAX8 as immunohistochemical markers for pancreatic neuroendocrine tumors. Endocr Pathol 2015;26:54–62.

74. Ebata T, Okuma Y, Nakahara Y, et al. Retrospective analysis of unknown primary cancers with malignant pleural effusion at initial diagnosis. Thorac Cancer 2016;7:39–43.

75. Crapanzano JP, Heymann JJ, Monaco S, et al. The state of cell block variation and satisfaction in the era of molecular diagnostics and personalized med-icine. Cytojournal 2014;11:7.

76. Gong Y, Joseph T, Sneige N. Validation of commonly used immunostains on cell-transferred cytologic specimens. Cancer Cytopathol 2005;105:158–64.

77. Ferguson J, Chamberlain P, Cramer HM, et al. ER, PR, and HER2 immunocytochemistry on cell-transferred cytologic smears of primary and meta-static breast carcinomas: a comparison study with formalin-fixed cell blocks and surgical biopsies. Di-agn Cytopathol 2013;41:575–81.

78. Fitzgibbons PL, Bradley LA, Fatheree LA, et al. Principles of analytic validation of immunohisto-chemical assays: guideline from the College of American Pathologists Pathology and Laboratory Quality Center. Arch Pathol Lab Med 2014;138:1432–43.

79. Sauter JL, Grogg KL, Vrana JA, et al. Young investi-gator challenge: validation and optimization for immunohistochemistry protocols for use on Cellient cell block specimens. Cancer Cytopathol 2016;124:89–99.

80. Horlings HM, van Laar RK, Kerst J-M, et al. Gene expression profiling to identify the histogenetic origin of metastatic adenocarcinomas of unknown primary. J Clin Oncol 2008;26:4435–41.

81. Monzon FA, Lyons-Weiler M, Buturovic LJ, et al. Multicenter validation of a 1,550-gene expression profile for identification of tumor tissue of origin. J Clin Oncol 2009;27:2503–8.

82. Ma XJ, Patel R, Wang X, et al. Molecular cla-ssification of human cancers using a 92-gene real-time quantitative polymerase chain reaction assay. Arch Pathol Lab Med 2006;130:465–73.

83. Talantov D, Baden J, Jatkoe T, et al. A quantitative reverse transcriptase-polymerase chain reaction assay to identify metastatic carcinoma tissue of origin. J Mol Diagn 2006;8:320–9.

84. Varadhachary GR, Talantov D, Raber MN, et al. Mo-lecular profiling of carcinoma of unknown primary and correlation with clinical evaluation. J Clin Oncol 2008;26:4442–8.

85. Lu J, Getz G, Miska EA, et al. MicroRNA expression profiles classify human cancers. Nature 2005;435(7043):834–8.

86. Bender RA, Erlander MG. Molecular classification of unknown primary cancer. Semin Oncol 2009;36:38–43.

87. Dolled-Filhart MP, Rimm DL. Gene expression array analysis to determine tissue of origin of carcinoma of unknown primary: cutting edge or already obsolete? Cancer Cytopathol 2013;121:129–35.

88. Stancel GA, Coffey D, Alvarez K, et al. Identification of tissue of origin in body fluid specimens using a gene expression microarray assay. Cancer Cytopa-thol 2012;120:62–70.

89. Matthew EM, Zhou L, Yang Z, et al. A multiplexed marker-based algorithm for diagnosis of carcinoma of unknown primary using circulating tumor cells. Oncotarget 2015;7(4):3662–76.

Pancreatic Cytology

Raza S. Hoda, MD, Martha B. Pitman, MD*

KEYWORDS

- Cytopathology • Fine-needle aspiration • Endoscopic ultrasound • Pancreas
- Pancreatic neoplasms • Pancreatic cysts

Key points

- The diagnostic approach to pancreaticobiliary disease requires a multidisciplinary team in which the cytopathologist plays a crucial role.
- Fine-needle aspiration, obtained by endoscopic ultrasound, is the diagnostic test of choice for pancreatic lesions.
- Preoperative clinical management depends on accurate cytologic assessment.
- Clinical history, imaging studies, cytology samples, and ancillary tests, including immunohistochemistry, biochemical analysis, and genetic sequencing, are integral to forming a complete diagnosis and guiding optimal patient management.
- Standardized reporting terminology improves communication about the diagnosis leading to better patient care.

ABSTRACT

The diagnostic approach to pancreaticobiliary disease requires a multidisciplinary team in which the cytopathologist plays a crucial role. Fine-needle aspiration, obtained by endoscopic ultrasound, is the diagnostic test of choice for pancreatic lesions. Preoperative clinical management depends on many factors, many of which rely on accurate cytologic assessment. Pancreaticobiliary cytology is wrought with diagnostic pitfalls. Clinical history, imaging studies, cytology samples, and ancillary tests, including immunohistochemistry, biochemical analysis, and genetic sequencing, are integral to forming a complete diagnosis and guiding optimal patient management. This article reviews clinical aspects and the diagnostic work-up of commonly encountered diagnostic entities within the field of pancreatic cytology.

OVERVIEW

Diseases of the pancreas include a variety of benign, premalignant, and malignant lesions resulting in a broad differential diagnosis. Preoperative diagnosis is imperative for appropriate patient management. The pathologist is a key member of the patient care team and must be well versed in the clinicopathologic profile of the various disease entities of the pancreas to provide accurate assessment.

Pancreatic lesions are typically characterized as either solid or cystic by imaging. Solid neoplasms are more common and often caused by adenocarcinoma. Cystic lesions are most frequently due to intraductal papillary mucinous neoplasms (IPMNs). Certain imaging features are helpful in stratification for risk malignancy, and patient management guidelines to this effect have been issued.[1,2] These international consensus guidelines, however, are

Department of Pathology, Massachusetts General Hospital, Harvard Medical School, 55 Fruit Street, Boston, MA 02114, USA
* Corresponding author.
E-mail address: mpitman@partners.org

Surgical Pathology 11 (2018) 563–588
https://doi.org/10.1016/j.path.2018.04.005
1875-9181/18/© 2018 Elsevier Inc. All rights reserved.

surgpath.theclinics.com

Abbreviations	
ACC	Acinar cell carcinoma
CEA	Carcinoembryonic antigen
ERCP	Endoscopic retrograde cholangiopancreatography
EUS	Endoscopic ultrasound
FNA	Fine-needle aspiration
IPMN	Intraductal papillary mucinous neoplasm
MCN	Mucinous cystic neoplasm
NGS	Next-generation sequencing
PanNET	Pancreatic neuroendocrine tumor
SPN	Solid-pseudopapillary neoplasm

only modestly sensitive and specific for identifying malignant lesions.[3,4] Serum biomarkers show promise in identifying malignant lesions but are insufficiently specific for management decisions.[5] Incisional pancreatic biopsies can miss the lesion entirely, carrying a high false-negative rate, and often incur significant complications, including hemorrhage, duodenal leakage, infection, and tumor seeding.[6] Endoscopic ultrasound–guided (EUS) fine-needle aspiration (FNA) allows for safe, sensitive, specific, and swift evaluation of pancreatic lesions. Accurate rapid on-site evaluation of cytologic material can reduce the false-negative rate of EUS-FNA. Likewise, biochemical and molecular analyses of pancreatic cyst fluid are important ancillary tests for accurate diagnosis of pancreatic cysts.[7–9]

EUS next-generation biopsy needles have greatly increased the yield of diagnostic material.[10] Moray™ microforceps (US Endoscopy, Mentor, OH), for example, allows for tissue sampling of the pancreatic cyst wall and offers a glimpse of the histologic features.[11,12] SharkCore™ core biopsy needles (Medtronic, Inc., Minneapolis, MN) can accurately assess for benign diseases, such as autoimmune pancreatitis, which traditional FNA samples can only suggest.[13] Moreover, microcores can be used for immunohistochemistry and molecular testing.[14–16]

Biliary strictures also present a diagnostic challenge. Imaging features and serum biomarkers can suggest but cannot definitively diagnose malignancy.[17,18] Endoscopic retrograde cholangiopancreatography (ERCP), a technique that combines luminal endoscopy and fluoroscopic imaging, can be used for the assessment of biliary and pancreatic duct obstructive lesions.

Such lesions can be due to the presence of calculi or to strictures caused by benign (typically chronic pancreatitis) or malignant (usually carcinoma) lesions. Exfoliative cytologic material obtained via ERCP can have a better yield than FNA.[19] Despite developments in sampling technology, bile duct brushing cytology shows high specificity but low sensitivity for malignancy.[20,21]

Ancillary tests, such as fluorescence in situ hybridization and next-generation sequencing (NGS), which can be performed on aspiration or exfoliative cytologic material, can assist in definitive diagnosis of malignancy.[22–24] These adjunctive tests are validated to detect mutant alleles at frequencies of at least 5% and thus require a tumor cellularity of at least 10%.

The terminology and reporting Papanicolaou Society of Cytopathology has published recommendations that stratifies risk of malignancy based on diagnostic categories and guidelines for management.[25–28] These recommendations provide a standardized reporting format designed to facilitate communication between clinicians and cytopathologists.[29] Details regarding various techniques for obtaining specimens and ancillary testing are included. Patient follow-up, with a multidisciplinary approach, is endorsed. Based on the Papanicolaou Society of Cytopathology guidelines, pancreatic FNAs can be stratified into 6 categories: (1) nondiagnostic, (2) negative (for malignancy), (3) atypical, (4) neoplastic (benign or other), (5) suspicious (for malignancy), and (6) positive (for malignancy).[28] **Table 1** delineates examples of specimen types within each division.

This article reviews clinical, radiological, cytologic and, when applicable, molecular aspects of the most common pancreatic diseases encountered in practice.

NORMAL FINDINGS AND CONTAMINANTS

Overinterpretation of benign tissue contaminants is of major diagnostic concern.[30] During EUS-FNA sampling, biopsy needles traverse either the gastric or duodenal wall and uninvolved pancreas in its approach. The pancreas is a parenchymal-rich, stromal-poor organ, readily yielding its benign components to biopsy. Mitsuhashi and colleagues[31] found normal gastric, duodenal, or pancreatic cells in more than 90% of EUS-FNA samples. In percutaneous approaches, principal contaminants are mesothelial cells, but colonic, renal, hepatic, splenic, and gastric tissues may also contaminate the specimen.

Table 1
Papanicolaou Society of Cytopathology system for reporting pancreaticobiliary cytology

Category	Examples of Diagnostic Entities
Nondiagnostic	• Acellular aspirate without evidence of a mucinous etiology • Gastrointestinal contamination
Negative (for malignancy)	• Benign pancreatic tissue • Acute pancreatitis • Chronic pancreatitis • Autoimmune pancreatitis • Pseudocyst • Lymphoepithelial cyst • Ectopic splenic tissue
Atypical	• Atypical cells suggestive of a neuroendocrine tumor
Neoplastic: benign	• Serous cystadenoma • Neuroendocrine microadenoma • Lymphangioma
Neoplastic: other	• Neuroendocrine tumor, well differentiated • IPMN, all grades of dysplasia • MCN, all grades of dysplasia • Solid-pseudopapillary neoplasm
Suspicious (for malignancy)	• Rare markedly atypical epithelial cells
Positive (for malignancy)	• Ductal adenocarcinoma, all variants • Cholangiocarcinoma • Acinar cell carcinoma • Neuroendocrine carcinoma, poorly differentiated • Pancreatoblastoma • Lymphoma • Metastatic malignancy

Adapted from Pitman MB, Centeno BA, Ali SZ, et al. Standardized terminology and nomenclature for pancreaticobiliary cytology: the Papanicolaou Society of Cytopathology guidelines. Diagn Cytopathol 2014;42:2–3; with permission.

Awareness of the needle trajectory and familiarity with the appearance of the usual suspects that contaminate pancreaticobiliary specimens are essential for accurate diagnostic interpretation.

The pancreas is primarily composed of exocrine acinar tissue arranged in lobules. Acinar cells

Key Features
BENIGN PANCREATIC PARENCHYMA

Cytologic features of benign acinar cells

Grapes on a vine cohesive cellular aggregates attached to fibrovascular stroma or dispersed in acinar clusters

Single polygonal scattered epithelial cells

Eccentrically placed, round nuclei with small nucleoli

Abundant granular cytoplasm

Cytologic features of benign ductal cells

Honeycomb, flat, cohesive sheets of evenly spaced epithelial cells

Round to oval nuclei with inconspicuous nucleoli

Moderate amount of finely granular, nonmucinous cytoplasm

secrete a wide variety of digestive enzymes. The latter drain into a central duct system. FNA samples of normal pancreas mainly yield acinar cells. Usually, the duct epithelium is sparsely represented. In contrast, bile duct brushings show mostly ductal cells and pancreatic acinar cells are usually absent. Cells picked up along the course of the needle tract (hitchhiking cells) can cause diagnostic difficulty.[32–36]

Nuclei of benign acinar cells are round with evenly distributed chromatin and micronucleoli, and their ample dense cytoplasm, appears granular blue-green (on Papanicolaou stain) or purple (on Diff-Quik stain). Borders of the acinar cells are typically sharp. Acinar cells can be arranged in small, cohesive, grapelike groups that center around a microlumen (grapes on a vine) (**Fig. 1**). Neoplastic acini form larger sheets and clusters vis-à-vis benign acini. When sampled by either FNA or ERCP, benign pancreatic ductal epithelium appears as large, cohesive, monotonous, flat sheets of evenly spaced cells with round, uniform nuclei, inconspicuous nucleoli a moderate amount of dense, nonmucinous cytoplasm, and well-defined borders conferring a honeycomb appearance (**Fig. 2**). Identification of intracytoplasmic mucin in ductal epithelia should raise concern for pancreatic intraepithelial neoplasia and well-differentiated adenocarcinoma. Gastric mucosa may also show intracytoplasmic mucin, although usually cup-shaped and apically oriented.[36]

Pitfalls
CONTAMINATION BY
BENIGN EPITHELIA

! Cytologic features of benign duodenal cells

Honeycomb, flat, cohesive sheets of cells; occasionally, papillary groups (villi)

Nonmucinous epithelial cells with brush border

Fried egg goblet cells and sesame seed lymphocytes sprinkled throughout the epithelial sheets

! Cytologic features of benign gastric cells

Small sheets and strips; occasionally, isolated single cells and gastric pits

Stripped, grooved nuclei, floating in thin mucin

Mucinous cytoplasm forming an apical cup

! Cytologic features of benign mesothelial cells

Honeycomb, flat sheet of cells, separated by intercellular windows

Grooved nuclei with even chromatin

Duodenal and gastric epithelial cells form a monolayer that can also display honeycomb arrangement. Duodenal enterocytes are nonmucinous and display a brush border (**Fig. 3**). Goblet cells stud the duodenal epithelium and appear to simulate fried eggs when fixed in alcohol. Also admixed are small intraepithelial lymphocytes, an appearance that has been likened to that of sesame seeds. Gastric surface foveolar cells have mucinous cytoplasm, often apically oriented. They can be arranged in small strips and sheets (**Fig. 4**). Isolated stripped, grooved nuclei of gastric foveolar epithelia may be encountered. These cells can be found floating in thin extracellular mucin—a diagnostic hint favoring gastric epithelium. Distinction between gastrointestinal epithelium from high-grade epithelial dysplasia is not problematic; however, a low-grade neoplastic process, such as branch-duct IPMN, may be indistinguishable from gastric contamination, because both are lined by foveolar-type cells. The distribution of cytoplasmic mucin can be a distinctive feature. In benign gastric foveolar cells, mucin is often limited to the upper one-third of the cell, whereas neoplastic cells typically have even distribution of mucin throughout the cytoplasm.

The anterior aspect of the pancreas is shrouded by the peritoneal mesothelium. In percutaneous biopsies, mesothelial cells may be picked up along the needle's path. Mesothelial cells share the flat honeycomb arrangement of benign ductal epithelium, and are distinguished. The former is distinguished by its distinctive intercellular windows.

SOLID PANCREATIC LESIONS

Pancreatic adenocarcinoma is the most significant and most common pancreatic neoplasm. Differential diagnosis of solid pancreatic neoplasms includes, but is not limited to, chronic pancreatitis (inclusive of autoimmune pancreatitis), pancreatic neuroendocrine tumor

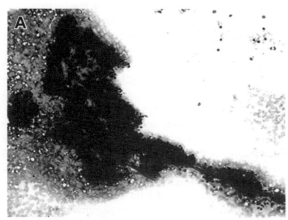
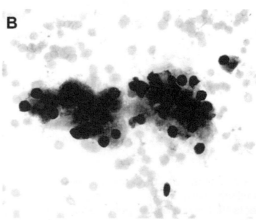

Fig. 1. (*A*) Benign pancreatic acinar cells have the appearance of grapes on a vine, at low magnification, because clusters of cells are arranged along loose vascular connective tissue (original magnification, ×20). (*B*) Acinar cells are polygonal in shape, with eccentrically placed round nuclei, small nucleoli and abundant granular cytoplasm, with a low nuclear-to-cytoplasmic ratio (original magnification, ×60). ([*A, B*] Direct smear, Diff-Quik stain).

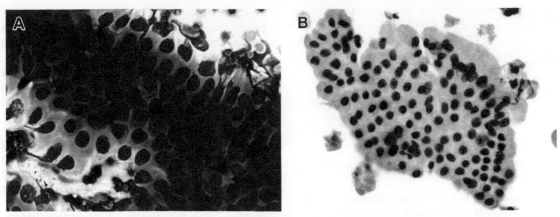

Fig. 2. Benign pancreatic ductal cells usually form large, flat, cohesive sheets of evenly spaced uniform nuclei that appear honeycomb-like ([A] Direct smear, Diff-Quik stain, original magnification, ×60; [B] ThinPrep Papanicolaou stain, original magnification, ×100).

(PanNET), acinar cell carcinoma (ACC), solid pseudopapillary neoplasm (SPN), ectopic splenic tissue, and metastatic neoplasms. Acute pancreatitis is typically diagnosed clinically with history, blood cell count, and serologic and imaging studies and thus is rarely biopsied. Symptoms of solid pancreatic lesions result from pancreatic and common bile duct obstruction and include nausea, vomiting, weight loss, and jaundice. Radiographic characteristics can be helpful in narrowing the differential diagnosis; however, features often overlap. Cytologically, these lesions may bear striking resemblance. Cell block preparations and immunohistochemistry can be useful in distinguishing these lesions. Such ancillary studies can be particularly helpful in distinguishing between the solid-cellular neoplasms—ACC, PanNET, SPN, and pancreatoblastoma. The clinicopathologic findings of solid pancreatic neoplasms are summarized in Table 2.

Fig. 3. Benign duodenal epithelial cells are non–mucin-secreting cells also arranged in large, flat, cohesive sheets of evenly spaced uniform nuclei with interspersed goblet cells that give a fried egg appearance (Cytospin, Papanicolaou stain, original magnification, ×20).

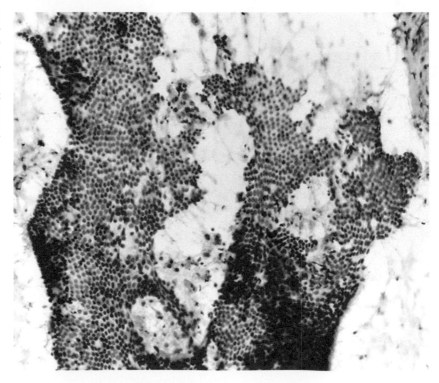

Key Features
CHRONIC PANCREATITIS

Scantily cellular specimen

Ductal epithelium in honeycomb sheets

Enlarged nuclei and prominent nucleoli

Low nuclear-to-cytoplasmic ratio

Mixed inflammatory cells, foamy histiocytes, fat necrosis, and calcifications

Inflamed stroma with lymphoplasmacytic infiltrate suggests autoimmune pancreatitis

Chronic pancreatitis represents the end-stage syndrome of different disorders. Etemad and Whitcomb developed the TIGAR-O system to categorize the 6 major predisposing risk factors to chronic pancreatitis: (1) toxic-metabolic, (2) idiopathic, (3) genetic, (4) autoimmune, (5) recurrent or severe acute pancreatitis, and (6) obstructive.[36] Toxic-metabolic etiologies—longstanding alcohol and tobacco use—are more common in men. Idiopathic and obstructive causes are more frequent in women.[37]

Chronic pancreatitis is characterized by irreversible parenchymal damage leading to tissue injury and scarring of acinar epithelium. In acute pancreatitis, the organ typically returns to its normal state; however, recurrent bouts may lead to chronic pancreatitis.

The fibrosis of chronic pancreatitis may form a mass, which can be radiologically indistinguishable from pancreatic adenocarcinoma. Its fibrotic nature makes FNA sampling difficult. Cytologic features are highlighted in (**Fig. 5**).

Autoimmune pancreatitis is a rare variant of chronic pancreatitis. The disease occurs more frequently in middle-aged men and may be associated with various inflammatory conditions, such as sclerosing cholangitis, Sjögren syndrome, and ulcerative colitis.[38,39] The disease has been divided into two types: type 1 and type 2. Type 1 autoimmune pancreatitis shows serologic and clinical features of IgG4-related disease.[40,41] Little is known regarding the underlying etiology of type 2 autoimmune disease.[42] Both types respond well to corticosteroid therapy, and neither requires surgical intervention. Imaging shows a characteristic sausage-like diffuse pancreatic enlargement and irregular segmental pancreatic duct stricture.[43] A markedly expansile fibrotic process may simulate carcinoma radiographically. Histology demonstrates fibrosis and marked periductal lymphoplasmacytic infiltration (**Fig. 6**). On EUS-FNA biopsies, fibrosis and fragments of cellular stroma admixed with inflammatory cells suggests autoimmune pancreatitis (**Fig. 7**).

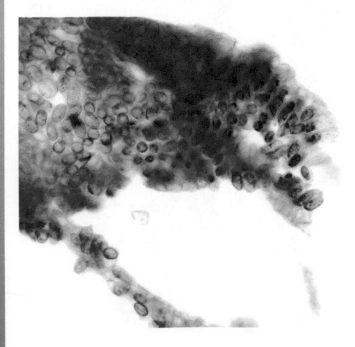

Fig. 4. Benign gastric epithelial cells display uniform, round nuclei and cup-shaped mucinous cytoplasm contained in the upper two-thirds of the cytoplasm (Cytospin, Papanicolaou stain, original magnification, ×100).

Key Features
DUCTAL ADENOCARCINOMA

Drunken honeycomb flat sheets of unevenly spaced, crowded ductal cells

Marked anisonucleosis and mitoses in high-grade cancers

Finely vacuolated, lacey-appearing intracytoplasmic mucin in low-grade cancers

Ductal adenocarcinoma accounts for 90% of pancreatic neoplasms and is a highly aggressive neoplasm with dismal prognosis. Overall 5-year survival rate is under 10%.[44] Typically, the disease occurs sporadically in older individuals and shows a slight male predilection (male-to-female ratio of 1.6:1). The etiology of ductal adenocarcinoma is unknown; however, smoking is a well-established risk factor. Several germline alterations (eg, Peutz-Jeghers syndrome, familial atypical multiple mole melanoma syndrome and familial pancreatitis) are associated with the disease. Presenting symptoms

Table 2
Clinicopathologic characteristics of solid pancreatic lesions

Diagnostic Entity	Demographics	Radiographic Findings	Cytologic Features	Immuno-histochemistry	Molecular Alterations
Ductal adeno-carcinoma	• Age: 60–70 y • F:M = 1:1.6	• Irregular, hypoechoic solid mass • Double-duct sign	• Drunken honeycomb • Cytoplasmic mucin	• p53 (strong nuclear + or total loss) • SMAD4 (nuclear loss)	• KRAS • TP53 • p16/CDKN2A • SMAD4
PanNET	• Age: 40–60 y • F:M = 1:1	• Round mass • Can have cystic change	• Solid-cellular smear pattern • Salt-and-pepper chromatin	• Chromogranin • Synaptophysin	• MEN1 • NF1 • TSC1/2 • VHL
ACC	Older men	• Round mass • Can have cystic change	• Solid-cellular smear pattern • Zymogen granules	• Trypsin • Chymotrypsin • BCL10	11p
SPN	• Age: 20–30 y • F:M = 9:1	• Round mass • Can have Solid and cystic change	• Solid-cellular smear pattern • Myxoid fibrovascular cores	• β-Catenin (nuclear +)	CTNNB1
Pancreato-blastoma	• Young children • F:M = 1:1	• Round mass • Large	• Solid-cellular smear pattern • Squamoid corpuscles	• Chymotrypsin • Chromogranin • Cytokeratin • Trypsin	11p
Ectopic splenic tissue	• Congenital accessory spleen (splenule) • Abdominal trauma or splenectomy (splenosis) • History of abdominal trauma or splenectomy	• Well-defined lesion • Round mass • Solitary (splenule) or multiple (splenosis) • Highly vascular lesion	• Small to medium-sized lymphocytes • Vessels	CD8	Not applicable
Metastases	• Generally older, with a history of malignancy	• Round • May mimic primary mass	• Most common is RCC • May mimic PanNET or low-grade PDAC	Depends on primary site	Depends on primary site

Abbreviations: +, indicates positive staining; F:M, female-to-male ratio; PDAC, pancreatic ductal adenocarcinoma; RCC, renal cell carcinoma.

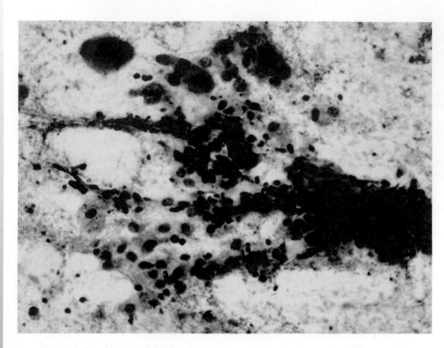

Fig. 5. Chronic pancreatitis shows inflammatory cells and histiocytes, some multinucleated, in a background of hemosiderin, fat necrosis and granular inflammatory debris (Direct smear, Papanicolaou stain, original magnification, ×60).

are nonspecific and include abdominal pain, jaundice, pruritus, sudden onset of diabetes mellitus, migratory thrombophlebitis (Trousseau syndrome), palpable gallbladder (Courvoisier sign), and unexplained weight loss. Cytologic diagnosis of ductal carcinoma is helpful in management, and confirmation of diagnosis even in unresectable cases may initiate neoadjuvant therapy.[45]

Ductal adenocarcinoma arises most often in the pancreatic head. Imaging studies show an ill-defined, irregular and hypoechoic mass. Pancreatic and bile duct strictures and downstream dilatation (double-duct sign) can occur due to mass effect, and this imaging feature is virtually pathognomonic of malignancy.[46]

Well-differentiated adenocarcinoma demonstrates nuclear crowding, overlapping of cells, loss of polarity, and uneven spacing of nuclei with loss of organization within the typical lattice-like pattern—the characteristic drunken

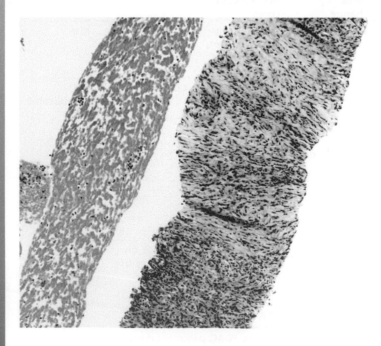

Fig. 6. This Shark core biopsy shows a lymphoplasmic infiltrate of the pancreatic tissue consistent with autoimmune pancreatitis. (Hematoxylin and eosin, original magnification, ×20).

Fig. 7. Autoimmune pancreatitis with acinar cells distributed singly and in clusters and cellular stromal fragments containing inflammatory cells (Direct smear, Papanicolaou stain, original magnification, ×40).

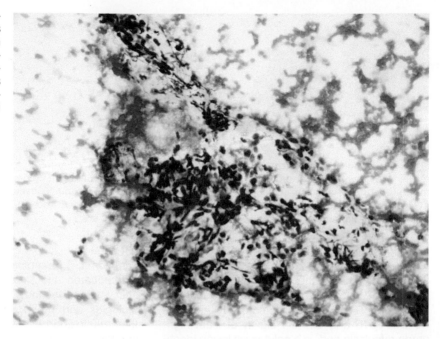

honeycomb appearance on cytology (**Fig. 8**). High-grade cells can be discohesive with pleomorphic nuclei, macronucleoli, hyperchromatic chromatin, marked anisonucleosis and nuclear membrane irregularities. Well-differentisted adenocarcinoma has abundant intracytoplasmic mucin, a deceptively low nuclear-to-cytoplasmic ratio, anisonucleosis (4:1), and with a distinctive lacey mucinous cytoplasmic appearnace in a single cluster (**Fig. 9**).

Immunohistochemistry can be helpful in challenging cases. Most ductal adenocarcinomas show diffuse nuclear staining or no staining (null type) for p53, and approximately half of cases demonstrate loss of SMAD4 nuclear expression (neither is encountered in chronic pancreatitis).[47–50] SMAD4 can also differentiate primary from metastatic carcinomas, because it is rarely lost in colonic, gynecologic tract, and pulmonary carcinomas.[50] *KRAS* mutations, *CDKN2A/p16*

Fig. 8. Ductal adenocarcinoma showing characteristic cytologic features with a drunken honeycomb appearance of cells in the sheet. The nuclei are pleomorphic, enlarged, irregular, with prominent nucleoli (Cytospin, Diff-Quik stain, original magnification, ×60).

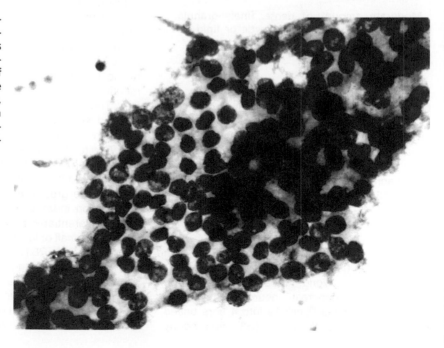

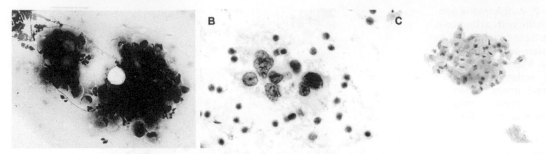

Fig. 9. (*A–C*) High-grade pancreatic adenocarcinoma shows more overt features of malignancy with pleomorphic nuclei with membrane irregularity, chromatin clearing and peripheral clumping, and abundant cytoplasmic mucin ([*A*] Direct smear, Diff-Quik, original magnification, ×60 [*B*] Cytospin, Papanicolaou stain, original magnification, ×100). (*C*) Well-differentiated adenocarcinoma with abundant lacey-appearing cytoplasmic mucin (Direct smear, Papanicolaou stain, original magnification, ×100).

deletions, *TP53* mutations, and *SMAD4* deletions are found by molecular analysis in most pancreatic adenocarcinomas. Although *KRAS* mutations may be detected in low-grade pancreatic intraepithelial neoplasia, *TP53* mutation and/or deletions of *CDKN2A/p16* and *SMAD4* signify at least high-grade dysplasia and, in a solid mass lesion identified on imaging, supports adenocarcinoma.[24,51]

> ### *Key Features*
> #### PANCREATIC NEUROENDOCRINE TUMOR
>
> Solid-cellular smear pattern of monotonous polygonal cells
>
> Uniform, round, eccentrically placed nuclei with salt-and-pepper chromatin
>
> Moderate amount of dense, finely granular cytoplasm; occasionally oncocytic or lipid-rich cytoplasm

PanNETs represent less than 2% of pancreatic neoplasms.[52] Most PanNETs occur sporadically in middle-aged patients. Many are nonfunctional and span less than 3 cm at presentation. Functional neoplasms can present earlier with symptoms of excess hormone production (eg, insulin hypersecretion leading to hypoglycemia). Approximately 15% of cases are associated with germline mutations.[53] These hereditary conditions include multiple endocrine neoplasia type I (*MEN1* gene), neurofibromatosis type 1 (*NF1* gene), tuberous sclerosis (either *TSC1* or *TSC2* genes), and von Hippel-Lindau (*VHL* gene) syndromes.[53–55]

The 2017 World Health Organization classification of pancreatic neuroendocrine neoplasms categorizes PanNETs into 4 tiers based on grade: 1 (G1), 2 (G2), 3 (G3), and poorly

differentiated pancreatic neuroendocrine carcinoma.[56] Emerging data suggest that well-differentiated and poorly differentiated pancreatic neuroendocrine neoplasms have distinct biologies and prognoses and require different therapeutic approaches.[57] On imaging, PanNETs appear as round enhancing masses.[58] Occasionally, they can present with cystic degeneration and may be confused with primary pancreatic cystic neoplasms (discussed later).

PanNETs are solid and hypercellular epithelial lesions with a minimal stromal component, unlike pancreatic adenocarcinomas, which generally elicit a dense desmoplastic stromal response. PanNET FNAs show numerous single polygonal cells with round, eccentric nuclei, coarse chromatin, inconspicuous nucleoli and variably dense cytoplasm (**Fig. 10**). The latter may appear oncocytic or vacuolated (lipid-rich). Cellular pleomorphism is common and grading of PanNETs cannot be based on purely cytologic features alone.[59] Proliferation index can provide prognostic information and is calculated by either mitotic count and/or Ki-67 immunohistochemistry. Ten high-power fields are scanned for mitoses and Ki-67 positivity. Grade 1 PanNETs have up to 1 mitotic figure or a Ki-67 index of less than 3%. Two to 20 mitoses or a Ki-67 index of 3% to 20% is seen in G2 PanNETs. Both G3 PanNETs and poorly-differentiated neuroendocrine carcinomas have greater than 20 mitoses and Ki-67 proliferation index of greater than 20 (**Fig. 11**). Poorly differentiated neuroendocrine carcinomas may be of small or large cell type and harbor mutations of *TP53*, *RB1*, and *KRAS*, whereas well-differentiated neuroendocrine tumors frequently exhibit *DAXX*, *ATRX*, and *MEN1*.[60,61] Gleeson and colleagues[61] found data that suggest *MEN1* alterations are an early event in the tumorigenesis of PanNETs. *ATRX/DAXX* portend a

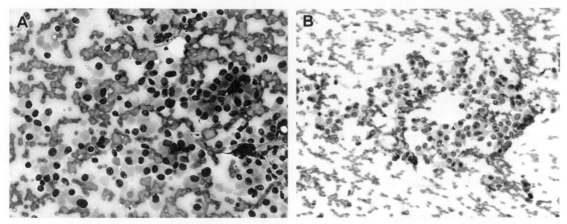

Fig. 10. (*A*, *B*) PanNETs show a sea of single polygonal plasmacytoid cells and with focal rosette formation. Cells show round, eccentric nuclei, coarse chromatin, inconspicuous nucleoli and variably dense cytoplasm, as well as stripped nuclei ([*A*] Direct smear, Diff-Quik, original magnification, ×40; [*B*] Direct smear, Papanicolaou stain, original magnification, ×40).

poor prognosis as mutations tend to occur later in the disease and are observed more in the metastatic setting.[61]

Well-differentiated PanNET, ACC, pancreatoblastoma, and SPNs are solid-cellular tumors that are rich in epithelium and poor in stroma. These tumors can resemble one other on cytology and histology. Immunohistochemistry is often in differentiating solid-cellular tumors. Synaptophysin, chromogranin, and CD56 highlight PanNETs. SPNs may also show expression for CD56, so caution should be used with the interpretation of this marker as the only marker supporting the diagnosis of PanNET.[62]

Key Features
ACINAR CELL CARCINOMA

Solid-cellular pattern

Irregular cell clusters with loss of benign grapes on a vine appearance

Stripped naked nuclei with smooth contours and prominent nucleoli

Variable amount of granular cytoplasm with zymogen granules which may be dispersed in the background from stripped cells

Even though acinar cells constitute most of the pancreas, ACC represents less than 2% of pancreatic neoplasms.[63] ACC typically occurs

in older male adults but can be frequently encountered in the pediatric population.[63,64] A prognosis of ACC is better than that of ductal adenocarcinoma but worse than PanNETs. Mean overall survival is approximately 4 years.[65]

Symptoms of ACC are related to mass effect and include abdominal pain, nausea, and weight loss. Sequelae of excessive pancreatic digestive enzyme production by neoplastic cells is the defining characteristic of ACC.[66] The tumor was first described in 1908 in a patient presenting with fever, polyarthritis, and subcutaneous nodular fat necrosis—related to lipase hypersecretion.[67,68]

ACC most commonly occurs in the pancreatic head. The tumor appears as a well-circumscribed, variably cystic, round mass and may resemble PanNET radiographically. ACC FNAs demonstrate a solid-cellular pattern with loose cell aggregates, acinar structures, and club-shaped cell aggregates and isolated polygonal cells with abundant granular cytoplasm (**Fig. 12**). Zymogen granules, released from disrupted cells, and the resultant naked nuclei may be noted in the background.

Diagnosis of ACC can be difficult on cytology, and misdiagnosis is common. Detection of acinar cell–specific enzymes—chymotrypsin, lipase, amylase, and trypsin—by immunohistochemistry supports the diagnosis of ACC.[69] The two most sensitive markers of ACC are chymotrypsin and trypsin.[69] Periodic acid–Schiff stain can highlight the intracytoplasmic zymogen granules. Cytogenetics reveal allelic loss on chromosome 11p.[70]

Key Features
SOLID-PSEUDOPAPILLARY NEOPLASM

Solid-cellular pattern

Papillae of neoplastic cells around myxoid fibrovascular cores

Round to oval cells with bean-shaped and Grooved nuclei with fine chromatin and inconspicuous nucleoli

Scant cytoplasm some with perinuclear vacuoles and hyalin globules

Background of hemorrhagic and necrotic debris, with foamy histiocytes

SPN, a tumor of low malignant potential, accounts for less than 2% of pancreatic neoplasms. SPN almost always occurs in young women but has been reported in older women and in men.[71] SPN occurs throughout the gland.

Radiographically, SPNs are generally circumscribed, round, solid, and cystic masses—much like PanNETs and ACCs. Hemorrhage in a cystic, nonseptate distal pancreatic mass of a younger woman suggests SPN.[68]

Cytologic samples display a solid-cellular pattern with abundance of monomorphic round to oval epithelial cells with grooved nuclei, inconspicuous nucleoli, and scant cytoplasm arranged around delicate fibrovascular cores (**Fig. 13**). The component of cystic SPNs may show background blood, foamy histiocytes, and necrotic debris. Diffuse, strong nuclear staining for β-catenin supports a diagnosis of SPN. Other solid-cellular neoplasms (ACC and pancreatoblastoma) may also show patchy positivity.[72] Cytokeratin is strongly positive in ACC and pancreatoblastoma whereas SPN often shows weak to negative staining for cytokeratin.[73] Immunohistochemistry for SOX-11, TFE3, LEF1, and AR [SRY-Box 11, transcription factor E3, lymphoid enhancer binding factor 1 and androgen receptor] has recently been shown to be helpful in diagnosing SPN.[74]

Key Features
PANCREATOBLASTOMA

Solid-cellular pattern

Clusters of acinar, neuroendocrine, and ductal cells

Squamoid corpuscle and primitive spindle cells

Rarely, heterologous elements (ie, cartilage)

Pancreatoblastoma comprises less than 0.5% of pancreatic neoplasms. It is the most common pediatric pancreatic malignancy and typically encountered in the first 10 years of life.[75] Adult cases are extraordinarily rare, with fewer than 40 reported cases.[75] Most are sporadic. In rare cases, there is an association with Beckwith-Wiedemann syndrome and familial adenomatous polyposis.[76] Pancreatoblastoma carries a dismal prognosis, albeit better than of ductal adenocarcinoma.[77]

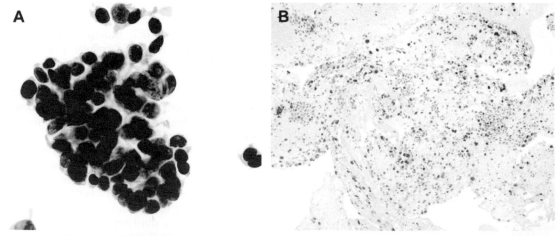

Fig. 11. (*A*) Poorly-differentiated pancreatic neuroendocrine carcinoma, small cell type shows nuclear hyperchromasia, crowding, molding, occasional nucleoli, and extremely scant cytoplasm (ThinPrep, Papanicolaou stain, original magnification, ×100). (*B*) Immunohistochemical stain for Ki-67 shows a high (>20) proliferation index (cell block, Ki-67 stain, original magnification, ×20).

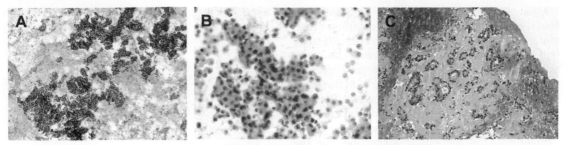

Fig. 12. ACC recapitulates normal acinar architecture; however, the neoplastic acini form solid and irregularly clusters shaped. Isolated cells and stripped naked nuclei are prominent compared to benign acinar tissue. Nuclei round to oval, smooth with prominent nucleoli. ([A, B] Direct smear, original magnification, ×20, Papanicolaou stain, original magnification, ×60; [C] cell block, hematoxylin-eosin stain, original magnification, ×20).

Pancreatoblastomas are characteristically large, ranging from 2 cm to 10 cm, and are well defined on imaging.[77] FNA shows a characteristic solid-cellular pattern. Acinar, neuroendocrine, and ductal cells are typically present, although acinar cells are most commonly encountered. Wilms tumor and neuroblastoma are in the differential diagnosis. Immunohistochemistry demonstrates the 3 populations in pancreatoblastoma—chymotrypsin for acinar cells, chromogranin for neuroendocrine cells, and cytokeratin for ductal cells. The distinguishing feature is the squamoid corpuscle that may express CK8, CK18, and CK 19 and cyclin D1.[72] Cytogenetics shows allelic loss on chromosome 11p.[76]

Pancreas is an unusual site for metastasis, which accounts for less than 2% of pancreatic neoplasms.[78] Accurate diagnosis of metastases

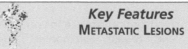

Key Features
METASTATIC LESIONS

Carcinomas most often metastasize to the pancreas

Most common metastasis is renal cell carcinoma; may appear years later and may mimic PanNET or PDAC

has dramatic disease management implications, such as avoidance of ineffective therapy, and heralds a hunt for a primary malignancy. Surgical resection of isolated metastasis carries low postoperative mortality.[78,79]

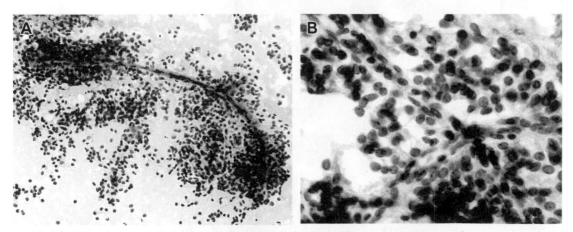

Fig. 13. (A) SPNs are composed of delicate vessels with a thin band of perivascular or myxoid stroma, surrounded by loosely arranged tumor cells and many isolated cells in the background (Direct smear, Diff-Quik stain, original magnification, ×20). (B) Delicate vessels with myxoid stroma are surrounded by loosely arranged tumor cells and isolated cells in the background. The nuclei are round to oval and bean shaped, with smooth or grooved contours, finely granular chromatin, inconspicuous nucleoli and delicate, cytoplasm ([B] Direct smear, Papanicolaou stain, original magnification, ×60).

Most secondary neoplasms are carcinomas. Renal cell carcinoma is the most common metastatic malignancy, representing approximately half of metastases.[79] Metastatic renal cell carcinomas are often metachronous and present as a solitary pancreatic mass.[80] Metastases may appear late (years, even decades) after primary diagnosis, and history may not be provided when evaluating the pancreatic lesion.[81] Conversely, the metastatic lesion may be the first sign of renal cell carcinoma.[81] FNA sampling shows large, polygonal cells with eccentric nuclei, prominent nucleoli, and vacuolated cytoplasm that may mimic a lipid-rich PanNET[82] (**Fig. 14**). Immunohistochemical positivity for PAX8 or adenocarcinoma supports a renal origin of the tumor.

Other neoplasms that metastasize to pancreas include lung and breast carcinomas.[79] In such circumstances, immunohistochemical stains for the suspected primary site should be used, that is, TTF-1 (thyroid transcription factor-1) for lung and GATA3 (GATA-binding protein 3) for breast.

| *Key Features* |
| ECTOPIC SPLENIC TISSUE |

Small to medium-sized lymphocytes

CD8+ splenic sinusoids

Splenic tissue may be found in the pancreas either as an accessory (splenule) or from trauma (splenosis) through autoimplantation. Accessory spleens are believed to form from incomplete fusion of splenic anlage and are found along the tracts of splenic vessels and ligaments.[83] The pancreatic tail is among the most common sites

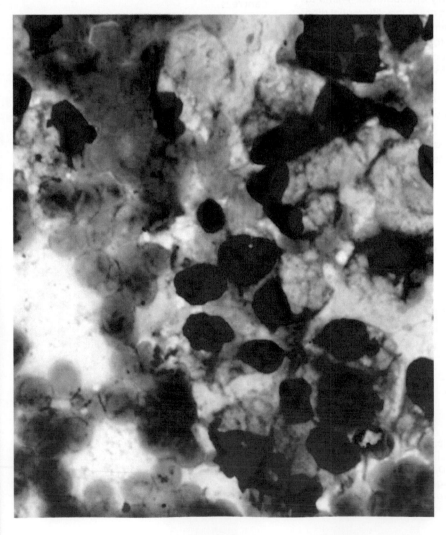

Fig. 14. Metastatic renal cell carcinoma shows eccentrically-placed irregular nuclei with moderately-abundant clear/vacuolated cytoplasm, morphologically similar to the primary renal cell carcinoma (Cytospin, Diff-Quik stain, original magnification, ×100).

of accessory spleen.[84] Splenosis results from autoimplantation of splenic tissue through abdominal trauma or splenectomy. Ectopic splenic tissue may pose a clinical challenge. Well-defined, solitary, and highly vascular accessory spleens may be mistaken radiographically for other solid mass-forming pancreatic lesions, such as PanNETs or metastatic renal cell carcinoma, and even may mimic lymphadenopathy.[84] Numerous small to medium-sized lymphocytes on FNA should raise the consideration of ectopic splenic tissue.[85] Immunohistochemistry on prepared cell blocks can be instrumental in confirming a diagnosis, because CD8 highlights the telltale splenic sinusoidal endothelial cells (**Fig. 15**).[86]

CYSTIC PANCREATIC LESIONS

Cystic pancreatic lesions present a conundrum to clinicians and challenge to cytopathologists. A multidisciplinary, multimodal diagnostic approach is recommended. Integrating clinical, radiological, cytomorphologic, biochemical and molecular information is essential for accurate preoperative diagnosis. It must be determined if the pancreatic cyst is mucinous or nonmucinous and if it is benign or malignant, because these factors bear implications for clinical management. Pseudocysts can be managed medically in most, and benign serous cystadenomas are surgically resected if large or symptomatic.[87] Management guidelines for suspected mucinous cysts are based on clinical and imaging findings. Small cysts, measuring less than 3 cm without high-risk features, may be conservatively managed. Patients with high-risk imaging features or with suspicious or malignant cytology are surgically managed. Patients with worrisome imaging features are evaluated by EUS-FNA.[2]

Pancreatic cyst cytology specimens often contain few to no epithelial cells. Ancillary tests, in particular biochemical and molecular studies, are integral in achieving actionable answers to clinically relevant questions about the cyst, that is, whether the cyst is mucinous or high risk. Cyst fluid analysis for amylase and carcinoembryonic antigen (CEA) levels can greatly enhance the sensitivity of EUS-FNA.[88,89] Genetic Analysis can highlight certain genetic alterations, like *KRAS*, which is a known mutation associated with neoplastic primary mucinous pancreatic cysts. The clinicopathologic findings of the most frequently seen cystic pancreatic neoplasms are summarized in **Table 3**.

Key Features
PSEUDOCYST

Nonmucinous cyst fluid; occasionally, contaminating mucin and gastrointestinal epithelium

Yellow pigment, resembling hematoidin

Acute and chronic inflammatory cells and histiocytes

Pseudocysts arise in the setting of autodigestive pancreatic parenchymal damage that occurs from the prolonged release and activation of pancreatic enzymes. This pattern of injury is most frequently a result of repeated bouts of severe, acute pancreatitis and is commonly associated with a longstanding history of alcohol abuse. Any risk factor of acute pancreatitis, however, including trauma

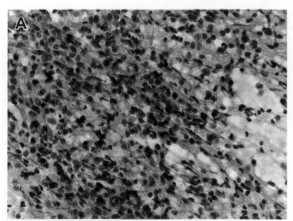
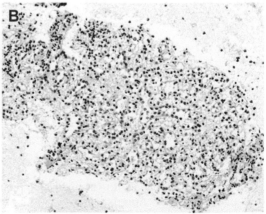

Fig. 15. (*A, B*). Ectopic splenic tissue demonstrates numerous small-to medium-sized lymphocytes ([*A*] smear, original magnification, ×40; [*B*] cell block, both hematoxylin-eosin stain, original magnification, ×20).

Table 3
Clinicopathologic characteristics of cystic pancreatic lesions

Diagnostic Entity	Demographics	Radiographic Findings	Cytologic Features	Cyst Fluid Analysis	Molecular Alterations
Pseudocyst	History of long-standing alcohol or abuse gallstones	• Thick-walled unilocular cyst • No septations or mural nodule	• Hypocellular, nonmucinous cyst fluid with inflammation • Yellow pigment	• High amylase • Low CEA	None identified
Serous cystadenoma	• Women > men • Mean age: 66 y	• Soap bubble pattern microcystic • Central, stellate scar • Larger cyst with septations (oligocystic)	• Sparsely cellular • Cuboidal cells with cytoplasmic glycogen	• Low amylase • Low CEA	VHL
Lymphoepithelial cyst	• F:M = 1:4 • Mean age: 56 y	• Round mass with solid or cystic appearance	• Abundant keratinous debris • Squamous cells • Cholesterol clefts • Background lymphocytes and histocytes	• High CEA	None identified
MCN	• F:M = 20:1 • Age: 40–50 y	• Solitary, thick-walled, multiloculated cyst • Body and tail mass in 95%	• Variable mucin, but thick, extracellular, colloid-like mucin supports neoplasia • Sparsely cellular	• Low or high amylase • High or low CEA	• KRAS • TP53[a] • CDKN2A loss[a] • SMAD4 loss[a]
Intraductal papillary mucinous neoplasm	• Mean age: 65 y • Men >women	• Thin-walled, unilocular to thinly septated cyst connected to the main pancreatic duct • High-risk features: main duct dilation of >10 mm, mural nodule or cyst wall mass • Pancreatic head most common location of branch-duct cyst	• Variale mucin but thick, extracellular, colloid-like mucin supports neoplasia • Variably cellular • Low-grade atypia: mucinous, columnar, or gastric-foveolar features • High-grade atypia: small (<12 μm) cells with increased nuclear-to-cytoplasmic ratio and abnormal chromatin	• High amylase • High or low CEA	• KRAS • GNAS • TP53[a] • P16/CDKN2A loss[a] • SMAD4 loss[a]

Abbreviation: F:M, female-to-male ratio.
[a] Indicates a high-risk cyst.

and surgery, can lead to the development of pseudocysts. Approximately 10% of patients with acute pancreatitis develop a pseudocyst.[90]

Pseudocysts, as their name suggests, are not true cysts and are collections of necrotic debris and pancreatic secretions surrounded by a thick, fibrous capsule, which lacks epithelial lining.

They may spontaneously resolve or rupture and cause numerous complications, such as obstruction and infection.[91] Their clinical management is variable and not well defined. On imaging, pseudocysts are unusually solitary, thick-walled, unilocular cysts.[92] They may vary in size and location within the pancreas but occur most commonly in the pancreatic tail.

Cytologically, the characteristic features include degenerative cyst debris with acute and chronic inflammatory cells, hemosiderin-laden macrophages (Fig. 16). No cyst-lining epithelial cells should be present, but contaminating gastrointestinal epithelia may be seen and are a diagnostic pitfall.

The differential diagnosis of a pseudocyst includes true pancreatic cysts. Patients with pseudocysts almost always have a history of pancreatitis. Biochemical analysis of aspirated cyst fluid may be helpful and amylase is consistently elevated in pseudocysts, typically in the thousands of units per liter. A cyst fluid with an amylase level less than 250 U/L is highly unlikely to be a pseudocyst.[93] CEA levels are typically undetectable or very low in pseudocysts. Mucinous cysts generally have CEA levels greater than 192 ng/mL. Molecular analysis should yield no mutations.

Key Features
SEROUS CYSTADENOMA

Sparsely cellular specimen

Clean or bloody background

Uniform cuboidal cells with small, smooth, round nuclei and with inconspicuous nucleoli

Finely vacuolated, nonmucinous cytoplasm

Hemosiderin-laden macrophages

Serous cystadenomas are the most common benign pancreatic cystic neoplasm, although they account for only 2% of pancreatic tumors.[94] Serous cystadenomas are more common in women (mean age of 66 years). There is an association with von Hippel-Lindau syndrome.[95] Most patients are asymptomatic but may present with nonspecific abdominal pain. Malignant serous cystadenocarcinomas exist have been rarely reported.[96]

Serous cystadenomas are subclassified on imaging by the number and size of cysts into microcystic, oligocystic, solid, and unilocular.[97]

The countless small cysts of the aptly named microcystic variant of serous cystadenoma give rise to the characteristic honeycomb, soap bubble pattern on imaging.[98] Additional radiographic features include a central, stellate scar, and calcifications. Oligocystic and unilocular variants may be indistinguishable from other cysts in the pancreas. The solid variant, which is most rare, may be misdiagnosed as a PanNET or carcinoma.

Cytologic samples are frequently paucicellular. Neoplastic cells are uniform, cuboidal cells with round nuclei with smooth contours, inconspicuous nucleoli and scant, finely vacuolated, nonmucinous cytoplasm (Fig. 17). Periodic acid–Schiff stain with and without diastase confirms the presence of cytoplasmic glycogen and excludes the presence of mucin, which can be performed on cellblock, core or forceps biopsy tissue (see Fig. 17). Cyst fluid analysis typically shows low levels of amylase and CEA (often <5 ng/mL). Molecular testing may reveal mutations in VHL gene and loss of 3p in sporadic and hereditary cases.[99]

Key Features
LYMPHOEPITHELIAL CYST

Abundant keratinous debris with nucleated and anucleated squamous cells

Cholesterol clefts

Background lymphocytes and histocytes

Lymphoepithelial cysts are extremely rare benign pancreatic lesions. There is a striking predilection for middle-aged men, with a male-to-female ratio of 4:1.[100] Lymphoepithelial cysts may occur anywhere within the pancreas and range from 1 cm to 17 cm in size.[101]

The radiographic findings are highly variable and nonspecific and may mimic other pancreatic lesions, appearing cystic, loculated, or solid (due to keratinous debris contents).[101] Furthermore, CEA levels may be markedly elevated, suggesting the more prevalent mucinous cyst (discussed later).[102] FNA sampling shows nucleated and anucleated squamous cells admixed with keratinous and cholesterol clefts (Fig. 18).[103] Histologically, it is a squamous-lined cyst with subepithelial nonneoplastic lymphoid tissue.

Key Features
MUCINOUS CYSTS: MUCINOUS CYSTIC NEOPLASM AND INTRADUCTAL PAPILLARY MUCINOUS NEOPLASM

Thick, colloid-like extracellular mucin is diagnostic.

Variable cellularity; often scant

Low-grade atypia (low-grade to intermediate-grade dysplasia): mucinous columnar to pseudostratified epithelium

High-grade atypia (high-grade dysplasia or adenocarcinoma): small cells (<12 μm duodenal enterocyte) with abnormal chromatin, irregular nuclear membrane, and increased nuclear-to-cytoplasmic ratio, often in a background of cellular necrosis

Mucinous cystic neoplasms (MCNs) and intraductal papillary neoplasms (IPMNs) are 2 distinct pancreatic mucinous cysts, which share common radiological and cytomorphologic features. These lesions are identified cystic precursors of invasive adenocarcinoma. They are both characterized by dysplastic mucinous epithelial lining cells and may be associated with carcinoma. The presence of invasive carcinoma chiefly drives prognosis.[104] On cytology, their diagnostic hallmark is the presence of thick, colloid-like extracellular mucin (**Fig. 19**).[105] The

cellular component of cyst fluid aspirations, however, is typically insufficient in quality and quantity to reliably distinguish these two entities, and the scant amount present may underestimate the histologic grade.[9] Correlation with clinical and imaging findings is often required for a specific diagnosis, which is relevant for appropriate management. Biochemical and molecular tests can help elucidate the etiology of the cystic lesion. CEA is the best test for determining a primary mucinous pancreatic cyst; a level of 192 ng/mL has an overall diagnostic accuracy of approximately 80%.[71,89] *KRAS* mutations support a neoplastic mucinous pancreatic cyst, and *GNAS* mutations support the diagnosis of an IPMN over an MCN.[106,107]

MCNs represent 5% of all pancreatic neoplasms on imaging studies and 25% of all resected cystic neoplasms.[108] They are found almost exclusively in women (with female-to-male ratio of 20:1) in the fourth and fifth decades of life.[109] Malignant cases are typically seen in women in their 60s.[104]

Radiographically, MCNs are solitary, round, septated cysts, which are circumscribed by a thick fibrous capsule.[110] They have a strong predilection for the pancreatic body and tail and can be large. MCNs generally do not communicate with the pancreatic ducts.

The defining feature of MCN is ovarian-type stroma found beneath its mucinous lining, and is only appreciated histologically. EUS-FNA samples of low-grade MCNs and IPMNs are scantily

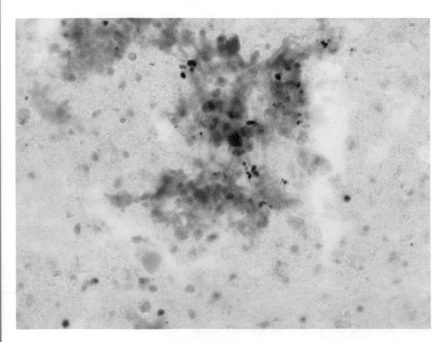

Fig. 16. Pseudocysts display acute and chronic inflammatory cells and yellow, hematoidin-like pigment in a background of degenerative amorphous cyst debris (SurePath, Papanicolaou stain, original magnification, ×60).

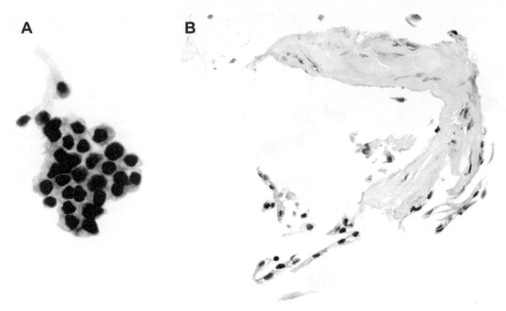

Fig. 17. (*A*) Neoplastic cells of serous cystadenomas appear as uniform, cuboidal cells with small, smooth, round nuclei, inconspicuous nucleoli and finely vacuolated cytoplasm on cytology (ThinPrep, Papanicolaou stain, original magnification, ×60). (*B*) Moray microforceps biopsy demonstrating the same neoplastic cells and cell wall of a serous cystadenoma ([*B*] Microforceps biopsy, hematoxylin-eosin stain, original magnification, ×20).

cellular and show single cells, small clusters, and flat sheets of bland glandular epithelial cells, displaying visible cytoplasmic mucin (see **Fig. 19**). Low-grade atypia may mimic contaminating gastrointestinal epithelia. Thick, viscous mucin, grossly and microscopically visible, supports the diagnosis of a mucinous cyst. Higher-grade cytologic atypia is defined by epithelial cells with nuclear crowding, loss of polarity, nuclear elongation or rounding, hyperchromasia, and increased nuclear-to-cytoplasmic ratio in small,

budlike cellular clusters or singly (**Fig. 20**). The treatment of choice for large, symptomatic MCNs is surgical. Distal pancreatectomy is a relatively easy procedure associated with low mortality, and preferred over lifelong imaging surveillance of a young woman. Whether MCNs less than 3 cm should be resected or clinically followed is currently debated.[111]

IPMNs account for approximately 5% of pancreatic neoplasms and 20% of neoplastic pancreatic cysts. Unlike MCNs, IPMNs affect older

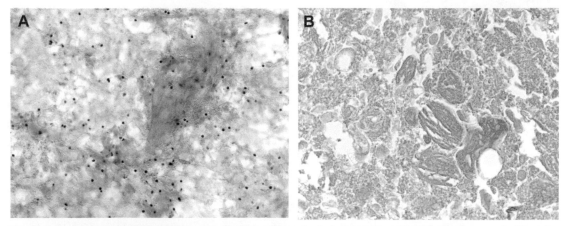

Fig. 18. (*A*) Lymphoepithelial cysts show nucleated and anucleated squamous cells with a background of lymphocytes (Direct smear, Papanicolaou stain, original magnification, ×20). (*B*) Abundant keratinous debris seen on a cell-block preparation (cell block, hematoxylin-eosin, original magnification, ×20).

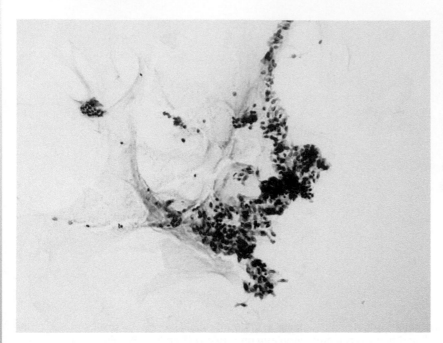

Fig. 19. The presence of thick, colloid-like extracellular mucin is the diagnostic hallmark of neoplastic mucinous cysts (either IPMN or MCN), as seen here in a case of low-grade intraductal papillary neoplasm (ThinPrep, Papanicolaou stain, original magnification, ×20).

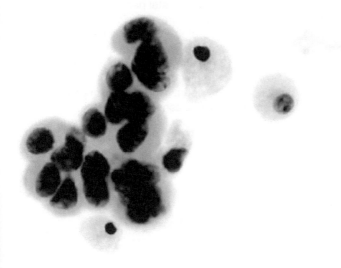

Fig. 20. This cluster of neoplastic cells shows the nuclear crowding, loss of polarity, nuclear irregularities, hyperchromasia and high nuclear-to-cytoplasmic ratio, seen in high-grade MCNs (ThinPrep, Papanicolaou stain, original magnification, ×60).

patients (mean age of 65 years), occur more frequently in men, are found in the pancreatic head, and lack ovarian-type stroma. Like MCNs, they are classified as premalignant or malignant, based on the identification of an invasive component, which is the ultimate prognostic factor. There are 3 main types of IPMNs, distinguished by the ducts involved (main duct, branch duct, or both). Branch-duct IPMNs typically behave better than main-duct and combined-type IPMNs.[112]

Radiographically, a markedly distended main pancreatic duct with multiple filling defects is a diagnostic feature of IPMN. The Fukuoka consensus guidelines stratify IPMNs into 3 risk groups, based entirely on imaging characteristics.[2] High-risk features include obstructive jaundice, enhancing solid component within cyst, and greater than or equal to 10 mm dilatation of the main pancreatic duct. Worrisome features are cysts greater than 3 cm, dilated main pancreatic duct measuring 5 mm to 9 mm, nonenhancing mural nodule, abrupt change in caliber of pancreatic duct with distal pancreatic atrophy, and regional lymphadenopathy. Detection of either high-risk stigmata or worrisome features warrants either resection or increased surveillance.

Pitman and colleagues[113] identified 5 cytologic criteria for diagnosing high-grade atypia in IPMNs, which include cell size less than a 12-μm enterocyte, increased nuclear-to-cytoplasmic ratio, nuclear membrane irregularities, abnormal chromatin pattern, and background cellular necrosis. These cytologic findings represent high-grade dysplasia or adenocarcinoma on histology. The group found that the 3 most accurate features for the identification of high-grade atypia were background necrosis, abnormal chromatin pattern, and an increased nuclear-to-cytoplasmic ratio.[113] The risk of malignancy of a cyst with a diagnosis of high-grade atypia is approximately 80%.[114]

Cytologic features of IPMNs with nonpapillary epithelium are indistinguishable from MCNs (discussed previously) (Fig. 21). It is important, however, to distinguish these 2 mucinous neoplasms because management differs. All MCNs are resected regardless of grade given the relative ease of the typical distal pancreatectomy in the usual middle-aged woman compared with the anxiety and lifelong surveillance of monitoring the tumor of malignant progression. IPMNs, on the other hand, more often occur in older patients with significant comorbidities and the risk of surgical resection must be balanced against the risk of malignancy. Most but not all branch-duct IPMNs are low risk and can be clinically followed. Currently, cytology is the best test for grading cysts that are not already high risk by imaging, but ancillary testing with molecular analysis is becoming an increasingly important tool in improving accuracy in risk assessment.[8,115,116]

FUTURE DIRECTIONS

Pancreaticobiliary cytology requires synthesis of clinical history, imaging studies, cytology samples, and ancillary tests, including immunohistochemistry, biochemical analysis, and genetic sequencing, for optimal patient management. The most common pancreatic neoplasms are challenging from clinical and cytologic standpoints. EUS-FNA shows high specificity approaching 100% in most studies.[117,118]

A **B**

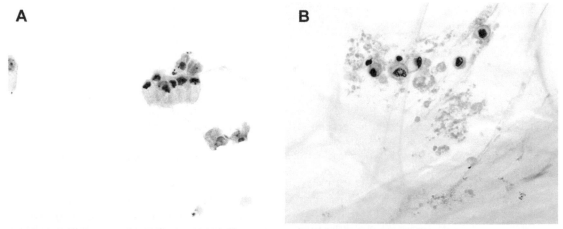

Fig. 21. (*A*) IPMNs appear cytomorphologically similar to MCNs, with benign-appearing mucinous epithelium, seen here in low-grade IPMNs (ThinPrep, Papanicolaou stain, original magnification, ×60). (*B*) High-grade cytologic features of small cells with abnormal chromatin, irregular nuclear membranes and increased nuclear-to-cytoplasmic ratio (Cytospin, Papanicolaou stain, original magnification, ×60).

Sensitivity is moderate, however, with relatively frequent false-negative diagnoses and indeterminate cytologic samples.[118] For solid-cellular neoplasms, much of the differential diagnosis relies on immunohistochemistry. Ultimately, genetic sequencing offers much promise in its ability to classify pancreatic cysts. With deeper understanding of the underlying pathogenesis of pancreatic disease, NGS potentially can reliably identify malignant lesions and provide molecular blueprints for targeted therapy.

REFERENCES

1. Tanaka M, Chari S, Adsay V, et al. International consensus guidelines for management of intraductal papillary mucinous neoplasms and mucinous cystic neoplasms of the pancreas. Pancreatology 2006;6:17–32.

2. Tanaka M, Fernández-del Castillo C, Adsay V, et al. International consensus guidelines 2012 for the management of IPMN and MCN of the pancreas. Pancreatology 2012;12:183–97.

3. Heckler M, Michalski CW, Schaefle S, et al. The Sendai and Fukuoka consensus criteria for the management of branch duct IPMN - a meta-analysis on their accuracy. Pancreatology 2017; 17:255–62.

4. Lee A, Kadiyala V, Lee LS. Evaluation of AGA and Fukuoka Guidelines for EUS and surgical resection of incidental pancreatic cysts. Endosc Int Open 2017;5:E116–22.

5. Yan T, Ke Y, Chen Y, et al. Serological characteristics of autoimmune pancreatitis and its differential diagnosis from pancreatic cancer by using a combination of carbohydrate antigen 19-9, globulin, eosinophils and hemoglobin. PLoS One 2017;12:e0174735.

6. Voss M, Hammel P, Molas G, et al. Value of endoscopic ultrasound guided fine needle aspiration biopsy in the diagnosis of solid pancreatic masses. Gut 2000;46:244–9.

7. Kadayifci A, Atar M, Wang JL, et al. Value of adding GNAS testing to pancreatic cyst fluid KRAS and carcinoembryonic antigen analysis for the diagnosis of intraductal papillary mucinous neoplasms. Dig Endosc 2017;29(1):111–7.

8. Jones M, Zheng Z, Wang J, et al. Impact of next-generation sequencing on the clinical diagnosis of pancreatic cysts. Gastrointest Endosc 2016; 83(1):140–8.

9. Pitman MB, Lewandrowski K, Shen J, et al. Pancreatic cysts: preoperative diagnosis and clinical management. Cancer Cytopathol 2010;118:1–13.

10. DiMaio CJ, Kolb JM, Benias PC, et al. Initial experience with a novel EUS-guided core biopsy needle (SharkCore): results of a large North American multicenter study. Endosc Int Open 2016;4:E974–9.

11. Attili F, Pagliari D, Rimbaş M, et al. Endoscopic ultrasound-guided histological diagnosis of a mucinous non-neoplastic pancreatic cyst using a specially designed through-the-needle microforceps. Endoscopy 2016;48(Suppl 1):E188–9.

12. Zhang ML, Arpin RN, Brugge WR, et al. Moray™ micro-forceps biopsy improves the diagnosis of specific pancreatic cysts. 106th Annual Meeting of the United States and Canadian Academy of Pathology. San Antonio (TX), March 4–10, 2017.

13. Bhattacharya A, Cruise M, Chahal P. Endoscopic ultrasound guided 22 gauge core needle biopsy for the diagnosis of autoimmune pancreatitis. Pancreatology 2018;18(2):168–9.

14. Brais RJ, Davies SE, O'Donovan M, et al. Direct histological processing of EUS biopsies enables rapid molecular biomarker analysis for interventional pancreatic cancer trials. Pancreatology 2012;12:8–15.

15. Chen AL, Misdraji J, Brugge WR, et al. Acinar cell cystadenoma: a challenging cytology diagnosis, facilitated by moray(®) micro-forceps biopsy. Diagn Cytopathol 2017;45:557–60.

16. Ishikawa T, Mohamed R, Heitman SJ, et al. Diagnostic yield of small histological cores obtained with a new EUS-guided fine needle biopsy system. Surg Endosc 2017;31:5143–9.

17. Qin LX, Tang ZY. Hepatocellular carcinoma with obstructive jaundice: diagnosis, treatment and prognosis. World J Gastroenterol 2003;9:385–91.

18. Kinoshita H, Tanimura H, Uchiyama K, et al. Prognostic factors of intrahepatic cholangiocarcinoma after surgical treatment. Oncol Rep 2002;9:97–101.

19. Sugiyama M, Atomi Y, Wada N, et al. Endoscopic transpapillary bile duct biopsy without sphincterotomy for diagnosing biliary strictures: a prospective comparative study with bile and brush cytology. Am J Gastroenterol 1996;91:465–7.

20. Barr Fritcher EG, Caudill JL, Blue JE, et al. Identification of malignant cytologic criteria in pancreaticobiliary brushings with corresponding positive fluorescence in situ hybridization results. Am J Clin Pathol 2011;136:442–9.

21. Avadhani V, Hacihasanoglu E, Memis B, et al. Cytologic predictors of malignancy in bile duct brushings: a multi-reviewer analysis of 60 cases. Mod Pathol 2017;30:1273–86.

22. Moreno Luna LE, Kipp B, Halling KC, et al. Advanced cytologic techniques for the detection of malignant pancreaticobiliary strictures. Gastroenterology 2006;131:1064e1072.

23. Liew ZH, Loh TJZ, Lim TKH, et al. Role of fluorescence in situ hybridization in diagnosing cholangiocarcinoma in indeterminate biliary strictures. J Gastroenterol Hepatol 2010;33(1):315–9.

24. Dudley JC, Zheng Z, McDonald T, et al. Next-generation sequencing and fluorescence in situ

hybridization have comparable performance characteristics in the analysis of pancreaticobiliary brushings for malignancy. J Mol Diagn 2016;18:124–30.

25. Adler D, Max SC, Al-Haddad M, et al. Clinical evaluation, imaging studies, indications for cytologic study, and preprocedural requirements for duct brushing studies and pancreatic FNA: the papanicolaou society of cytopathology recommendations for pancreatic and biliary cytology. Diagn Cytopathol 2014;42:325–32.

26. Layfield LJ, Ehya H, Filie AC, et al. Utilization of ancillary studies in the cytologic diagnosis of biliary and pancreatic lesions: the Papanicolaou Society of Cytopathology guidelines for pancreatobiliary cytology. Diagn Cytopathol 2014;42:351–62.

27. Pitman MB, Centeno BA, Ali SZ, et al. Standardized terminology and nomenclature for pancreaticobiliary cytology: the Papanicolaou Society of Cytopathology guidelines. Diagn Cytopathol 2014;42:338–50.

28. Pitman MB, Layfield LJ. The papanicolaou society of cytopathology system for reporting pancreaticobiliary cytology. New York: Springer; 2015.

29. Perez-Machado MA. Pancreatic cytology: standardised terminology and nomenclature. Cytopathology 2016;27:157–60.

30. Young NA, Mody DR, Davey DD. Misinterpretation of normal cellular elements in fine-needle aspiration biopsy specimens: observations from the College of American Pathologists interlaboratory comparison program in non-gynecologic cytopathology. Arch Pathol Lab Med 2002;126:670–5.

31. Mitsuhashi T, Ghafari S, Chang CY, et al. Endoscopic ultrasound-guided fine needle aspiration of the pancreas: cytomorphological evaluation with emphasis on adequacy assessment, diagnostic criteria and contamination from the gastrointestinal tract. Cytopathology 2006;17:34–41.

32. Layfield LJ, Jarboe EA. Cytopathology of the pancreas: neoplastic and nonneoplastic entities. Ann Diagn Pathol 2010;14:140–51.

33. Jhala NC, Jhala DN, Chhieng DC, et al. Endoscopic ultrasound-guided fine-needle aspiration. A cytopathologist's perspective. Am J Clin Pathol 2003;120:351–67.

34. Nawgiri RS, Nagle JA, Wilbur DC, et al. Cytomorphology and B72.3 labeling of benign and malignant ductal epithelium in pancreatic lesions compared to gastrointestinal epithelium. Diagn Cytopathol 2007;35:300–5.

35. Nagle J, Wilbur DC, Pitman MD. The cytomorphology of gastric and duodenal epithelium and reactivity to B72.3: a baseline for comparison to pancreatic neoplasms aspirated by EUS-FNAB. Diagn Cytopathol 2005;33:381–6.

36. Etemad B, Whitcomb DC. Chronic pancreatitis: diagnosis, classification, and new genetic developments. Gastroenterology 2001;120:682–707.

37. Yadav D, Lowenfels AB. The epidemiology of pancreatitis and pancreatic cancer. Gastroenterology 2013;144:1252–61.

38. Detlefsen S, Klöppel G. IgG4-related disease: with emphasis on the biopsy diagnosis of autoimmune pancreatitis and sclerosing cholangitis. Virchows Arch 2018;472(4):545–56.

39. Kamisawa T, Funata N, Hayashi Y, et al. A new clinicopathological entity of IgG4-related autoimmune disease. J Gastroenterol 2003;38:982–4.

40. Weindorf SC, Frederiksen JK. IgG4-related disease: a reminder for practicing pathologists. Arch Pathol Lab Med 2017;141:1476–83.

41. Onweni C, Balagoni H, Treece JM, et al. Autoimmune pancreatitis type 2: case report. J Investig Med High Impact Case Rep 2017;5, 2324709617734245.

42. Zhang J, Jia G, Zuo C, et al. (18)F- FDG PET/CT helps differentiate autoimmune pancreatitis from pancreatic cancer. BMC Cancer 2017;17:695.

43. Palazzo M, Palazzo L, Aubert A, et al. Irregular narrowing of the main pancreatic duct in association with a wall thickening is a key sign at endoscopic ultrasonography for the diagnosis of autoimmune pancreatitis. Pancreas 2015;44:211–5.

44. Siegel RL, Miller KD, Jemal A. Cancer statistics. CA Cancer J Clin 2017;2017(67):7–30.

45. Tang K, Lu W, Qin W, et al. Neoadjuvant therapy for patients with borderline resectable pancreatic cancer: a systematic review and meta-analysis of response and resection percentages. Pancreatology 2016;16:28–37.

46. Low G, Panu A, Millo N, et al. Multimodality imaging of neoplastic and nonneoplastic solid lesions of the pancreas. Radiographics 2011;31:993–1015.

47. Blackford A, Serrano OK, Wolfgang CL, et al. SMAD4 gene mutations are associated with poor prognosis in pancreatic cancer. Clin Cancer Res 2009;15:4674–9.

48. Kurahara H, Maemura K, Mataki Y, et al. Impact of p53 and PDGFR-β expression on metastasis and prognosis of patients with pancreatic cancer. World J Surg 2016;40:1977–84.

49. Tascilar M, Skinner HG, Rosty C, et al. The SMAD4 protein and prognosis of pancreatic ductal adenocarcinoma. Clin Cancer Res 2001;7:4115–21.

50. Ali S, Cohen C, Little JV, et al. The utility of SMAD4 as a diagnostic immunohistochemical marker for pancreatic adenocarcinoma, and its expression in other solid tumors. Diagn Cytopathol 2007;35:644–8.

51. Fabbri C, Gibiino G, Fornelli A, et al. Team work and cytopathology molecular diagnosis of solid pancreatic lesions. Dig Endosc 2017;29:657–66.

52. Lee DW, Kim MK, Kim HG. Diagnosis of pancreatic neuroendocrine tumors. Clin Endosc 2017;50:537–45.

53. Mortaji P, Morris KT, Samedi V, et al. Pancreatic neuroendocrine tumor in a patient with a TSC1

variant: case report and review of the literature. Fam Cancer 2018;17(2):275–80.

54. Auernhammer CJ, Spitzweg C, Angele MK, et al. Advanced neuroendocrine tumours of the small intestine and pancreas: clinical developments, controversies, and future strategies. Lancet Diabetes Endocrinol 2018;6(5):404–15.

55. Minnetti M, Grossman A. Somatic and germline mutations in NETs: implications for their diagnosis and management. Best Pract Res Clin Endocrinol Metab 2016;30:115–27.

56. Lloyd R, Osamura RY, Kloppel G, et al. WHO classification of tumours of endocrine organs. 4th edition. Lyon (France): IARC Press; 2017.

57. Raj N, Valentino E, Capanu M, et al. Treatment response and outcomes of grade 3 pancreatic neuroendocrine neoplasms based on morphology: well differentiated versus poorly differentiated. Pancreas 2017;46:296–301.

58. Dromain C, Déandréis D, Scoazec JY, et al. Imaging of neuroendocrine tumors of the pancreas. Diagn Interv Imaging 2016;97:1241–57.

59. Sigel CS, Krauss Silva VW, Reid MD, et al. Assessment of cytologic differentiation in high-grade pancreatic neuroendocrine neoplasms: a multiinstitutional study. Cancer 2018;126(1):44–53.

60. Klöppel G. Neuroendocrine neoplasms: dichotomy, origin and classifications. Visc Med 2017;33(5): 324–30.

61. Gleeson FC, Voss JS, Kipp BR, et al. Assessment of pancreatic neuroendocrine tumor cytologic genotype diversity to guide personalized medicine using a custom gastroenteropancreatic next-generation sequencing panel. Oncotarget 2017;8:93464–75.

62. Ahmed A, VandenBussche CJ, Ali SZ, et al. The dilemma of "indeterminate" interpretations of pancreatic neuroendocrine tumors on fine needle aspiration. Diagn Cytopathol 2016;44:10–3.

63. Klimstra DS, Heffess CS, Oertel JE, et al. Acinar cell carcinoma of the pancreas. A clinicopathologic study of 28 cases. Am J Surg Pathol 1992;16:815–37.

64. Wisnoski NC, Townsend CM Jr, Nealon WH, et al. 672 patients with acinar cell carcinoma of the pancreas: a population-based comparison to pancreatic adenocarcinoma. Surgery 2008;144: 141–8.

65. Schmidt CM, Matos JM, Bentrem DJ, et al. Acinar cell carcinoma of the pancreas in the United States: prognostic factors and comparison to ductal adenocarcinoma. J Gastrointest Surg 2008;12: 2078–86.

66. Holen K, Klimstra DS, Hummer A, et al. Clinical characteristics and outcomes from an institutional series of acinar cell carcinoma of the pancreas. J Clin Oncol 2002;20:4673–8.

67. Berner O. Subkutane fettgewebsnekose. Virchow Arch Path Anat 1908;193:510–8.

68. Stauffer JA, Asbun HJ. Rare tumors and lesions of the pancreas. Surg Clin North Am 2018;98:169–88.

69. Sigel CS, Klimstra DS. Cytomorphologic and immunophenotypical features of acinar cell neoplasms of the pancreas. Cancer Cytopathol 2013;121: 459–70.

70. Abraham SC, Wu TT, Hruban RH, et al. Genetic and immunohistochemical analysis of pancreatic acinar cell carcinoma: frequent allelic loss on chromosome 11p and alterations in the APC/beta-catenin pathway. Am J Pathol 2002;160:953–62.

71. Limaiem F, Mestiri H, Mejri S, et al. Solid pseudopapillary neoplasm of the pancreas in two male patients: gender does not matter. Pan Afr Med J 2017;27:283.

72. Tanaka Y, Kato K, Notohara K, et al. Significance of aberrant (cytoplasmic/nuclear) expression of beta-catenin in pancreatoblastoma. J Pathol 2003;199: 185–90.

73. Bardales RH, Centeno B, Mallery JS, et al. Endoscopic ultrasound-guided fine-needle aspiration cytology diagnosis of solid-pseudopapillary tumor of the pancreas: a rare neoplasm of elusive origin but characteristic cytomorphologic features. Am J Clin Pathol 2004;121:654–62.

74. Kim EK, Jang M, Park M, et al. LEF1, TFE3, and AR are putative diagnostic markers of solid pseudopapillary neoplasms. Oncotarget 2017;8:93404–13.

75. Vilaverde F, Reis A, Rodrigues P, et al. Adult pancreatoblastoma - case report and review of literature. J Radiol Case Rep 2016;10:28–38.

76. Abraham SC, Wu T, Klimstra DS, et al. Distinctive molecular genetic alterations in sporadic and familial adenomatous polyposis-associated pancreatoblastomas. Am J Pathol 2001;159:1619–27.

77. Dhebri AR, Connor S, Campbell F, et al. Diagnosis, treatment and outcome of pancreatoblastoma. Pancreatology 2004;4:441–51.

78. Bokhari A, Tiscornia-Wasserman PG. Cytology diagnosis of metastatic clear cell renal cell carcinoma, synchronous to pancreas, and metachronous to thyroid and contralateral adrenal: report of a case and literature review. Diagn Cytopathol 2017;45:161–7.

79. El Hajj II, LeBlanc JK, Sherman S, et al. Endoscopic ultrasound-guided biopsy of pancreatic metastases: a large single-center experience. Pancreas 2013;42:524–30.

80. Gilani SM, Tashjian R, Danforth R, et al. Metastatic renal cell carcinoma to the pancreas: diagnostic significance of fine-needle aspiration cytology. Acta Cytol 2013;57:418–22.

81. Cheng SK, Chuah KL. Metastatic renal cell carcinoma to the pancreas: a review. Arch Pathol Lab Med 2016;140:598–602.

82. Alomari AK, Ustun B, Aslanian HR, et al. Endoscopic ultrasound-guided fine-needle aspiration

diagnosis of secondary tumors involving the pancreas: an institution's experience. Cytojournal 2016;13:1.

83. Bhutiani N, Egger ME, Doughtie CA, et al. Intrapancreatic accessory spleen (IPAS): a single-institution experience and review of the literature. Am J Surg 2017;213:816–20.

84. Pandey A, Pandey P, Ghasabeh MA, et al. Accuracy of apparent diffusion coefficient in differentiating pancreatic neuroendocrine tumour from intrapancreatic accessory spleen. Eur Radiol 2018;28(4):1560–7.

85. Rodriguez E, Netto G, Li QK. Intrapancreatic accessory spleen: a case report and review of literature. Diagn Cytopathol 2013;41:466–9.

86. Hwang HS, Lee SS, Kim SC, et al. Intrapancreatic accessory spleen: clinicopathologic analysis of 12 cases. Pancreas 2011;40:956–65.

87. Sahani DV, Kambadakone A, Macari M, et al. Diagnosis and management of cystic pancreatic lesions. AJR Am J Roentgenol 2013;200:343–54.

88. Cizginer S, Turner BG, Bilge AR, et al. Cyst fluid carcinoembryonic antigen is an accurate diagnostic marker of pancreatic mucinous cysts. Pancreas 2011;40:1024–8.

89. Oh SH, Lee JK, Lee KT, et al. The combination of cyst fluid carcinoembryonic antigen, cytology and viscosity increases the diagnostic accuracy of mucinous pancreatic cysts. Gut Liver 2017;11:283–9.

90. Banks PA, Bollen TL, Dervenis C, et al, Acute Pancreatitis Classification Working Group. Classification of acute pancreatitis–2012: revision of the Atlanta classification and definitions by international consensus. Gut 2013;62:102–11.

91. Rasch S, Nötzel B, Phillip V, et al. Management of pancreatic pseudocysts-a retrospective analysis. PLoS One 2017;12:e0184374.

92. Finkelmeier F, Sturm C, Friedrich-Rust M, et al. Predictive value of computed tomography scans and clinical findings for the need of endoscopic necrosectomy in walled-off necrosis from pancreatitis. Pancreas 2017;46:1039–45.

93. van der Waaij LA, van Dullemen HM, Porte RJ. Cyst fluid analysis in the differential diagnosis of pancreatic cystic lesions: a pooled analysis. Gastrointest Endosc 2005;62:383–9.

94. Valsangkar NP, Morales-Oyarvide V, Thayer SP, et al. 851 resected cystic tumors of the pancreas: a 33-year experience at the Massachusetts General Hospital. Surgery 2012;152:S4–12.

95. Findeis-Hosey JJ, McMahon KQ, Findeis SK. Von Hippel-Lindau disease. J Pediatr Genet 2016;5:116–23.

96. King JC, Ng TT, White SC, et al. Pancreatic serous cystadenocarcinoma: a case report and review of the literature. J Gastrointest Surg 2009;13:1864–8.

97. Reid MD, Choi H, Balci S, et al. Serous cystic neoplasms of the pancreas: clinicopathologic and molecular characteristics. Semin Diagn Pathol 2014;31:475–83.

98. Zaheer A, Pokharel SS, Wolfgang C, et al. Incidentally detected cystic lesions of the pancreas on CT: review of literature and management suggestions. Abdom Imaging 2013;38:331–41.

99. Lilo MT, VandenBussche CJ, Allison DB, et al. Serous cystadenoma of the pancreas: potentials and pitfalls of a preoperative cytopathologic diagnosis. Acta Cytol 2017;61:27–33.

100. Mege D, Grégoire E, Barbier L, et al. Lymphoepithelial cyst of the pancreas: an analysis of 117 patients. Pancreas 2014;43:987–95.

101. Borhani AA, Fasanella KE, Iranpour N, et al. Lymphoepithelial cyst of pancreas: spectrum of radiological findings with pathologic correlation. Abdom Radiol (NY) 2017;42:877–83.

102. Raval JS, Zeh HJ, Moser AJ, et al. Pancreatic lymphoepithelial cysts express CEA and can contain mucous cells: potential pitfalls in the preoperative diagnosis. Mod Pathol 2010;23:1467–76.

103. VandenBussche CJ, Maleki Z. Fine-needle aspiration of squamous-lined cysts of the pancreas. Diagn Cytopathol 2014;42:592–9.

104. Crippa S, Bassi C, Salvia R, et al. Low progression of intraductal papillary mucinous neoplasms with worrisome features and high-risk stigmata undergoing non-operative management: a mid-term follow-up analysis. Gut 2017;66:495–506.

105. Centeno BA, Stelow EB, Pitman MB. Pancreatic cytohistology. Cambridge (England): Cambridge UP; 2015.

106. Theisen BK, Wald AI, Singhi AD. Molecular diagnostics in the evaluation of pancreatic cysts. Surg Pathol Clin 2016;9:441–56.

107. Wu J, Matthaei H, Maitra A, et al. Recurrent GNAS mutations define an unexpected pathway for pancreatic cyst development. Sci Transl Med 2011;3:92ra66.

108. Farrell JJ. Prevalence, diagnosis and management of pancreatic cystic neoplasms: current status and future directions. Gut Liver 2015;9:571–89.

109. Griffin JF, Page AJ, Samaha GJ, et al. Patients with a resected pancreatic mucinous cystic neoplasm have a better prognosis than patients with an intraductal papillary mucinous neoplasm: a large single institution series. Pancreatology 2017;17:490–6.

110. Reddy RP, Smyrk TC, Zapiach M, et al. Pancreatic mucinous cystic neoplasm defined by ovarian stroma: demographics, clinical features, and prevalence of cancer. Clin Gastroenterol Hepatol 2004;2:1026–31.

111. Basar O, Brugge WR. My treatment approach: pancreatic cysts. Mayo Clin Proc 2017;92:1519–31.

112. Tanaka M. Thirty years of experience with intraductal papillary mucinous neoplasm of the pancreas: from discovery to international consensus. Digestion 2014;90:265–72.

113. Pitman MB, Centeno BA, Daglilar ES, et al. Cytological criteria of high-grade epithelial atypia in the cyst fluid of pancreatic intraductal papillary mucinous neoplasms. Cancer Cytopathol 2014; 122:40–7.

114. Hoda RS, Arpin R, Rosenbaum MW, et al. Risk of malignancy in pancreatic cysts with high-grade atypical cytology. 106th Annual Meeting of the United States and Canadian Academy of Pathology. San Antonio (TX), March 4–10, 2017.

115. Rosenbaum MW, Jones M, Dudley JC, et al. Next-generation sequencing adds value to the preoperative diagnosis of pancreatic cysts. Cancer Cytopathol 2017;125:41–7.

116. Singhi AD, McGrath K, Brand RE, et al. Preoperative next-generation sequencing of pancreatic cyst fluid is highly accurate in cyst classification and detection of advanced neoplasia. Gut 2017. https://doi.org/10.1136/gutjnl-2016-313586.

117. Gillis A, Cipollone I, Cousins G, et al. Does EUS-FNA molecular analysis carry additional value when compared to cytology in the diagnosis of pancreatic cystic neoplasm? A systematic review. HPB (Oxford) 2015;17:377–86.

118. Kameta E, Sugimori K, Kaneko T, et al. Diagnosis of pancreatic lesions collected by endoscopic ultrasound-guided fine-needle aspiration using next-generation sequencing. Oncol Lett 2016;12:3875–81.

Updates in Cervical Cytology
The 90-Year-Long Journey from Battle Creek to Today

Catherine J. Roe, MD, Krisztina Z. Hanley, MD*

KEYWORDS

- Pap test • HPV testing • ASCCP guidelines • The Bethesda System • HPV vaccine

Key points

- Major improvements have been made to the "Pap test" since Papanicolaou first introduced exfoliative cytology for the diagnosis of cervical cancer and its precursors.
- Discovery of causal association between cervical cancer and human papilloma virus (HPV) infection opened the door for molecular tests for detection of HPV DNA.
- Several immunomarkers have been studied to increase the sensitivity and specificity of cervical cytology for detection of high-grade squamous intraepithelial lesion.
- A standardized terminology and reporting system, The Bethesda System, was first implemented in 1988 and has undergone 4 revisions.
- Advancements in cervical cancer screening, detection, and reporting led to implementation of the 2012 consensus guidelines for the management of women with abnormal cervical cancer screening test.

ABSTRACT

Ninety years ago, at the Battle Creek conference, Papanicolaou introduced cervical exfoliative cytology. Since then, the "Pap test" has come a long way. The discovery of a causal relationship between cervical carcinoma and HPV infection opened the door for molecular testing and immunomarkers for HPV. The Clinical Laboratory Improvement Amendments, 1988, established quality assurance and quality control programs to monitor performance of cytology laboratories. The Bethesda System for reporting cervical cytology laid the foundations for cervical cytology education, implementation of management guidelines, and further research on cervical carcinogenesis. HPV vaccine penetration in both genders remains 62% or less.

UPDATE ON CERVICAL CANCER SCREENING AND REPORTING

CERVICAL CANCER SCREENING IN THE UNITED STATES

Statistics

The National Cancer Institute (NCI) Surveillance, Epidemiology, and End Results (SEER) Program

Authors have nothing to disclose.

Department of Pathology and Laboratory Medicine, Emory University School of Medicine, 1364 Clifton Road Northeast, Atlanta, GA 30322, USA

* Corresponding author. Department of Pathology and Laboratory Medicine, Emory University Hospital, Room H-187, 1364 Clifton Road Northeast, Atlanta, GA 30322.

E-mail address: khanley@emory.edu

compiles a statistics fact sheet composed of survival statistics, prevalence, stage at diagnosis, and changes over time regarding cervical cancer.[1] According to their data, in 2014 there were an estimated 256,078 women living with cervical cancer in the United States, and approximately 0.6% of women will be diagnosed with cervical cancer at some point in their lifetime. The risk factors for development of cervical cancer correlate with the risk factors for acquiring human papillomavirus (HPV), which include number of sexual partners and immunocompromised states.

There were an estimated 12,820 new cases of cervical cancer in 2017 (0.8% of all new cancer cases), and 4210 deaths as a result (0.7% of all cancer deaths). Compared with other cancer cases and subsequent deaths, cervical cancer comprises a small subset. The number of deaths from cervical cancer over all races was 2.3 women per 100,000 per year from 2010 to 2014. Looking specifically at races, the number was highest for African American women at 3.8 per 100,000 women dying of cervical cancer and lowest for Asian/Pacific Islanders at 1.7 women per 100,000. Many more women, however, are diagnosed with cervical cancer than die as a result of it. Based on 2010 to 2014 cases, the number of new cases of cervical cancer was 7.4 per 100,000 women per year, with 49 being the median age of diagnosis. Regarding extent at diagnosis, almost half (45.7%) of cervical cancers are detected early. Diagnosis at a low stage has a 5-year survival of 91.5%, evincing the numerical distinction between the number of women with new diagnoses of cervical cancer and those who die from the disease.

Based on 2007 to 2013 data, the overall 5-year survival for cervical cancer is 67.1%.[2] According to the SEER Program statistical analysis, rates for new cervical cancer cases have not changed significantly over the past 10 years, but death rates have been falling on average 0.8% each year over 2005 to 2014.[1] Attempts to combat the rate of cervical cancer include screening compliance and concurrent development and adherence to appropriate screening guidelines. Additional factors include HPV testing and cervical cytology detection and diagnosis, along with HPV vaccine utilization and efficacy.

Compliance with Screening

Within the past 3 years, an estimated 14 million women aged 21 to 65 had not been screened for cervical cancer. Watson and colleagues,[3] using 2015 National Health Interview Survey data to examine recent cervical cancer screening practices, found that 81.1% of eligible women reported having a Pap test within 3 years. Women without a usual source of income, women without health care, and recent immigrants to the United States had lower odds of being up to date with screening.[4,5] These studies highlight the factors that make adherence to screening guidelines difficult, such as lack of access to health care and low income.

It is additionally problematic that the United States has no national cervical cancer screening program. Screening is then opportunistic, as evidenced by studies showing low income and lack of access to health care prevent women from being up to date with screening. There is also an issue with providers not necessarily following updated screening guidelines, as well as algorithms that might be deemed confusing to follow. Additionally, without a national screening program conveying an overlying message, women may receive varying viewpoints from providers regarding cervical cancer screening and prevention.[2] Such issues delineate the trends causing declines in cervical cancer screening compliance, which is falling below the *Healthy People 2020* goal of 93%.[6]

CERVICAL CANCER SCREENING GUIDELINES: RECENT UPDATES

BASIC PRINCIPLES

The objectives of screening for cervical cancer are to prevent morbidity and mortality from the disease and prevent overtreatment of precursor lesions that will most likely regress. When cervical cancer screening guidelines were established, the emphasis was placed on detecting persistent high-risk HPV (hr-HPV) infection, cervical intraepithelial neoplasia 3 (CIN3), CIN2 in older women, and persistent CIN2 or CIN3. Fundamentals of cervical cancer screening are based on accepting minimal risk, because no screening test is 100% sensitive, and because zero risk cannot be achieved. The optimal balance between benefit and harm is achieved by screening at the least frequent interval. Women with a comparable risk for cancer (CIN3) should be managed similarly, regardless of how the risk is assessed. In 2001, The American Society of Colposcopy and Cervical Pathology (ASCCP) initiated the implementation of a comprehensive, evidence-based consensus guidelines for the clinical management of women diagnosed with abnormal cervical cytology. Since then, several revisions of these guidelines were implemented, as knowledge on the biology of cervical cancer in various age groups has expanded.

Co-testing (Pap and hr-HPV), hr-HPV genotyping, recommendations on post-colposcopy follow-up, and management of women with abnormal cervical cytology between ages 21 to 24 expanded the 2006 guidelines and were incorporated in the new 2012 ASCCP guidelines.[7] **Box 1** is a summary of updates incorporated into the 2012/2014 ASCCP cervical cancer screening guidelines. These guidelines incorporate both cervical cytology and HPV testing in different combination (reflex testing vs co-testing) and are tailored to patients' age and specific patient population (immunocompromised, pregnant, and exposed to diethylstilbestrol in utero).

CERVICAL CYTOLOGY

CHANGES TO IMPROVE SENSITIVITY AND SPECIFICITY

The Papanicolaou test (Pap test) is the most widely accepted and applied cancer screening test, and due to its popularity there has been a dramatic decline in cervical cancer in the United States.[8] The Pap test was named after Georgios Papanicolaou, who studied exfoliative cytology on alcohol-fixed vaginal and cervical specimens. He first announced his method of examining vaginal smears, now commonly known as the "Pap test," at the 1928 Battle Creek conference in Michigan. The basic principles of the Pap test are based on Papanicolaou's meticulous microscopic examinations and descriptions of cytologic characteristics of normal squamous and glandular cells of cervix and a systematic classification of cells at intermediate stages between normal and malignant. Reported sensitivity of conventional Pap test for the detection of $\geq$CIN2+ is 51%, with specificity of 66.6%.[9]

Liquid-based cytology (LBC) is an alternative to conventional Pap smears, and currently most of the screening in the United States is done with LBC.[10] The US Food and Drug Administration (FDA) approved the ThinPrep Pap test (Hologic, Marlborough, MA) in 1996, which uses a methanol-based fixative (PreserveCyt). Cell are homogenized, transferred to a filter via suction, and blotted to a glass slide, resulting in a 20-mm-diameter circular deposit of cells. The SurePath (previously known as Auto-Cyte Prep; BD TriPath, Burlington, NC) was FDA approved in 1999. The transport vial used in these collection methods contains ethanol. An aliquot of the homogenized sample is placed on a density column, and after centrifugation the cells are placed into a chamber and placed on an adhesive slide ultimately yielding a 13-mm circular cellular material.

Box 1
Summary of changes in cervical cancer screening and management according to the 2012 American Society of Colposcopy and Cervical Pathology guidelines

1. Cervical cancer screening should begin at age 21, regardless of age of sexual onset

2. Pap test "alone" in ages 21–29 every 3 years, human papillomavirus (HPV) testing is not used as a screening test

3.. Screening interval for women 30–64 years of age is recommended every 5 years with co-testing or with Pap alone every 3 years

4. Women with HPV-negative atypical squamous cell of undetermined significance should continue screening according to age-specific guidelines

5. Women with positive HPV and negative Pap should be followed with either co-testing at 12 months, or referred to colposcopy if HPV 16/18 genotyping is positive

6.. Screening should stop at age 65 for women with prior adequate negative screening and no history of cervical intraepithelial neoplasia 2 (CIN2) or worse in the past 20 years

7. Screening should stop following total hysterectomy (removal of cervix) if no history of prior CIN2 or worse

8. Screening recommendations are the same in the HPV-vaccinated population

9.. Women with negative cytology but lacking endocervical cells can be managed without early repeat

10. Cytology reported as unsatisfactory requires repeat even if HPV negative

Adapted from Massad LS, Einstein MH, Huh WK, et al. 2012 updated consensus guidelines for the management of abnormal cervical cancer screening tests and cancer precursors. Obstet Gynecol 2013;121(4):832; with permission.

Studies have shown several great advantages of LBC compared with conventional Pap smears, including uniform cellular distribution, better morphologic preservation and visualization, cleaner background, ability to capture nearly all cellular material and presence of more representative (randomized) cell pattern on each slide.[10–14] Both LBC and conventional smears are acceptable for cervical cancer screening and studies have shown no significant difference in relative detection rate, sensitivity, and specificity for the diagnosis of CIN2 or higher.[10] Performance of LBC for the detection of lesions are sensitivity of 42.0% to 73.0% and specificity of 61.6% to 80.1% based on results from the Addressing The Need for Advanced HPV Diagnostics (ATHENA) trial.[15] These advantages of LBC, as well as advancements in computer technology, are the major factors that led to the development of automated screening techniques in cervical cytology. The 2 pillars of automated cervical cancer screening include selection of slides that require a manual review and identification of cells or area on the slide with high probability of abnormality and referred to further human review.

Several studies have shown improved sensitivity, specificity, and productivity for cytologic detection of cervical abnormalities using automated screening methods.[14,16–19] The combination of LBC and computerized automated screening significantly improves accuracy and productivity. The FocalPoint and Focal PointGS (BD/Tripath, Burlington, NC) is a computerized scanning device for both slide analysis (scoring) and location-guided screening, and can be used for both quality control (QC) application and primary screening. The Cytyc ThinPrep Imaging System (Hologic, Marlborough, MA) was FDA approved in 2003. The basic principle of this computer-based slide analysis is the utilization of a Papanicolaou-like stain that is stoichiometric for the DNA contents of the nuclei and identification of cells with abnormal DNA content. The system identifies 22 "high-probability" fields of view for cytotechnologist examination. Factors associated with increased sensitivity of automated computer-assisted cervical cytology screening methods include increased identification of small single cells and hyperchromatic groups, increased detection of low-grade squamous intraepithelial lesion (LSIL), and darker and more vivid staining of nuclei. High correlation of high-grade squamous intraepithelial lesion (HSIL) detected by automated screening techniques with subsequent biopsy results reflects accuracy and high positive predictive value.[14] Understanding the role of hr-HPV types in the pathogenesis of cervical cancer led to

development of various molecular platforms for detection of hr-HPV and subsequent incorporation of molecular testing into cervical cancer screening guidelines. Reported sensitivity of hr-HPV testing is between 88.2% and 90.1% for the detection of $\geq$CIN2+.[20]

Ancillary Studies

Rationale behind using immunomarkers in cervical cytology

Molecular alterations caused by HPV infection of cervical epithelial cells have been investigated as potential targets for immunohistochemistry as an adjunct tool for cervical cancer screening. Theoretically, the 2 major goals the use of immunomarkers could accomplish are (1) increase the accuracy of HSIL detection and (2) identify cases of atypical squamous cell of undetermined significance (ASC-US) and LSIL that will progress to HSIL or invasive cancer. Applications of these biomarkers on residual material from LBC vial have been investigated by several study groups.[21–25] Dysregulation of the cell cycle by integration of hr-HPV viral DNA into the host genome results in continuous expression of E6 and E7 oncoproteins. E6 binds p53, which results in degradation and loss of expression of p53-responsive genes. E7 binds and inactivates pRb, which ultimately leads to release of active E2F and activation of S-phase genes in the epithelial basal layer. The 2 most important activated S-phase genes are p16^{INK4A} and p14^{ARF}. As a result, the p16^{INK4A} feedback loop is bypassed, leading to prolonged activation of E2F and p14^{ARF} overexpression results in inactivation of MDM2, and loss of regulation of p53.

Most commonly used immunomarkers in cervical cytology

Based on the effects of hr-HPV on cell cycle control, the most extensively studied immunomarkers are p16^{INK4A}, MIB-1, BD-ProExC and capsid protein L1. P16^{INK4A} is the most studied and widely used surrogate marker for hr-HPV infection. It is an effective immunomarker for detection of HSIL both in cytologic and histologic preparations. Routine application of p16^{INK4A} in cytologic preparations is challenging due to lack of standardized criteria for positive staining results (nuclear vs nuclear and cytoplasmic), lack of minimal threshold for positivity, and positivity in benign epithelia due to metaplasia and atrophy.[22,24,25]

MIB-1 antibody detects Ki-67 antigen, which is present in all phases of the cell cycle of proliferating cells. In normal squamous epithelium, MIB-1 labeling is restricted to parabasal and basal cell layers. HPV infection results in activation of the cell cycle, which is reflected by increased nuclear MIB-1 labeling. MIB-1 alone has limited utility on cytology preparation, and is better used in combination with p16^{INK4A}. Several studies have concluded that p16^{INK4A} and MIB-1 dual stains improve the accuracy of HSIL detection on LBC and cell block samples.[22,25] The combination of these immunomarkers is also routinely used on histologic preparations to differentiate atrophy from HSIL. BD-ProExC is a cocktail of 2 monoclonal antibodies that target expression of minichromosome maintenance proteins and TOP2A.[23] Parabasal cells of atrophy and metaplastic glandular cells show nuclear expression of ProExC, which can be a pitfall on cytologic preparations. Patchy positivity has also been reported in benign/menstrual endometrial cells.[24] Sensitivity of BD-ProExC for the detection of HSIL is 92% and specificity is 84%.[24,25] Major capsid protein L1 of HPV is expressed in the early productive phase of HPV infection and is later lost during carcinogenesis. Therefore, L1 has the highest level of expression in LSIL and is negative in HSIL due to integration of viral DNA into the host genome.[22,26] Loss of L1 expression also can be seen in latent HPV infection. Combination of p16^{INK4A} and L1 on HPV DNA–positive cytologic samples has been evaluated as a prognostic marker based on the following combination of results: in L1 negative, p16 negative cases viral DNA is present without replication or altering the cell cycle (no dysplasia); L1 positive, p16 negative indicated productive HPV infection without alteration of cell cycle; L1 positive, p16 positive pattern reflects productive infection and alteration of cell cycle and indicated early dysplasia; L1 negative, p16 positive result reflects latent infection or integration of viral DNA and alteration of cell cycle, therefore "advanced" dysplasia.[21]

Quality assurance programs Cytology laboratories must establish and follow written policies and procedures for a comprehensive quality assurance (QA) program. The Clinical Laboratory Improvement Amendments of 1988 set specific standards for cytology, especially Pap tests. Highlights from the regulations list for cytology include workload limits for cytotechnologists, QC procedures (5-year retrospective rescreening, 10% prospective rescreen of negative Pap cases, and cytologic-histologic correlation), pathologist's review of all abnormal cervico-vaginal smears, all nongynecologic specimens, proficiency testing, and unannounced specialized surveys. The 2 major goals of cyto-histologic correlation in cervical pathology are (1) to confirm and resolve Pap and cervical biopsy discrepancies that will impact patient management; and (2) to monitor and improve quality of interpretation by any given laboratory. The rules for cytology QC encompass slide staining, workload limits, and result reporting. More detailed information on QA and QC regulations on cytology laboratory and procedures is available at https://www.cdc.gov/mmwr/preview/mmwrhtml/00016177.htm.

The College of American Pathologists (CAP) recommends that laboratories monitor their ASC/SIL ratio, which is an independent parameter of the laboratories' patient population (disease prevalence). The recommended ratio is between the 5th and 95th percentile, which is 0.7 to 3.4 (median 1.5) for laboratories using ThinPrep cervical cytology, according to the 2006 CAP survey.[27]

LIMITATIONS OF CERVICAL CANCER SCREENING

The widespread use of conventional cervical cytology in countries with well-organized screening programs have resulted in significant decrease in cervical cancer mortality.[8] Traditional cytology-based screening for cervical cancer identifies high-grade precursor lesions that can be treated, and has been used for decades with some success. Despite significant improvements in preparation methods used in cervical cytology and major advancement in technology, the Pap smear still suffers from relatively low sensitivity and interobserver and interlaboratory reproducibility, and cervical cancer remains a significant health concern for several reasons. Interpretation of cervical cytology is subjective, with significant interlaboratory variation in the rate of cytologic abnormalities influenced by the prevalence of disease. Conclusions from the ATHENA (Addressing The Need for Advanced HPV diagnostics) trial, a large interlaboratory study using LBC cervical cytology, showed a strong correlation between a laboratory's overall abnormal rate and sensitivity of cytology. Sensitivity to detect high-grade precursor lesions ranged from 42% (lowest abnormality rate laboratory) to 73% (highest abnormality rate laboratory).[28,29] Additionally, there is significant interobserver variability in the interpretation of cervical cytology. The ASC-US category is a well-known source of disagreement, with only 43% agreement between first review versus QC group review according to the ASCUS-LSIL triage study (ALTS).[29] Similarly, only 47% agreement between primary review versus QC review was achieved for cases in the HSIL category. The high sensitivity of HPV molecular tests to detect ≥CIN2+ lesions is well-known, and it ranges from 88.4% to 90.1%,[15] which is on average 35.7% higher than cytology alone.[10]

Infection by hr-HPV is very common at the time of onset of sexual activity, with the highest prevalence reported in women younger than 25 years of age. Most (80%) hr-HPV infections are transient and spontaneously clear within 2 years, which explains the lower specificity (54.7%–58.4%) of hr-HPV molecular tests for the detection of ≥CIN2+.[15]

THE BETHESDA SYSTEM FOR REPORTING CERVICAL CYTOLOGY: FROM 1988 TO 2014

A variety of nonstandardized terminology and poorly reproducible terms were used in reporting cervical cytology results before implementation of The Bethesda System (TBS) for reporting cervical cytologic diagnoses on 1988. The goal of this uniform reporting system was to provide an effective communication among cytopathologists and referring clinicians, facilitate cytologic-histologic correlation, and further research on the biology and epidemiology of cervical carcinogenesis. The first edition of TBS in 1988 outlined and implemented the 3 major components of cervical cytology reports: (1) evaluation of specimen adequacy, (2) optional general categorization (interpretation), and (3) descriptive diagnosis.[30] A 2-tiered system was used for reporting HPV-associated squamous lesions: LSIL and HSIL. The use of term "atypia" was recommended for both for squamous and glandular cells only if the cause of atypia was unclear (undetermined). A few years later, in 1991, NCI sponsored a follow-up meeting to refine and further standardize reporting and terminology for cervical cytology. The first Bethesda Atlas was published in 1994, which also included interim management guidelines for women with abnormal cervical cytology.[30] The ALTS study provided groundbreaking results not only in the management of women with equivocal cervical cytology results but also in cervical carcinogenesis, which ultimately had major impact in clinical practice habits.[29] Reflex molecular testing for hr-HPV was implemented to triage women with ASC-US cytology, which resulted in up to 50% reduction in colposcopic referrals. The third revision of TBS in 2001 was mainly driven by practice changes and advances in technology and science. Major changes included the replacement of ASC-US by ASC, addition of adenocarcinoma in situ as a distinct category, further subclassifications in the category of atypical glandular cell to reflect concern for neoplasia, and specify glandular cell type (endometrial vs endocervical).[31] Widely available educational methods were implemented such as The Bethesda print atlas, Bethesda Web atlas, and the Web-based Bethesda Interobserver Reproducibility Study to improve consensus and interobserver variability and to identify diagnostic categories with poor agreement. Clinical management of women with abnormal cervical cytology was harmonized with reporting terminology as a result of a multidisciplinary consensus conference organized by ASCCP. The latest 2014 TBS revision was undertaken to reflect decades of experience gained from using liquid-based cervical cytology, use of co-testing, and recently implemented primary hr-HPV testing.[32] Changes related to TBS terminology included (1) age of reporting benign-appearing endometrial cells was changed from 40 to 45, and (2) no new category was created for squamous lesions with LSIL and cells suggestive of concurrent HSIL. The third enhanced edition of the Bethesda Atlas was expanded with more text and illustrations, and additional chapters on adjunctive testing, anal cytology (epidemiology, collection devices, adequacy criteria, high-resolution anoscopy), computer-assisted screening, and cervical cancer risk assessment. A large spectrum of cytologic findings is illustrated by both conventional and liquid-based preparations, including classic examples and common diagnostic dilemmas. Updates on specimen adequacy in certain situations, such as assessment of cellularity in specimens obtained after radiation, obscuring substances (lubricant), and the effect of adequacy on HPV testing are also included.

HUMAN PAPILLOMAVIRUS TESTING UPDATES

GENERAL CONSIDERATIONS

As almost all cases of cervical precancerous (CIN2, CIN3) and cancerous lesions are associated with 14 hr-HPV genotypes (16, 18, 31, 33, 35, 39, 45, 51, 52, 56, 58, 59, 66, and 68), HPV16 and 18 being the most oncogenic. Several studies have confirmed that infection with HPV 31 and 33 also carry significant risk for developing CIN3+ and that most adenocarcinomas are caused by HPV types 18 and 45.[33] High oncogenicity of HPV16 and 18 is attributed to proteins of early genes E6 and E7 that derail normal cell cycle by interfering with tumor suppressor gene p53 (E6) and pRb (E7). Prevalence of hr-HPV infection is the highest in women younger than 25, with a smaller increase in women 40 years of age.[34] Approximately 80% of hr-HPV infections will clear within 2 years. In women with persistent hr-HPV infection of at least 12 months, the risk of developing ≥CIN2+ is 21%.[34] Molecular tests for detection of nucleic acid from hr-HPV serotypes are highly sensitive (92%–95%) with a negative predictive value of 99.58%.[15] Therefore, the combination of Pap and hr-HPV tests provides valuable information for the management of women with increased risk for ≥CIN2+, and in the same time reassures women with negative results of their very low cancer risk. The role of E6 and E7 genes in cervical carcinogenesis is well-established and their overexpression correlates with HPV genome integration. Studies have shown that testing for oncogenic E6/E7 mRNA from hr-HPV has a sensitivity comparable to hr-HPV DNA-based tests for detection of ≥CIN2+ lesions with improved specificity.[35] **Table 1** summarizes the characteristics of currently commercially available FDA-approved HPV testing methodologies in the United States. All of these assays use residual material or a small (1 mL) aliquot from LBC vial and therefore are suitable platforms for HPV testing according to the ASCCP guidelines.

The most commonly identified hr-HPV types in CIN2+ lesions are HPV 16, 18, and 45, and HPV16 and 18 account for more than 70% of cervical cancers. Current guidelines recommend cotesting (hr-HPV testing and cytology) for women 30 years of age and older. Women with negative cytology and positive for hr-HPV should undergo repeat co-testing in 12 months. The alternative option for these women is genotyping for HPV16/18 to identify a subset of women who have the highest risk for developing ≥CIN2+ to be referred to immediate colposcopy.

CO-TESTING AND REFLEX TESTING

The 2012 updated consensus guidelines for management of abnormal cervical cancer screening test and cancer precursors incorporate the use of validated and FDA-approved HPV assays with similar performance characteristics. Testing is restricted to high-risk HPV types (16, 18, 31, 33, 35, 39, 45, 51, 52, 56, 58, and 59) with a clinically valid cutoff to optimize the detection of precancerous or cancerous lesions, and to provide maximum reassurance to women who are not at risk and can be followed at long intervals. Compared with cervical cytology, HPV testing is 20% to 40% more sensitive to detect CIN2 or worse lesions, and has more than 90% sensitivity for detection of CIN3 or worse lesions, with a specificity of 5% to 10% less than cytology. hr-HPV testing is recommended to triage women with ASC-US cytology (reflex testing) and as an adjunct test to cytology for women 30 years and older (co-testing).

There are several cervical cancer screening strategies that use co-testing (cytology and hr-HPV testing) or reflex testing for hr-HPV, which are summarized in **Table 2**.

Potential limitations of co-testing include cost and complicated managerial algorithms, which can be difficult to follow. The 2012 ASCCP guidelines include 18 different algorithms for the management of women with abnormal cervical cytology, and for each patient the results of both tests (cytology and HPV test) have to be taken into account.[7]

HUMAN PAPILLOMAVIRUS TESTING AS A PRIMARY SCREENING METHOD

hr-HPV testing as a primary screening modality for cervical cancer has already been implemented in several countries, including Australia and the Netherlands, where hr-HPV testing is also used as a surveillance test in women treated for CIN. Potential benefits and advantages of primary hr-HPV testing include higher sensitivity and earlier detection of CIN3, lower cost, and more simplified management of patients with abnormal results. The ATHENA was the first large prospective study in the United States evaluating the HPV molecular test as a primary screening test for cervical cancer. The basic principle behind the HPV primary screening strategy is that HPV types 16 and 18 together cause approximately 70% of cervical cancers. HPV 16 is more often seen in squamous lesions, and HPV 18 is frequently seen in glandular lesions. When HPV testing is used as a primary screening method for cervical cancer, HPV 16/18–positive women are referred to colposcopy, and cytology becomes a reflex test or a triage test for non–16/18 HPV–positive patients. Women from the latter group are referred to colposcopy if their cytology returns as ASC-US or worse. Conclusions from the ATHENA study show that HPV primary screening has increased sensitivity for the detection of CIN3+ in women older than 25 years, compared with cytology and combination of cytology and HPV testing. As more women get HPV vaccination, there is an anticipated decrease in HPV 16/18–associated lesions and prevalence of disease in the future. These changes will result in decreased sensitivity of cervical cytology and potentially make cytologic interpretation even more challenging.

HUMAN PAPILLOMAVIRUS–NEGATIVE CERVICAL CANCER

Infection with hr-HPV is a necessary step in the development of most cervical squamous cell carcinoma and its precursors. The classic high-risk types are HPV 16 and HPV 18, and classic low-risk types are HPV 6 and HPV 11. There are, however, types of cervical carcinomas that are not HPV-associated, which include clear cell adenocarcinoma, mesonephric adenocarcinoma, gastric-type adenocarcinoma, minimal deviation

Table 1
Currently commercially available FDA-approved HPV testing methodologies in the United States

Test	Manufacturer	HPV Types Detected	Method	Option for Genotyping	Automation	Internal Control	Specimen Volume	Analytical Sensitivity	Potential Disadvantages
Hr-HC2	Qiagen (Hilden, Germany)	Pooled detection of 13 hr-HPV[b]	Signal amplification ELISA	No	Dilution and pipetting only	None	4 mL	5000 DNA copies	Cross hybridization with lr-HPV and hr-HPV types, false-positive results if pBR322 present
Cervista	Hologic, Marlborough, MA	Pooled detection of 14 hr-HPV[c]	Invader chemistry DNA genomic sequences of L1, E6, and E7 HPV	Yes HPV 16/18	Highly automated	Human histone gene 2	2 mL	1250–7500 DNA copies	Cross reactivity with HPV 67, 70,[a] HPV 33, 35, 56, and 59 cannot be reliably detected at 5000 copies
Aptima	Hologic Marlborough, MA	Qualitative detection of E6/E7 mRNA from 14 hr-HPV[c]	Transcription mediated amplification	Yes HPV 16, 18/45	Fully automated	Positive and negative controls	1 mL	200 mRNA copies	Cross reactivity with lr-HPV 26, 67, 70, 82
Cobas	Roche Molecular Diagnostics, Branchburg, NJ	L1 region of 14 hr-HPV[c] genome	Real-time PCR	Yes, simultaneous for HPV 16, 18	Fully automated	Human β-globin	1 mL	600 copies of DNA	Sample needs to be prealiquoted before cytology processing

Abbreviations: E6/7, early genes 6 and 7; ELISA, enzyme-linked immunosorbent assay; FDA, Food and Drug Administration; HC2, hybrid capture 2 for hr-HPV; HPV, human papillomavirus; hr-HPV, high-risk human papilloma virus; L1, late gene 1; lr-HPV, low-risk human papilloma virus; PCR, polymerase chain reaction.
[a] HPV 67 and 70 have no known cervical cancer risk association.
[b] 13 hr-HPV types include: 16, 18, 31, 33, 35, 39, 45, 51, 52, 56, 58, 59 and 68.
[c] 14 hr-HPV types include: 16, 18, 31, 33, 35, 39, 45, 51, 52, 56, 58, 59, 66 and 68.

Data from Laudadio J. Human papillomavirus detection: testing methodologies and their clinical utility in cervical cancer screening. Adv Anat Pathol 2013;20(3):158–67.

Table 2
Comparison of different combinations of cytology and HPV testing for cervical cancer screening

Primary Test	Secondary Test	Threshold for Colposcopy	Age Range	Sensitivity, %	False-Positive Rate, %	Included in 2012 ASCCP Guidelines
1. Cytology	Reflex HPV testing for ASC-US	ASC-US HPV+ or >ASC-US	21 or older	51.4	12.0	Yes
2. HPV and Pap test (co-testing)	N/A	ASC-US HPV+ or >ASC-US	30 or older	51.4	12.0	Yes
3. HPV with 16/18 genotyping and Pap test (co-testing)	N/A	ASC-US HPV+, >ASC-US, NILM HPV 16/18+	30 or older	67.5	18.0	Yes
4. HPV with 16/18 genotyping and Pap test (co-testing)	N/A	LSIL or NILM/ASC-US with HPV16/18+	30 or older	61.8	15.2	Yes
5. HPV with reflex Pap test	Pap test	HPV+ ASC-US		47.5	8.2	No
5. HPV with 16/18 genotyping	Pap test if HPV 16/18−	HPV 16/18+ or ASC-US Pap	30 or older	63.6	14.3	No

Abbreviations: ASCCP, American Society of Colposcopy and Cervical Pathology; ASC-US, atypical squamous cell of undetermined significance; HPV, human papillomavirus; LSIL, low-grade squamous intraepithelial lesion; N/A, not applicable; NILM, negative for intraepithelial lesion and malignancy; +, positive; −, negative.

Adapted from Cox JT, Castle PE, Behrens CM, et al. Comparison of cervical cancer screening strategies incorporating different combinations of cytology, HPV testing, and genotyping for HPV 16/18: results from the ATHENA HPV study. Am J Obstet Gynecol 2013;208(3):184.e7; with permission.

adenocarcinoma (adenoma malignum), and a subset of serous carcinomas.[36] Because of the high sensitivity (97%–98%) of the currently used and clinically validated HPV tests for detection of CIN3, the very small portion on CIN3 lesions that test negative for HPV are presumed to represent false-negative samples.[37] Often these samples test positive for HPV with a different molecular method. Other less common causes of false-negative results include non–hr-HPV types as a causative agent, such as HPV 73 and 82, or limitations in the detection HPV 52.[37] Detection of HPV 52 by the Liner Array-HPV assay is done using probes that cross-hybridize with probes specific for HPV 33, 35, and 58 and is confirmed only if there is no hybridization with probes specific for HPV 33, 35, and 58. Otherwise, concurrent infection with HPV 52, and the 3 aforementioned genotypes cannot be detected.[38]

Glandular lesions demonstrate limitations in cervical cytology as well as in HPV testing. Oncogenic HPV-negative results are more common in adenocarcinomas and cancers that are in a more advanced stage and higher grade.[39] The CAP Interlaboratory Comparison Program in Cervical

Cytology showed false-negative rates of 11.7% for adenocarcinoma in situ and 8.9% for adenocarcinoma.[40] These false-negative rates and negative HPV results demonstrate the difficulty of detecting and diagnosing these lesions.

IMPACT ON HUMAN PAPILLOMAVIRUS VACCINATION ON CERVICAL CANCER SCREENING

There are currently 3 licensed HPV vaccines: Cervarix, which protects against types 16 and 18; Gardasil, which protects against types 6, 11, 16, and 18; and Gardasil 9, which covers additional types 31, 33, 45, 52, and 58. The vaccination protocol consists of 3 doses at intervals of 0, 2, and 6 months. HPV vaccination was implemented in 2006 for girls and in 2011 for boys in the United States. Studies have shown compliance issues in following through with all 3 doses of the vaccine for both genders. Coverage with ≥1 dose of the vaccine has increased from 53.0% for girls and 8.3% for boys in 2011 to 62.8% for girls and 49.8% for boys in 2015 (ages 13–17 years). As of

2015, 41.9% of adolescent girls had received all 3 doses of the vaccine.[41]

Vaccine penetrance differs among countries due to vaccine delivery systems. Canada, Australia, and England have school-based vaccine delivery systems with national insurance.[42] The United States, however, relies on doctors' offices and public and private insurance for vaccine access. Additional issues in vaccination revolve around not only access and cost, but social and interpersonal attitudes. Concerns regarding vaccination safety and association with increased incidence of sexually transmitted infections have been mitigated through multiple studies.[43]

Increased vaccination, however, presents an interesting diagnostic dilemma in cervical cancer screening in that a reduction in the prevalence of high-risk HPV types is expected to cause a decrease in positive predictive value of cervical cancer screening. This decrease in positive predictive value could potentially cause more false positives and consequently overtreatment. A change in the epidemiology of cervical cancer from vaccination is also not expected for decades due to the lag time between HPV infection acquisition and development of malignancy.[44]

REFERENCES

1. National Cancer Institute. 2014. Available at: https://seer.cancer.gov/statfacts/html/cervix.html. Accessed May 12, 2017.
2. National Health Interview Survey, 2015. Public-use Data File and Documentation: National Center for Health Statistics, Centers for Disease Control and Prevention. 2016. Available at: http://www.cdc.gov/nchs/nhis/. Accessed May 12, 2017.
3. Watson M, Benard V, King J, et al. National assessment of HPV and Pap tests: changes in cervical cancer screening, National Health Interview Survey. Prev Med 2017;100:243–7.
4. Tangka FK, Howard DH, Royalty J, et al. Cervical cancer screening of underserved women in the United States: results from the National Breast and Cervical Cancer Early Detection Program, 1997-2012. Cancer Causes Control 2015;26(5):671–86.
5. Tsui J, Saraiya M, Thompson T, et al. Cervical cancer screening among foreign-born women by birthplace and duration in the United States. J Womens Health (Larchmt) 2007;16(10):1447–57.
6. Healthy People 2020 [internet]. Washington, DC: U.S. Department of Health and Human Services. Office of Disease Prevention and Health Promotion; 2016. Available at: https://www.cdc.gov/nchs/healthy_people/hp2020/hp2020_data_issues.htm.
7. Massad LS, Einstein MH, Huh WK, et al. 2012 updated consensus guidelines for the management of abnormal cervical cancer screening tests and cancer precursors. Obstet Gynecol 2013;121(4):829–46.
8. Benard VB, Watson M, Saraiya M, et al. Cervical cancer survival in the United States by race and stage (2001-2009): findings from the CONCORD-2 study. Cancer 2017;123(Suppl 24):5119–37.
9. Karimi-Zarchi M, Peighmbari F, Karimi N, et al. A comparison of 3 ways of conventional pap smear, liquid-based cytology and colposcopy vs cervical biopsy for early diagnosis of premalignant lesions or cervical cancer in women with abnormal conventional pap test. Int J Biomed Sci 2013;9(4):205–10.
10. Whitlock EP, Vesco KK, Eder M, et al. Liquid-based cytology and human papillomavirus testing to screen for cervical cancer: a systematic review for the U.S. Preventive Services Task Force. Ann Intern Med 2011;155(10):687–97. W214–5.
11. Ronco G, Cuzick J, Pierotti P, et al. Accuracy of liquid based versus conventional cytology: overall results of new technologies for cervical cancer screening: randomised controlled trial. BMJ 2007;335(7609):28.
12. Ronco G, Giorgi-Rossi P, Carozzi F, et al. Efficacy of human papillomavirus testing for the detection of invasive cervical cancers and cervical intraepithelial neoplasia: a randomised controlled trial. Lancet Oncol 2010;11(3):249–57.
13. Siebers AG, Klinkhamer PJ, Grefte JM, et al. Comparison of liquid-based cytology with conventional cytology for detection of cervical cancer precursors: a randomized controlled trial. JAMA 2009;302(16):1757–64.
14. Halford JA, Batty T, Boost T, et al. Comparison of the sensitivity of conventional cytology and the ThinPrep Imaging System for 1,083 biopsy confirmed high-grade squamous lesions. Diagn Cytopathol 2010;38(5):318–26.
15. Wright TC Jr, Stoler MH, Behrens CM, et al. Interlaboratory variation in the performance of liquid-based cytology: insights from the ATHENA trial. Int J Cancer 2014;134(8):1835–43.
16. Chivukula M, Saad RS, Elishaev E, et al. Introduction of the Thin Prep Imaging System (TIS): experience in a high volume academic practice. CytoJournal 2007;4:6.
17. Bolger N, Heffron C, Regan I, et al. Implementation and evaluation of a new automated interactive image analysis system. Acta Cytol 2006;50(5):483–91.
18. Davey E, Irwig L, Macaskill P, et al. Cervical cytology reading times: a comparison between ThinPrep Imager and conventional methods. Diagn Cytopathol 2007;35(9):550–4.
19. Lozano R. Comparison of computer-assisted and manual screening of cervical cytology. Gynecol Oncol 2007;104(1):134–8.
20. Laudadio J. Human papillomavirus detection: testing methodologies and their clinical utility in cervical cancer screening. Adv Anat Pathol 2013;20(3):158–67.

21. Yoshida T, Sano T, Kanuma T, et al. Immunochemical analysis of HPV L1 capsid protein and p16 protein in liquid-based cytology samples from uterine cervical lesions. Cancer 2008;114(2):83–8.

22. Yu L, Wang L, Zhong J, et al. Diagnostic value of p16INK4A, Ki-67, and human papillomavirus L1 capsid protein immunochemical staining on cell blocks from residual liquid-based gynecologic cytology specimens. Cancer Cytopathol 2010;118(1):47–55.

23. Alaghehbandan R, Fontaine D, Bentley J, et al. Performance of ProEx C and PreTect HPV-Proofer E6/E7 mRNA tests in comparison with the hybrid capture 2 HPV DNA test for triaging ASCUS and LSIL cytology. Diagn Cytopathol 2013;41(9):767–75.

24. Ge Y, Mody DR, Smith D, et al. p16(INK4a) and ProEx C immunostains facilitate differential diagnosis of hyperchromatic crowded groups in liquid-based Papanicolaou tests with menstrual contamination. Acta Cytol 2012;56(1):55–61.

25. Pinto AP, Degen M, Villa LL, et al. Immunomarkers in gynecologic cytology: the search for the ideal 'biomolecular Papanicolaou test'. Acta Cytol 2012; 56(2):109–21.

26. Griesser H, Sander H, Hilfrich R, et al. Correlation of immunochemical detection of HPV L1 capsid protein in pap smears with regression of high-risk HPV positive mild/moderate dysplasia. Anal Quant Cytol Histol 2004;26(5):241–5.

27. Eversole GM, Moriarty AT, Schwartz MR, et al. Practices of participants in the College of American Pathologists interlaboratory comparison program in cervicovaginal cytology, 2006. Arch Pathol Lab Med 2010;134(3):331–5.

28. Cox JT, Castle PE, Behrens CM, et al. Comparison of cervical cancer screening strategies incorporating different combinations of cytology, HPV testing, and genotyping for HPV 16/18: results from the ATHENA HPV study. Am J Obstet Gynecol 2013; 208(3):184.e1-11.

29. Stoler MH, Schiffman M, Atypical Squamous Cells of Undetermined Significance-Low-grade Squamous Intraepithelial Lesion Triage Study Group. Interobserver reproducibility of cervical cytologic and histologic interpretations: realistic estimates from the ASCUS-LSIL Triage Study. JAMA 2001;285(11):1500–5.

30. Nayar R, Wilbur DC. The Bethesda System for reporting cervical cytology: a historical perspective. Acta Cytol 2017;61(4–5):359–72.

31. Solomon D, Davey D, Kurman R, et al. The 2001 Bethesda System: terminology for reporting results of cervical cytology. JAMA 2002;287(16):2114–9.

32. Nayar R, Wilbur DC. The Pap test and Bethesda 2014. Cancer Cytopathol 2015;123(5):271–81.

33. Kjaer SK, Frederiksen K, Munk C, et al. Long-term absolute risk of cervical intraepithelial neoplasia grade 3 or worse following human papillomavirus infection: role of persistence. J Natl Cancer Inst 2010;102(19):1478–88.

34. Rodriguez AC, Schiffman M, Herrero R, et al. Rapid clearance of human papillomavirus and implications for clinical focus on persistent infections. J Natl Cancer Inst 2008;100(7):513–7.

35. Reid JL, Wright TC Jr, Stoler MH, et al. Human papillomavirus oncogenic mRNA testing for cervical cancer screening: baseline and longitudinal results from the CLEAR study. Am J Clin Pathol 2015;144(3): 473–83.

36. McCluggage WG. New developments in endocervical glandular lesions. Histopathology 2013;62(1): 138–60.

37. Petry KU, Cox JT, Johnson K, et al. Evaluating HPV-negative CIN2+ in the ATHENA trial. Int J Cancer 2016;138(12):2932–9.

38. Monsonego J, Cox JT, Behrens C, et al. Prevalence of high-risk human papilloma virus genotypes and associated risk of cervical precancerous lesions in a large U.S. screening population: data from the ATHENA trial. Gynecol Oncol 2015;137(1):47–54.

39. Hopenhayn C, Christian A, Christian WJ, et al. Prevalence of human papillomavirus types in invasive cervical cancers from 7 US cancer registries before vaccine introduction. J Low Genit Tract Dis 2014; 18(2):182–9.

40. Davey DD, Neal MH, Wilbur DC, et al. Bethesda 2001 implementation and reporting rates: 2003 practices of participants in the College of American Pathologists Interlaboratory Comparison Program in Cervicovaginal Cytology. Arch Pathol Lab Med 2004;128(11):1224–9.

41. Lehtinen M, Apter D. Gender-neutrality, herd effect and resilient immune response for sustainable impact of HPV vaccination. Curr Opin Obstet Gynecol 2015;27(5):326–32.

42. Fisher H, Audrey S, Mytton JA, et al. Examining inequalities in the uptake of the school-based HPV vaccination programme in England: a retrospective cohort study. J Public Health (Oxf) 2014;36(1): 36–45.

43. Zhu Y, Wang Y, Hirschhorn J, et al. Human papillomavirus and its testing assays, cervical cancer screening, and vaccination. Adv Clin Chem 2017; 81:135–92.

44. Massad LS, Einstein M, Myers E, et al. The impact of human papillomavirus vaccination on cervical cancer prevention efforts. Gynecol Oncol 2009;114(2): 360–4.

Diagnostic Advances in Urine Cytology

Juan Xing, MD[a], Jordan P. Reynolds, MD[b],*

KEYWORDS

• Bladder cancer • Paris system • Urothelial carcinoma

Key points

- The Paris system for reporting urinary cytology is the most current classification method and it is based on both cytologic criteria and consensus on reporting schemes.

- The major diagnostic criterion for determining high-grade urothelial carcinoma is increased nuclear-to-cytoplasmic ratio, and the minor criteria include nuclear hyperchromasia, nuclear irregularity, and clumped chromatin.

- There are many benign entities that may mimic urothelial carcinoma, therefore leading to overdiagnosis.

- Ancillary testing is currently used with fluorescence in situ hybridization (UroVysion [Des Planes, IL]), the most commonly used test. Further validation is needed for ancillary testing for routine use in screening and detection of bladder cancer.

ABSTRACT

The utility of urine cytology has shifted from the identification of red blood cells, crystals, or parasites to its currently used role of detection of cancer cells exfoliated in urine samples. A variety of ancillary tests have been developed to complement the diagnostic ability of urine cytology. Furthermore, urine testing will continue to evolve as the pathogenesis of genitourinary tract diseases in depth is understood. This article focuses on the diagnostic advances in urine cytology from the cytomorphological perspective, past and current reporting schemes, and the application of ancillary testing in urine samples.

microscopic examination conducted by cytopathologists.[1] Using urine cytology to detect cancer cells was first introduced by Dr Hermann Lebert in 1845 and Dr Vilem D. Lamble in 1856.[2,3] Dr William R. Sanders subsequently contributed to this subject in 1864.[4] Detection of cancer cells using urine cytology, however, did not gain mainstream popularity until 1945 after Drs George Papanicolaou and Victor F. Marshall[5] published their original work. Since then, urine cytology for identifying cancer cells has been integrated into routine urologic diagnosis and continues to play an important role in the diagnosis of urothelial carcinoma. Currently, urine cytology is still the best available test for diagnosing, screening, and monitoring bladder cancer and referred to as "good old cytology" by Dr DeMay.[2]

HISTORY OF URINE CYTOLOGY

Examination of urine is one of the oldest medical tests and has evolved from visual fluid inspection by ancient Egyptians and Greeks to routine

PAST URINE CYTOLOGY DIAGNOSTIC CRITERIA AND REPORTING SCHEMES

Although examination of urine has been used in medicine for centuries, the detailed

Disclosure Statement: The authors have nothing to disclose.

[a] University of Pittsburgh Medical Center, UPMC Shadyside Hospital, 5150 Centre Avenue, POB2, Suite 201.2, Pittsburgh, PA 15232, USA; [b] Cleveland Clinic Foundation, Pathology and Laboratory Medicine Institute, Cleveland Clinic, 9500 Euclid Avenue, Cleveland, OH 44195, USA
* Corresponding author.
E-mail address: reynolj4@ccf.org

Surgical Pathology 11 (2018) 601–610
https://doi.org/10.1016/j.path.2018.06.001

surgpath.theclinics.com

cytomorphological description of cancer cells and reporting system were not proposed until Drs Papanicolaou and Marshall published their original work in 1947.[5,6] They studied cytologic findings of 240 cases and correlated the results with histologic diagnoses and found that urine cytology had high positive predictive value for urothelial carcinoma. The diagnostic criteria originally described included nuclear abnormalities, such as enlargement, anisonucleosis, hyperchromasia, coarse chromatin pattern, and prominence of nucleolus; cytoplasmic changes, including basophilia; and vacuolization as well as significant changes in their shape and size compared with their normal counterparts. In addition, a classification scheme consisting of 5 classes for reporting urine cytology was also proposed by Dr Papanicolaou: (1) absence of abnormal or atypical cells; (2) atypical cells present but without abnormal features; (3) cells with abnormal features but not sufficiently pathognomonic; (4) fair number of pathognomonic cells and cell clusters; and (5) large number of conclusive cells and cell clusters. Although the classification system was proposed, rigorous cytologic criteria for each specific category were not defined in this reporting scheme.

Although Dr Papanicolaou established the fundamental role of urine cytology in diagnosing bladder cancer, Dr Leopold G. Koss[7] made subsequent numerous contributions to the fields of urine cytology and cytopathology in general. Among his notable works, Koss first began to correlate the cytopathology and histopathology. He described the cytomorphologic features of urine cytology based on the 1973 World Health Organization classification of bladder cancer and pointed out that diagnosing of bladder cancers should depend on both architectural and nuclear abnormalities.[8] He also observed that it was extremely difficult to diagnose low-grade papillary tumors unless papillary fragments with fibrovascular cores were present.[9] The cytomorphologic features supporting malignancy included variable size and configuration with a very high nucleus-to-cytoplasmic (N:C) ratio, nuclear hyperchromasia, irregular nuclear membranes, abnormal chromatin texture, and high cellularity. Among them, hyperchromasia was the most important diagnostic feature.[9] He also addressed the issue of atypical urothelial cells and subclassified them into atypical 1 cells (ATY1) with hyperchromasia and predominantly round or oval contours and atypical 2 cells (ATY2) with hyperchromias and nuclear membrane irregularity. Based on his observation, Koss proposed his classification scheme: (1) benign cells; (2) ATY1 cells and few clusters; (3) clusters, nuclear elongation, and few

ATY2 cells; and (4) malignant tumor cells and many ATY2 cells. The first 2 classes corresponded to histologic benign conditions. Class 3 corresponded to histologic low-grade neoplasms (eg, papilloma and grade 1 papillary carcinoma) and class 4 to high-grade carcinomas (eg, grades 2 and 3 papillary carcinoma and carcinoma in situ).

A few recent urine cytology classification schemes have also been proposed in the literature (Table 1).[10–13] Murphy and colleagues[10] suggested a classification system in 1984. They described morphologic features that might be useful for identifying low-grade urothelial tumors in addition to the features of high-grade neoplasms. They observed that papillary and loose clusters, increased cellularity, eccentric nuclear location with more granular chromatin pattern, 1 or 2 nuclear indentions, and lack of prominent nucleoli were often associated with low-grade lesions. There was lack of consensus, however, on these features. Later, Ooms and Veldhuizen[11] proposed another classification scheme in 1993 and reported that more single cells and greater nuclear atypia were associated with increased tumor grade. In 2004, the Papanicolaou Society of Cytopathology Task Force published recommendations for reporting urine cytology in a format similar to the 2001 Bethesda System for reporting cervical cytology.[12] The Johns Hopkins Hospital template was published in 2013. They observed that the most common morphologic features that were associated with increased risk for high-grade urothelial carcinoma included hyperchromasia, irregular nuclear borders, increased N:C ratio, and anisonucleosis whereas hyperchromasia was the strongest predictor.[13,14]

Nevertheless, none of these reporting schemes gained broad acceptance due to lack of validated diagnostic criteria for each specific category and lack of consensus for indeterminant diagnoses.[15] The indeterminant diagnostic category may cause unnecessary stress to patients and create management dilemmas for clinicians. Therefore, there was a crucial need to develop a standardized terminology with specific diagnostic criteria in urine cytology.

THE PARIS SYSTEM FOR REPORTING URINARY CYTOLOGY

The Paris system for reporting urinary cytology (TPSRUC) was initiated at the 2013 International Congress of Cytology in Paris and the final work was published in 2016.[16] The multidisciplinary

Table 1
Summary of previously proposed reporting systems for urine cytology in the literature

Urine Cytology Classification			
Murphy (1984)	**Ooms (1993)**	**Papanicolaou Society of Cytopathology (2004)**	**Hopkins Template (2013)**
Negative/reactive	Negative cytology	I. Adequacy statement	No urothelial atypia or dysplasia
Dysplastic cells	Atypical cells	II. General categorization	Atypical urothelial cells of uncertain significance
Suspicious for malignancy	Suspicious for malignancy	Negative	Atypical urothelial cells, cannot exclude high-grade carcinoma
Malignant tumor cells	Neoplastic cells present	Epithelial cell abnormality	Urothelial carcinoma
Low-grade neoplasm	Grade 1 carcinoma	III. Descriptive diagnosis	low-grade urothelial carcinoma
High-grade neoplasm	Grade 2 carcinoma	Negative	high-grade urothelial carcinoma
Squamous cell carcinoma	Grade 3 carcinoma	Infectious agents	Inadequate
Undifferentiated malignant tumor	Carcinoma in situ	Nonspecific inflammatory changes	
Nonepithelial neoplasm	Squamous cell carcinoma	Cellular changes associated with chemotherapy or radiation	
	Adenocarcinoma	Epithelial cell abnormality	
	Small cell carcinoma	Atypical	
	Others	Low-grade urothelial carcinoma	
		High-grade urothelial carcinoma	
		Squamous cell carcinoma	
		Adenocarcinoma	
		IV. Others	

task force included cytopathologists, surgical pathologists, and urologists.

Compared with other reporting schemes, TPSRUC acknowledges the suboptimal sensitivity of diagnosing low-grade lesions by urine cytology as well as the distinct pathogenesis of low-grade and high-grade urothelial neoplasms. TPSRUC is focused on detecting more clinically significant lesions—for example, high-grade urothelial carcinoma. Based on this fundamental principle, TPSRUC created the following diagnostic categories: (1) adequacy; (2) negative for high-grade urothelial carcinoma; (3) atypical urothelial cells; (4) suspicious for high-grade urothelial carcinoma; (5) high-grade urothelial carcinoma; (6) low-grade urothelial neoplasia; and (7) other malignancies. Diagnostic criteria were described for each specific category (**Table 2**) and an adequacy algorithm was recommended based on available literature, evidence-based studies, and expert consensus. Applying these criteria to each specimen helps to justify using each diagnostic category. For example, **Fig. 1** demonstrates cells with hyperchromasia and nuclear irregularity with clumpy chromatin (minor criteria). Due to the ample amount of cytoplasm present, however, the N:C ratio falls in the 0.5 to 0.7 range. These cells are best classified under the "suspicious for high-grade urothelial carcinoma" category. **Fig. 2** illustrates 3 examples having all of the features necessary to render a diagnosis of "positive for high-grade urothelial carcinoma," including an N:C ratio of 0.7, hyperchromasia, nuclear irregularity, and coarse chromatin.

Although classification systems have been applied in the past, as described previously and in **Table 1**, TPSRUC is the first standardized terminology for urinary cytology that is evidence based and consensus based. It is also the first reporting scheme that defines specific diagnostic criteria for each individual category and recommends an adequacy algorithm. Recent studies have been

Table 2
Diagnostic criteria of the Paris system for reporting urinary cytology

Atypical Urothelial Cells	Suspicious for High-Grade Urothelial Carcinoma	High-Grade Urothelial Carcinoma	Low-Grade Urothelial Neoplasia
Major criterion (required) N:C ratio >0.5 Minor criteria (1 required) Hyperchromasia Irregular nuclear membranes Irregular clumpy chromatin	Major criterion (required) N:C ratio, at least 0.5–0.7 Hyperchromasia Minor criteria (1 required) Marked irregular nuclear membranes Irregular clumpy chromatin Less than 5–10 abnormal cells	Major criterion (required) N:C ratio >0.7 Hyperchromasia Marked irregular nuclear membranes Coarse chromatin More than 5–10 abnormal cells	3-D cellular papillary clusters with fibrovascular cores, including capillaries

From Rosenthal DL, Wojcik E, Kurtycz DF. The Paris system for reporting urinary cytology. New York: Springer; 2016; with permission.

performed to validate this new classification system and have demonstrated better performance with lower atypical rates and high reproducibility with improved risk stratification for the development of high-grade urothelial carcinoma.[17,18]

CORRELATION WITH CYSTOSCOPY FINDINGS

Although gross features of the urine sample are not important, the cystoscopic findings of the urologist are and should be correlated with cytologic examination. Visualization of a papillary lesion may support a papillary urothelial carcinoma.

Erythematous areas may indicate the presence of carcinoma in situ. Image enhancing techniques, such as use of blue light (or hexaminolevulinate) or white light may aid the urologist in findings subtle flat lesions. Previously resected areas may present as a scar on cystoscopy.

CYTOMORPHOLOGIC EXAMINATION AND DIFFERENTIAL DIAGNOSIS

The normal urine cytology specimen may consist of a wide variety of normal cellular elements, such as squamous cells, urothelial cells, umbrella

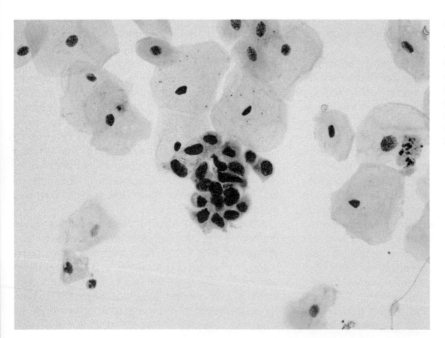

Fig. 1. Papanicolaou stain ×40: The N:C ratio is between 0.5 and 0.7; however, the cells in question demonstrate nuclear irregularity and hyperchromasia with clumped chromatin. This should be classified as high-grade urothelial carcinoma.

Fig. 2. (*A–C*) Papanicolaou stain ×40: these examples each demonstrate all of the cytologic features necessary to render a diagnosis of "positive for high-grade urothelial carcinoma," as described by the Paris system: N:C ratio of greater than 0.7, marked nuclear irregularity, hyperchromasia, and clumped chromatin.

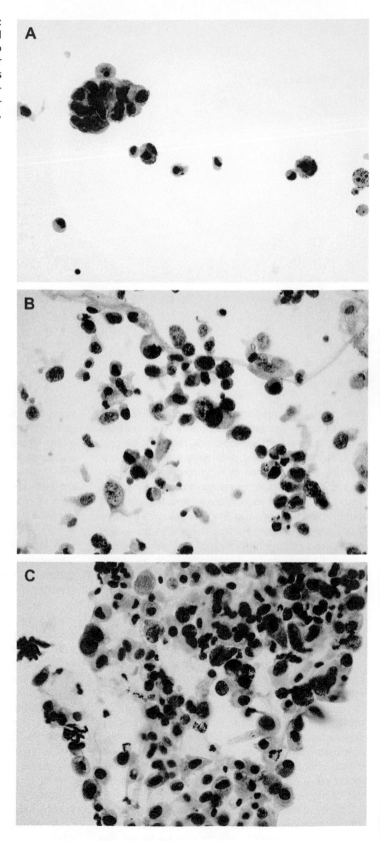

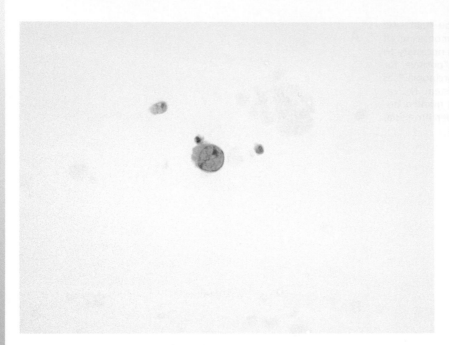

Fig. 3. Papanicolaou stain ×40: this urothelial cell is infected by polyoma virus and demonstrates nuclear enlargement with an increased N:C ratio. The cobweb-like inclusions are present in the nuclear membrane.

cells, and inflammatory cells. Extracellular elements, such as proteinaceous casts, corpora amylacea, and bacterial colonies, may also be present. Normal urothelial cells have a small nucleus without irregularity or hyperchromasia and they may appear in groups or as single cells. Superficial umbrella cells can show more bizarre features and exhibit binucleation with pleomorphism but maintain a low N:C ratio. Benign cells have an evenly distributed chromatin pattern. Urine samples obtained via instrumented methods, such as catheterization or bladder washing (barbotage), typically have higher cellularity compared with voided samples. Clusters of cells in papillary formations may be more prominent in these samples, but they lack a fibrovascular core characteristic of papillary carcinomas.

As discussed previously, the microscopic features of urothelial carcinoma have been documented historically and have since been honed to specific diagnostic criteria. The 4 findings most commonly found in urothelial carcinoma are increased N:C ratio, nuclear irregularity, clumped chromatin, and nuclear hyperchromasia. Use of digital imaging to measure nuclear size and N:C ratio further demonstrated that N:C ratio is predictive of high-grade urothelial carcinoma.[19]

There are many non-neoplastic entities that may mimic features worrisome for urothelial carcinoma. Viral cytopathic effects can be found, the most common of which is polyomavirus cellular change. Viral inclusions characterized by nuclear enlargement, glassy homogeneous appearance, and organized cobweb-like stranding of the nuclear material is present (**Fig. 3**). Ancillary techniques are available, including the SV40 immunocytochemistry stain, as well as fluorescence in situ hybridization (FISH) for BK virus. Polymerase chain reaction (PCR) testing to assess viral load. Infection with other viruses, such as herpesvirus and cytomegalovirus, may exhibit viral cytopathologic effects.[2] Other reactive cellular changes may also occur in the setting of treatment of another malignancy.[20] Chemotherapeutic agents and radiation may cause cytomegaly and nuclear atypia in benign urothelial cells. Architectural changes, especially papillary structures, can pose a diagnostic challenge in urine cytology. Benign urothelial tissue fragments appearing as papillary clusters caused by urolithiasis, indwelling catherization, or instrumented urine specimens may be overinterpreted as neoplasia.[21] Presence of a true fibrovascular core and correlation with the biopsy findings can be helpful in diagnosing low-grade urothelial neoplasms. For cases of definitive malignancy, clinical correlation may be necessary in some cases to exclude direct invasion from prostate, uterine, or colorectal primaries or even distant metastases from other primary sites.

Differential Diagnosis
BENIGN MIMICKERS OF UROTHELIAL CARCINOMA

- Reactive changes
  - Squamous metaplasia
  - Changes associated with cystitis cystica
- Viral
  - Cytomegalovirus, polyomavirus, herpesvirus
- Iatrogenic
  - Chemotherapy effect
  - Bacillus Calmette-Guérin treatment-related effect
  - Radiation changes

Differential Diagnosis
PAPILLARY STRUCTURES IN URINE

- Instrumentation effect
  - Bladder washing
  - Ureteral brushing
  - Long term in dwelling catheterization
- Urinary stones
  - Bladder calculi
  - Upper tract stones
- Low-grade urothelial neoplasm

Differential Diagnosis
NONUROTHELIAL MALIGNANCIES

- Tumors present via direct invasion
  - Prostatic
  - Endometrial
  - Colorectal
- Tumors present via distant metastases
  - Melanoma
  - Lung cancer
  - Others

DIAGNOSTIC UTILITY OF URINE CYTOLOGY

Urine cytology has been credited as an easy, safe, and inexpensive test with high specificity for diagnosing high-grade urothelial carcinoma; however, its sensitivity is not optimal, especially for low-grade urothelial carcinoma. Prior to TPSRUC, many cytologic features of low-grade carcinomas have been described but have not been validated and these account for a high rate of indeterminate diagnoses. Many ancillary tests have been developed to overcome the suboptimal sensitivity associated with urine cytology but demonstrate similar performance.

The main goal of TPSRUC is to detect high-grade urothelial carcinoma. By separating low-grade lesions from categories specific for high-grade urothelial carcinoma, the authors anticipate the urine cytology will continue to maintain its high specificity, and TPSRUC will help improve the sensitivity and reduce the rate of indeterminant diagnoses. In the era of molecular pathology, more advanced ancillary studies will likely be developed; meanwhile, urine cytology will continue to be the main test for diagnosing, screening, and monitoring patients with bladder cancers.

ANCILLARY TECHNIQUES IN URINE CYTOLOGY

FLUORESCENCE IN SITU HYBRIDIZATION (UroVysion)

Urine cytology is highly useful for detecting high-grade urothelial carcinomas. Urine cytology has a high specificity (80%–95%) for detecting high-grade carcinomas but a low sensitivity (20%–50%). Because the sensitivity and negative predictive value of screening urine cytology are so low, ancillary tests that would increase detection of carcinoma would make urine cytology more effective as a screening test.

Cytogenetically, urothelial carcinoma is an aneuploid cancer, harboring multiple copies of abnormal chromosomes. Prior to FISH, digital imaging analysis used morphometric analysis of DNA content with Feulgen staining. Aneuploid cells were detected by their higher DNA content. Currently, FISH uses molecular probes to detect DNA content of urothelial cells. Centromere enumeration probes for chromosomes 3, 7, and 17 label the chromosomal centromere. The presence of more than 2 signals within a cell confirms the presence of aneuploidy. Each institution/laboratory may have varying guidelines and cutoffs regarding what is considered positive or negative for aneusomy.

The 4′6-diamidino-2-phenylindole (DAPI) stain is used to visualize the nucleus. Benign urothelial cells will show a homogeneous staining pattern, demonstrating an even chromatin distribution within a cell with normal DNA content. Conversely, tumor cells show large nuclei and a clumped, coarse chromatin pattern. This reflects an aneuploid cell with coarse chromatin distribution and nuclear irregularity, similar to the findings of urothelial carcinoma cytology. These cells can be detected by fluorescence microscopy either manually by a molecular technologist or cytotechnologist. Automated screening systems are also available.

On identification of an abnormal cell on DAPI staining, analysis of the different probes is done by changing the filter. Centromere enumeration probes directed toward the chromocenter of chromosomes 3 (red), 7 (green), and 17 (aqua) reflect the number of copies of chromosomes. Gold is locus-specific for 9p21. In many laboratories, cytotechnologists, who are already trained to screen for abnormal cells on bright field microscopy, can be trained to detect probes through the various filters and perform a count. Molecular technologists are also highly skilled for interpretation of this test. Automated systems can save on technologist time. Ultimately, the final interpretation is signed out by a pathologist.[22] FISH in the upper urothelial tract should be interpreted with caution, because of the possibility of false positive cases. Tetrasomic cells in the upper tract are more frequently found due to more mitotically active cells present in the upper tract and pelvis. Tetrasomic cases should be interpreted as suspicious for malignancy but not as positive. In addition, concomitant urothelial carcinoma of the bladder may lead to a false-positive result.[23]

ImmunoCyt/uCyt+

ImmunoCyt/uCyt+ (DiagnoCure, Quebec City, Quebec, Canada) testing is an immunocytochemical assay-based technique to detect bladder cancer in urine. There are 3 monoclonal antibodies that detect distinct targets: M344, LDQ10, and 19A211. Cell membrane fluorescence for high-molecular-weight glycosylated carcinogenic embryonic antigen (19A211—red) and bladder cancer mucin-like antigens (LDQ10, M344—green) are evaluated. The presence of 5 or more positive cells confirms a positive diagnosis. ImmunoCyt has approximately 2-fold sensitivity for detecting bladder cancer compared with urine cytology but lower specificity. An advantage of ImmunoCyt/uCyt+, in addition to its overall high sensitivity, is that it is more sensitive in detecting low-grade tumors because M344 is expressed by 70% of noninvasive papillary urothelial carcinomas. One disadvantage is low specificity of the test. Benign prostatic hyperplasia and bladder calculi may cause false-positive results. Urine specimens derived from ileal conduits may also exhibit false positivity because small bowel epithelial cells are positive for carcinoembryonic antigen.[21]

OTHER ASSAYS

Recent findings on telomerase have added intrigue to molecular diagnostics in urine cytology. Telomerase is an RNA that adds telomeres to DNA ends, which increases the integrity of DNA and can allow for immortalization of the DNA. PCR-based

Table 3
Urine-based markers for diagnosis of bladder cancer

UroVysion	ImmunoCyt (Bladder Cancer Immunofluorescence Assay)	Telomerase	Fibroblast Growth Factor Receptor	Bladder Tumor Antigen	Nuclear Matrix Protein 22 (NMP22)
FISH test to assess for aneuploid tumor cells Sensitivity 70%–80% Specificity 80%–85%	Cocktail of antibodies to detect tumor cells in urine Approved for surveillance in conjunction with urine cytology Sensitivity 80% 85% Specificity 30%–40%	hTERT Sensitivity —70%–100% Specificity —60%–70%	Found to be commonly mutated in low-grade urothelial carcinomas Sensitivity —39%–78% Specificity —96%–100%	Dipstick-based test detecting complement factor H-related protein Sensitivity 50% for low-grade UC Specificity— lower	Dipstick-based test detecting family of proteins involved with DNA replication and nuclear structural support Sensitivity 34.6%–100% Specificity 49.5%–65%[24]

testing is available for urine specimens. It carries a sensitivity between 70% and 100% and a specificity of 60% to 70%.[24] A test for human telomerase reverse transcriptase (hTERT), a catalytic subunit of telomerase, has recently been developed; however, further studies are ongoing to test its utility.

Fibroblast growth factor (FGF) controls many cellular proliferative functions by binding to their transmembrane tyrosine-kinase receptors (FGFRs). FGF signaling is altered in a high proportion of bladder cancers and has been found commonly mutated in low-grade urothelial carcinoma. Fibroblast receptor growth factor receptor 3 (*FGFR*) mutations have a positive predictive value of 95% in patients with no history of transitional cell carcinoma.[25] Real-time PCR on urine samples was shown to have a sensitivity of 39% to 78% and specificity of 96% to 100% for detection of urothelial carcinoma. FGFR3 testing on urine cytology remains a promising future endeavor.[23] Integration of further urinary biomarker testing will require well-developed protocols and retrospective and prospective trials to entrench themselves in the role of detection and screening going forward.

Table 3 summarizes the ancillary tests discussed as well as additional proposed assays of bladder tumor antigen and NMP22.

SUMMARY

Overall, although urine cytology is highly specific for detecting high-grade urothelial carcinoma, there is low sensitivity for detecting such tumors and an even lower sensitivity for detecting low-grade tumors. The use available ancillary tests as an adjunct to cytologic examination may help provide clinical guidance for patient treatment, especially for urine cytology samples that are diagnostically equivocal. Urine cytology continues to be a cost-effective test for screening, diagnosis, and surveillance of urothelial tract malignancies.

REFERENCES

1. Berger D. A brief history of medical diagnosis and the birth of the clinical laboratory. Part 4–Fraud and abuse, managed-care, and lab consolidation. MLO Med Lab Obs 1999;31:38–42.
2. Demay RM. The art and science of cytopathology: 2nd edition. 2nd edition. Chicago: ASCP Press; 2012.
3. Antic T, RD. The fascinating history of urine examination. J Am Soc Cytopathology 2014;3:135–6.
4. Long SR, Cohen MB. Classics in cytology. V.: William Sanders and early urinary tract cytology. Diagn Cytopathol 1992;8:135–6.
5. Papanicolaou GN, Marshall VF. Urine sediment smears as a diagnostic procedure in cancers of the urinary tract. Science 1945;101:519–20.
6. Papanicolaou GN. Cytology of the urine sediment in neoplasms of the urinary tract. J Urol 1947;57:375–9.
7. Koss L. Diagnostic cytpathology and its histopathologic basis. Philadelphia: Lippincott Company; 2006.
8. Mostofi FKSL, Torloni H. Histologic typing of urinary bladder tumors. Geneva (Switzerland): World Health Organization; 1973.
9. Koss LG, Hoda RS. Koss's cytology of the urinary tract with histopathologic correlations. New York: Springer; 2012.
10. Murphy WM, Soloway MS, Jukkola AF, et al. Urinary cytology and bladder cancer. The cellular features of transitional cell neoplasms. Cancer 1984;53:1555–65.
11. Ooms EC, Veldhuizen RW. Cytological criteria and diagnostic terminology in urinary cytology. Cytopathology 1993;4:51–4.
12. Layfield LJ, Elsheikh TM, Fili A, et al. Review of the state of the art and recommendations of the Papanicolaou Society of Cytopathology for urinary cytology procedures and reporting: the Papanicolaou Society of Cytopathology Practice Guidelines Task Force. Diagn Cytopathol 2004;30:24–30.
13. Rosenthal DL, Vandenbussche CJ, Burroughs FH, et al. The Johns Hopkins Hospital template for urologic cytology samples: part I-creating the template. Cancer Cytopathol 2013;121:15–20.
14. VandenBussche CJ, Sathiyamoorthy S, Owens CL, et al. The Johns Hopkins Hospital template for urologic cytology samples: parts II and III: improving the predictability of indeterminate results in urinary cytologic samples: an outcomes and cytomorphologic study. Cancer Cytopathol 2013;121:21–8.
15. Owens CL, Vandenbussche CJ, Burroughs FH, et al. A review of reporting systems and terminology for urine cytology. Cancer Cytopathol 2013;121:9–14.
16. Rosenthal DL, Wojcik E, Kurtycz DF. The Paris system for reporting urinary cytology. New York: Springer; 2016.
17. Cowan ML, Rosenthal DL, VandenBussche CJ. Improved risk stratification for patients with high-grade urothelial carcinoma following application of the Paris System for Reporting Urinary Cytology. Cancer Cytopathol 2017;125:427–34.
18. Wang Y, Auger M, Kanber Y, et al. Implementing The Paris System for Reporting Urinary Cytology results in a decrease in the rate of the "atypical" category and an increase in its prediction of subsequent high-grade urothelial carcinoma. Cancer Cytopathol 2018;126:207–14.
19. Hang JF, Charu V, Zhang ML, et al. Digital image analysis supports a nuclear-to-cytoplasmic ratio cutoff value of 0.5 for atypical urothelial cells. Cancer Cytopathol 2017;125:710–6.

20. Wojcik EM. What should not be reported as atypia in urine cytology. J Am Soc Cytopathology 2015;4: 30–6.

21. Onur I, Rosenthal DL, VandenBussche CJ. Benign-appearing urothelial tissue fragments in noninstrumented voided urine specimens are associated with low rates of urothelial neoplasia. Cancer Cytopathol 2015;123:180–5.

22. Halling KC, King W, Sokolova IA, et al. A comparison of cytology and fluorescence in situ hybridization for the detection of urothelial carcinoma. J Urol 2000; 164:1768–75.

23. Reynolds JP, Voss JS, Kipp BR, et al. Comparison of urine cytology and fluorescence in situ hybridization in upper urothelial tract samples. Cancer Cytopathol 2014;122:459–67.

24. Lamarca A, Barriuso J. Urine telomerase for diagnosis and surveillance of bladder cancer. Adv Urol 2012;2012:693631.

25. Miyake M, Sugano K, Sugino H, et al. Fibroblast growth factor receptor 3 mutation in voided urine is a useful diagnostic marker and significant indicator of tumor recurrence in non-muscle invasive bladder cancer. Cancer Sci 2010;101:250–8.

Adult Renal Neoplasms
Cytology, Immunohistochemistry, and Cytogenetic Characteristics

Jaylou Velez-Torres, MD, Luiz Paulo Guido, MD,
Merce Jorda, MD, PhD, MBA*

KEYWORDS

• Fine needle aspiration • FNAC • Kidney tumors • Small renal masses • SRM

Key points

- The combined use of core biopsy (CB) and fine-needle aspiration cytology (FNAC) as diagnostic methods of renal neoplasms is expanding in clinical practice, especially in small renal masses.
- The combined used of CB and FNAC plays a pivotal role in therapeutic decision-making in patients with renal neoplasms.
- Grouping the renal neoplasms in differential diagnostic groups helps in choosing specific immunohistochemical markers and reaching an accurate diagnosis.

ABSTRACT

Tissue sampling of renal masses is traditionally performed using percutaneous sonographic or CT guidance core biopsy (CB) with or without touch preparation cytology and/or fine-needle aspiration cytology (FNAC). The combined used of CB and FNAC is expanding in clinical practice, especially in small renal masses and plays a pivotal role in therapeutic decision making. Grouping the renal neoplasms in differential diagnostic groups helps in choosing specific immunohistochemical markers and reaching an accurate diagnosis.

OVERVIEW

Tissue sampling of renal masses is traditionally performed using percutaneous sonographic or CT guidance core biopsy (CB) with or without touch preparation cytology and/or fine-needle aspiration cytology (FNAC). By imaging, renal lesions are divided in 2 distinct groups: cystic and solid. The Bosniak renal cyst classification further categorizes renal cysts into benign, complex, undetermined, and malignant and they are rarely sampled.[1] Solid renal masses have been conventionally evaluated by its imaging characteristics and, if indicated, further sampling for tissue and/or cytologic interpretation is obtained. Indications for diagnostic procedure in renal lesions include infectious diseases; undetermined radiologic findings for the diagnosis of malignancy; untreatable malignancy or metastasis; treatment planning, including surveillance; and percutaneous ablation by either cryotherapy or radiofrequency.[2–5]

During the past decades, improvement in imaging technology has increased the detection and characterization of renal masses, with up to 80% of renal cell carcinomas (RCCs) incidentally detected during radiological work-up. At time of surgery, 70% to 90% of solid renal lesions proved to be RCCs and, consequently, an enhancing renal neoplasm by imaging studies has been

Disclosure Statement: Nothing to disclose.
Department of Pathology and Laboratory Medicine, University of Miami Miller School of Medicine, 1400 Northwest 12th Avenue, Miami, FL 33136, USA
* Corresponding author.
E-mail address: Mjorda@med.miami.edu

Surgical Pathology 11 (2018) 611–631
https://doi.org/10.1016/j.path.2018.06.003

considered a sufficient indication for surgery.[6,7] Recent studies, however, have demonstrated that up to 30% of detected renal lesions are benign, depending on lesion size,[8–10] or they represent indolent low-grade malignancies.[11–13] Small renal masses (SRMs) (<4 cm) have been increasingly detected and the patients may be candidates for conservative and minimally invasive therapies.[14–19] Most of the SRMs are incidental and patient management is largely based on pathologic diagnosis. In a Surveillance, Epidemiology, and End Results analysis, including 19,932 patients with localized RCC, 84% of SRMs proved to be indolent tumors.[13] Furthermore, the largest increase in incidentally detected SRMs has occurred in elderly patients, where the option for surveillance may be attractive because they are at higher risk for other health hazards.[20] Consequently, an early diagnosis of SRMs is highly beneficial for patient management.

CORE BIOPSY VERSUS FINE-NEEDLE ASPIRATION CYTOLOGY

Tissue or cytologic sampling of renal lesions is performed using percutaneous sonographic or CT-guided CB or FNAC. This has proved a useful technique to classify SRMs as benign or malignant and into different RCC subtypes, considering that some forms may respond differently to specific targeted therapies. In addition, cytologic evaluation of renal lesions can be obtained by endoscopic ultrasound-guided FNAC.[14–19] Endoscopic ultrasound-guided FNAC is associated with lower risk of needle seeding in comparison to percutaneous FNAC, and it can be extremely useful in the sampling of anterior renal tumors, whereas those located at the posterior aspect of the kidney may be better sampled by the percutaneous method.[8] Percutaneous FNAC is a safe, rapid, and widely accepted procedure and it is highly used in other abdominal organs.[21] FNAC, in comparison to CB, is relatively less invasive, cost effective, and amenable to immediate assessment and can guide the radiologist for accurate targeting using rapid on-site evaluation. FNAC can have a high value, yielding diagnosis in most of the cases,[21] and can separate benign from malignant neoplasms in more than 90% of cases with histologic classification of tumor type possible in 87% of tumors.[22] Nondiagnostic or inadequate specimens are largely due to sampling error and occur in approximately 30% of cases. On the other hand, FNAC of renal tumors has been used in advanced-stage disease, in patients with poor surgical status and/or with prior history of other malignancy, and in cases of discrepant clinical presentation and CT findings.[15,23–28] On most occasions, FNAC is placed on smears with or without collection of material for cell block preparation. Both alcohol-fixed smears and cell blocks are suitable for immunocytochemical and cytogenetic analysis. Liquid-based cytologic preparation, on the other hand, is a safe and valuable diagnostic tool used in many organs. Due to inexperience with this method, however, which alters the morphology, diagnosing renal tumors remains a challenge for the cytopathologist.[29] Considering all discussed previously, the use of percutaneous renal CB and/or FNAC is expanding in clinical practice and plays a pivotal role in therapeutic decision making. Both FNAC and CB demonstrate excellent diagnostic accuracy when diagnosing malignancy demonstrating synergistic results. In a previous study, the combination of FNAC and CB was found to significantly improve the diagnostic rate when compared with the use of FNAC alone (92% vs 72%; $P<.05$) and was better than CB alone (92% vs 87%).[30] The accuracy of FNAC alone distinguishing benign from malignant renal masses ranges from 73% to 94%.[31] FNAC cytology correctly subclassifies RCC in 74% of cases.[32] FNAC samples, however, may reduce the ability to differentiate between non–clear cell RCC (CCRCC) subtypes.[33] When pathologic characteristics are insufficient to accurately diagnose carcinoma or to issue a tumor subclassification, ancillary techniques, such as immunohistochemistry (IHC) and cytogenetics, seem to improve the diagnostic accuracy of both CB and FNAC.[33,34]

NORMAL ELEMENTS IN FINE-NEEDLE ASPIRATION CYTOLOGY OF KIDNEY

Although reviewing cytology smears belonging to FNAC cytology of kidney, it is common to find normal elements, such as glomeruli, proximal tubular cells, and distal tubular cells. Glomeruli, at low power, may mimic the papillae seen in papillary RCC (PRCC). They are globular structures with highly cellular globular content; however, the endothelial cells lining the capillary loops are seen at the extreme edge of many glomeruli. In RCCs, the nucleus is rounder than in endothelial cells, and the cytoplasm almost always extends peripherally beyond the nucleus.

Proximal tubular cells may be present and consist of sheets of cells with abundant granular cytoplasm, round bland nuclei, and easily seen small nucleoli. The cell membrane is commonly torn, due to the process of ripping from the tubules, and the granules may appear to be spilling out of the cells. These cells may resemble oncocytoma cells and some cases of PRCC and chromophobe RCC. The FNAC of these tumors, however, is characteristically much more cellular, with papillary tumors forming papillae and spherules, and the chromophobe tumors may present binucleated tumor cells. The proximal tubular epithelial cells are present in loose aggregates, which may show tubule formation. Distal tubular cells may be seen singly or in cohesive sheets (up to approximately 20 cells) with scant clear to slightly nonvacuolated granular cytoplasm and small round nuclei with or without very small nucleoli, closely resembling tumor cells of either low-grade CCRCC or PRCC. The distal tubular cells have scant cytoplasm, making the cell membrane difficult to identify. The most important point to remember is that to differentiate aggregates of normal tubular cells from low-grade renal neoplasms, the increased cellularity present in the latter is crucial to make the correct diagnosis.

RENAL NEOPLASMS: CYTOLOGIC, IMMUNOCYTOCHEMICAL, AND GENETIC CHARACTERISTICS

The new 2016 World Health Organization (WHO) classification of renal tumors refers to subtypes that have been named based on predominant cytoplasmic features, architectural features, anatomic location of tumors, and correlation with a specific renal disease background as well as molecular alterations pathognomonic for RCC subtypes.[35]

BENIGN NEOPLASMS

The most frequent solid benign renal tumors occurring in adults and currently listed in the WHO 2016 classification are renal cell tumors, including papillary adenoma and oncocytoma; metanephric adenoma; mesenchymal tumors, including angiomyolipoma (AML); and mixed epithelial and stromal tumors (MEST). Other benign renal neoplasms currently listed in the WHO 2016 classification, occur either mainly in children or are mainly cystic in nature and rarely needled.

Papillary Adenoma

Until 2015, papillary adenoma was defined as tumors measuring 0.5 cm. The WHO 2016 classification defines papillary adenomas as unencapsulated tumors with papillary or tubular architecture, low WHO/International Society of Urological Pathology (ISUP) grade, and a diameter of 1.5 cm or less. The decision to increase the cutoff size was based on available data showing that unencapsulated grades 1 to 2 tumors have no capacity to metastasize.[36] A diagnosis of papillary adenoma based on needle biopsy or cytology should be made with extreme caution because the presence of any capsule or grade heterogeneity may not be visualized. Even if cell block is available, the cytomorphology, immunophenotype, and cytogenetics characteristics of the lesion are indistinguishable from low-grade PRCCs, and a diagnosis of papillary adenoma should only be made with the knowledge of the lesion size obtained by imaging methods.

Oncocytoma

Oncocytoma accounts for 3% to 5% of all renal neoplasms.[37] Tumors grossly present as a well-circumscribed lesion with the same color as the adjacent cortex, ranging from mahogany brown to pale. Tumor cells are arranged in rounded nests. Cytologic features are among the major defining criteria of renal oncocytoma. Oncocytoma cells usually have voluminous, densely eosinophilic cytoplasm; nuclei are uniform and round, typically lacking binucleation (**Fig. 1A, B**), in contrast to the notched raisinoid nuclei with detailed chromatin seen in chromophobe RCC (ChrRCC).[38] Oncocytoma may show degenerative atypia with large, often multinucleated cells with smudgy hyperchromatic nuclei and poorly preserved chromatin detail (see **Fig. 1B**). Large bizarre nuclei may be occasionally found, with marked size variation and hyperchromatic, with a somewhat smudged chromatin but without prominent nucleoli (**Fig. 1C**). Mitoses are rare or absent.[38] Despite these characteristic cytologic features, diagnosis of oncocytoma by FNAC may be controversial, especially considering that some RCCs may display areas with oncocytic features. In contrast to oncocytoma, smears of RCCs are typically highly cellular and the cells are easily dissociated, yielding numerous single cells and loosely cohesive small clusters of up to approximately 10 monomorphic tumor cells, abundant eosinophilic granular cytoplasm, well-defined cell membranes, frequent binucleation, and round nuclei with small but distinct nucleoli.[37] Hyaline globules may be present. The oncocytoma tumor cells resemble proximal tubular epithelial cells, hepatocytes, CCRCC, and eosinophilic ChrRCC.

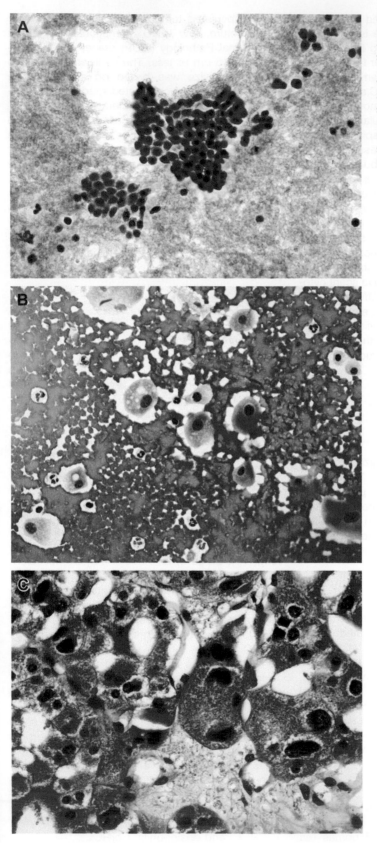

Fig. 1. Oncocytoma. (*A*) The cells are uniform with eosinophilic cytoplasm and round nuclei (Papanicolaou-stained smear; original magnification ×40). (*B*) The cells are voluminous with eosinophilic cytoplasm, uniform and round nuclei (Papanicolaou-stained smear; original magnification ×60). (*C*) Degenerative atypia with large, often multinucleated cells with smudgy hyperchromatic nuclei (cell block; original magnification ×60).

IHC can be of help if a cell block or multiple smears are available. A common problem faced by pathologists is distinguishing between a renal oncocytoma and an eosinophilic variant of ChrRCC, even though most of these cases can be distinguished from each other by careful evaluation of the nuclear features.[39] The cells of renal oncocytoma exhibit membranous CD117 immunoreactivity.[40] Oncocytoma is also positive for HNF1β and S100A1 in a significantly greater proportion than ChrRCCs.[41] Characteristically, CK7 immunostaining is negative in oncocytomas.[40] ChrRCCs have similar immunoreactivity for CD117 than oncocytoma, but, in addition, this tumor expresses CK7 diffusely in a membranous distribution.[42] Unfortunately, the eosinophilic variant of ChrRCC can have low expression of CK7, with the possibility of generating a pitfall. Fluorescence in situ hybridization (FISH) studies on core needle and FNAC samples may improve the overall accuracy of diagnosis in needle biopsies/cytology samples, especially in SRMs.[34,43–45] Chromosomal aberrations in oncocytoma have been described as loss of 3p21 without gain of 5q, t:(11q3) rearrangement and loss of chromosome 1.[33]

It is currently recommended that renal tumors with these cytomorphologic features and the staining characteristics of an oncocytoma be diagnosed as renal oncocytic neoplasms with a comment listing the differential diagnosis.

Metanephric Adenoma

Metanephric adenoma is a benign lesion that commonly occurs in women during the fifth decade of life. Smears are cellular and consist of small short papillae, small tubules, and loose sheets of cells with scant cytoplasm, round nuclei, and fine chromatin with inconspicuous nucleoli. The chromatin resembles that seem in papillary carcinoma of thyroid. The tumor comprises tubules and papillae, forming glomeruloid bodies lined by uniformly bland cells, with occasional psammoma bodies (**Fig. 2**). Tumors have *BRAF* V600E mutations.[46,47] The lesional cells are positive for WT-1, CD57, and mutant-specific antibodies for BRAF V600E; tumors are negative for EMA and CK7. Both IHC and cytogenetic features are helpful in distinguishing metanephric adenoma from low-grade PRCC. Finally, epithelial-predominant Wilms tumor cannot be

Fig. 2. Metanephric adenoma. The cells display scant cytoplasm, round nuclei, inconspicuous nucleoli, and psammoma bodies (Papanicolaou-stained smear; original magnification ×60).

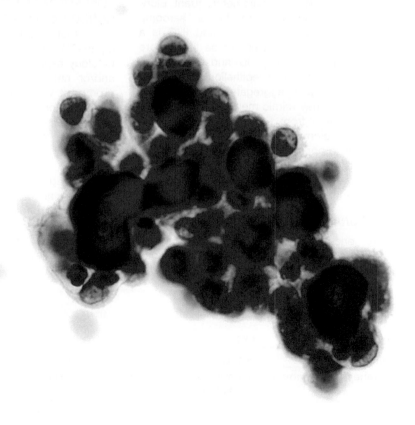

distinguished from metanephric adenoma by cyto-morphology alone[40] (**Table 1**).

Angiomyolipoma

AML is composed of 3 elements, including blood vessels, mature fat, and smooth muscle cells, with moderate to severe nuclear atypia. Tumors are common in young adults in the context of tuberous sclerosis, in a multiple and bilateral presentation. Tumors also occur sporadically in young and middle-aged women, usually as solitary tumors. This tumor type is seldom aspirated because it demonstrates characteristic imaging features, although the fat-poor variant is an exception and is frequently aspirated because it cannot be distinguished from other renal neoplasms by imaging studies. The smears of the fat-poor variant of AML show large groups of elongated and round cells in cohesive cell groups that resemble cellular stroma, with rare single cells (**Fig. 3**A). At high power, the cells are smooth muscle, which can be elongated, round, bland, or even markedly atypical. The atypia pattern may vary, commonly consisting of markedly enlarged, darkly hyperchromatic, generally with round nuclei. The cytoplasm may be difficult to appreciate in most specimens, often stringy or crystalline rather than granular or vacuolated. Large clear vacuoles may be present, representing fat, but are not frequent. Elongated cells raise concern for a sarcoma diagnosis or sarcomatoid RCC, and IHC is a valuable tool in these cases. These lesions are positive for HMB-45 (**Fig. 3**B) and negative for epithelial markers. The epithelioid variant of AML demonstrates aggregates of epithelioid cells only and may mimic melanoma. AML must be differentiated from RCC, liposarcoma, leiomyoma, and leiomyosarcoma. For the epithelioid variant, it is important to consider melanoma and adrenocortical carcinoma. Staining with EMA, pan-keratin, and HMB-45 is advisable to address this differential diagnosis[40] (**Table 2**).

Mixed Epithelial and Stromal Tumors

MESTs encompass a spectrum of tumors, including predominantly cystic tumors (adult cystic nephroma) and tumors that are more solid. Adult cystic nephroma was previously classified as a separate entity from MEST. Based on similar age and gender distributions and a similar histochemical profile, adult cystic nephroma is now classified within this spectrum of MEST. In contrast to adult cystic nephroma, pediatric cystic nephroma is a distinct entity with specific DICER1 mutations.[48]

MEST can mimic RCC and typically presents as an isolated mass. Adult cystic nephroma form and classical MEST present similar cytologic features, further supporting its joint classification.[37] The smears are paucicellular, consisting of single cells without large groups, with clear to vacuolated cytoplasm, occasionally displaying atypical cells with irregular nuclear membrane and prominent nucleoli or, less commonly, spindle cells. If cell block or CB is available, the characteristic arrangement of cysts and cellular stroma may help distinguishing these cells from CCRCC. If only smears are available, paucicellular samples should be diagnosed as atypical or suspicious rather than positive to avoid a misdiagnosis and erroneous patient management.

MALIGNANT NEOPLASMS

Clear Cell Renal Cell Carcinoma

CCRCC represents 65% to 70% of all RCCs. Genetic analysis shows mutations in VHL gene (3p25–26) or chromosome 3p losses.[37] The cytology aspirates are hypercellular with bloody and/or necrotic background, in occasions of prominent vasculature (**Fig. 4**A). The cells have abundant or finely vacuolated cytoplasm with round centrally located nuclei (**Fig. 4**B, C) and may have prominent nucleoli (**Fig. 4**D). The nuclei may also be eccentrically located giving the cell a plasmacytoid appearance (**Fig. 4**E) Higher-grade tumors have more isolated cells and less vacuolated cytoplasm and can show rhabdoid morphology (**Fig. 4**F).

The differential diagnosis includes benign tubular cells, macrophages, adrenocortical cells, hepatocytes, and other variants of RCC.

Table 1
Differential diagnosis: papillary renal cell carcinoma versus metanephric adenoma

Tumor Type	CK7	AMACR	WT-1	CD57	BRAF V600E
Solid papillary RCC	Positive	Positive	Negative	Negative	Negative
Metanephric adenoma	Negative or isolated cells	Negative	Positive, nuclear	Positive	Positive

Fig. 3. AML. (*A*) The cells are elongated and/or round, in cohesive cell groups that resemble cellular stroma (Papanicolaou-stained smear; original magnification ×60). (*B*) AML. The cells are positive for HMB-45 by IHC (HMB-45 stain on smear; original magnification ×60).

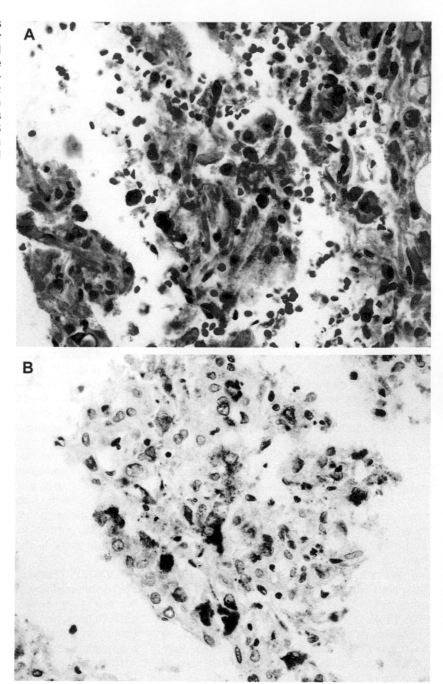

Aspirates of benign renal tubular cells may simulate low-grade CCRCC. The aspirate is scant and shows small flat groups of cells without vacuolated cytoplasm or branching vessels. Macrophages are usually isolated cells with kidney-shaped nuclei and vacuolated cytoplasm without atypia. Adrenocortical cells are smaller and have a fine bubbly cytoplasm; typically, the cells lose their cytoplasm and are present as bare nuclei in a background of debris. Hepatocytes have a uniformly granular cytoplasm with centrally placed nuclei.

The differential diagnosis clear cell tubulopapillary renal cell carcinoma includes all renal tumors composed predominantly of clear cells: clear cell PRCC (or clear cell tubulopapillary

Table 2
Differential diagnosis of tumors composed predominantly of clear cells

Tumor Type	Carbonic Anhydrase IX	CK7	CD117	Cathepsin K	HMB-45
CCRCC	Positive, diffuse membranous	Negative	Negative	Negative	Negative
Clear cell PRCC	Positive, cuplike	Positive	Negative	Negative	Negative
Chromophobe RCC	Negative	Positive, cytoplasmic	Positive, membranous	Negative	Negative
Epithelioid-AML	Negative	Negative	Negative	Positive, cytoplasmic	Positive, cytoplasmic
MiTF-TFE tumors					
Xp11 family	Variable but focal	Negative	Variable	Positive (50%), cytoplasmic	Negative
t(6;11)	Variable but focal	Negative	Negative	Positive, cytoplasmic	Positive (always focal)

Abbreviations: c, cytoplasmic; m, membranous.

RCC), ChrRCC, epithelioid AML, and MiTF-TFE tumors. IHC can be a helpful aid. CCRCC are positive for carbonic anhydrase IX (CAIX) (**Fig. 4**G), a transmembrane member of the carbonic anhydrase family of genes, and has a role in CO_2 transport and in regulation of pH. It is under the regulation of the hypoxia-inducible factor, which is invariably dysregulated in CCRCC. For this reason, CAIX is characteristically overexpressed in these tumors diffusely and in a membranous pattern. Only membranous and not cytoplasmic staining should be taken into consideration.[49,50] Decreased expression may be seen in high-grade tumors. In addition, CCRCC commonly expresses epithelial markers, such as AE1/AE3, CAM5.2, and epithelial membrane antigen (EMA). CCRCC do not express CK7, CD117, or cathepsin K HMB-45[40] (see **Table 2**).

Several patterns of chromosomal aberrations have been described in cytologic samples from CCRCC: loss of 3p2; loss of 3p21 with gain of 5q; loss of 3p (3p25 and 3p21); loss of 3q and gain of 5q; loss of chr3 without 2 or more typical chromophobe RCC (ChrRCC) losses; gain of chr5 without gain of chr17 and 3; or 2 or more typical ChrRCC losses.[33]

Papillary Renal Cell Carcinoma

The PRCC tumor accounts for 7% to 15% of all RCCs.[37] The cytology aspirates are hypercellular with abundant papillary structures. Some investigators distinguish type 1 and type 2 PRCC. Type 1 tumors show papillae covered by a single layer of small bland cuboidal cells with uniform round nuclei (**Fig. 5**A). Type 2 tumors show papillae covered by large eosinophilic cells with enlarged nuclei and prominent nucleoli (**Fig. 5**B). The cytoplasm may be clear, eosinophilic, or granular. Abundant intracytoplasmic hemosiderin may be present. Psammoma bodies are rarely seen.

The differential diagnosis of PRCC includes papillary adenoma and other neoplasms with a significant papillary component: CCRCC with papillary growth, clear cell PRCC, and MiTF-TFE–associated neoplasms. The tumor cells of PRCC are positive for CK7, AMACR, renal cell common antigen, and CD10. They are usually negative for CAIX, cathepsin K, 34bE12, and TFE3/TFEB[40] (**Table 3**). In rare occasions, smears from an oncocytoma may mimic low-grade PRCC; however, they usually lack the papillary architecture. Oncocytoma cells are negative for CK7 in contrast to low-grade PRCC. Papillary adenomas are indistinguishable on cytologic material.

The most common genetic abnormalities of PRCC are trisomy 7 and trisomy 17 and loss of chromosome Y.[37]

Chromophobe Renal Cell Carcinoma

The ChrRCC tumor represents approximately 3% to 5% of all RCCs and bears and excellent prognosis.[37] The aspirates are hypercellular and consist of groups of round or polygonal cells with abundant cytoplasm and sharply defined cell borders (plant cell appearance) with hyperchromatic wrinkled nuclei (**Fig. 6**A) with perinuclear clearing (koilocytoid cells). Binucleation is

Fig. 4. CCRCC. (*A*) Hypercellular smear with prominent vasculature (Papanicolaou-stained smear; original magnification ×60); (*B*) cells with abundant, finely vacuolated cytoplasm with round centrally located nuclei (Papanicolaou-stained smear; original magnification ×60); (*C*) cells with abundant, finely vacuolated cytoplasm with round centrally located nuclei (cell block; original magnification ×40); (*D*) cells with prominent nucleoli (Papanicolaou-stained smear; original magnification ×60); (*E*) plasmacytoid nuclear appearance (Papanicolaou-stained smear; original magnification ×40); (*F*) isolated cells with rhabdoid morphology (Papanicolaou-stained smear; original magnification ×60); and (*G*) CAIX diffusely positive in a membranous pattern (CAIX immunostaining on cell block; original magnification ×40).

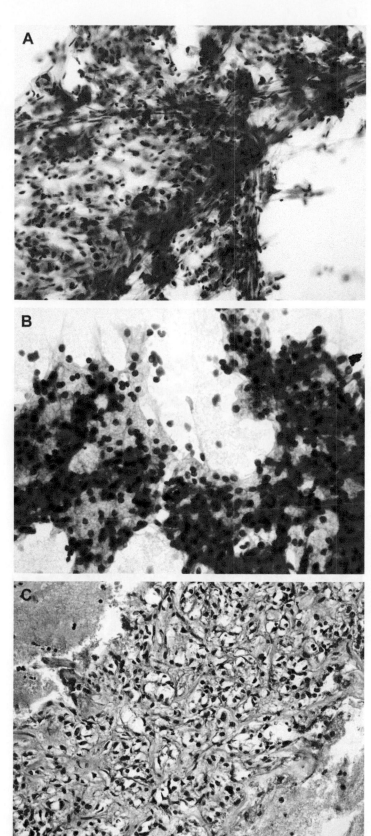

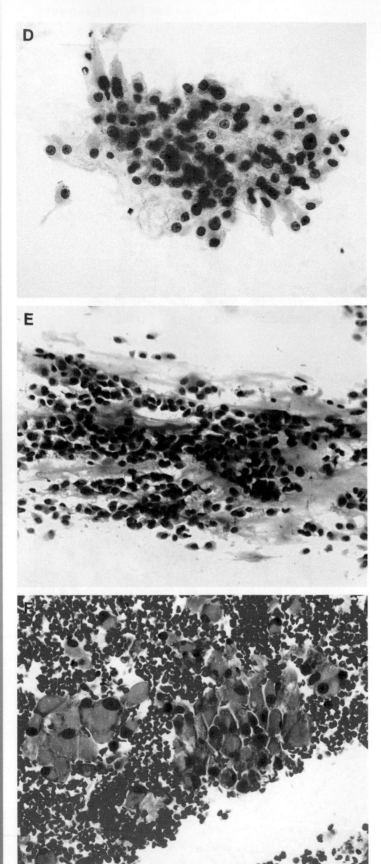

Fig. 4. (continued).

Fig. 4. (continued).

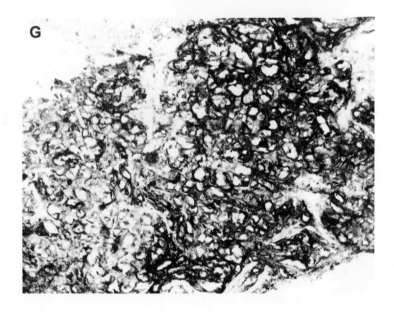

common (**Fig. 6**B). Cell blocks show cords of tumor cells with distinct cytoplasmic borders, abundant granular cytoplasm, perinuclear clearing, and dark hyperchromatic chromatin.

The immunocytochemical profile of this tumor is characteristic, expressing CK7 and CD117, but lacks expression for CAIX,[49] HMB-45, and cathepsin K[40] (**Table 4**). Also, the cells stain diffusely positive in a cytoplasmic pattern with Hale colloidal iron stain.

The differential diagnosis includes tumors with predominant clear cell features (see **Table 2**) and the eosinophilic variant of ChrRCC with tumors with predominant oncocytic features (see **Table 4**). Oncocytoma have round nuclei without koilocytic changes and are negative for CK7 and Hale colloidal iron. HNF1β and S100A1 are both more likely to be positive in oncocytoma and are negative in most ChrRCCs.[41] CCRCCs have abundant or finely vacuolated cytoplasm with a round centrally located nuclei with prominent nucleoli in contrast to the hyperchromatic wrinkled nuclei of ChrRCC and is usually negative for CK7 and CD117.[40]

ChrRCC is associated with extensive chromosomal losses usually affecting chromosomes 1, 6, 10, 13, 17, and 21.[37]

Mucinous Tubular and Spindle Cell Carcinoma

Originally described as a morphologic variant of CCRCC, now mucinous tubular and spindle cell carcinoma is identified as a different entity.[51] The epithelial-appearing cells are usually low cuboidal with small amounts of the amphophilic

to eosinophilic cytoplasm and low-grade nuclei. In the spindle cells, the nuclei are morphologically like those in the tubular areas. Myxoid stroma is present in a majority of the cases, although occasional tumors may be mucin-poor.[51] Uncommon features that may be seen include presence of foamy macrophages, necrosis, papillary formations, and focal clear cells and rarely oncocytic tubules.[51]

The immunocytochemical profile is similar to the one seen in PRCC. The cells are positive for CK7, AMACR, renal cell common antigen, and CD15 in both tubular and spindle cell areas. CD10 may be focally positive.[51]

Clear Cell Papillary (or Clear Cell Tubulopapillary) Renal Cell Carcinoma

Clear cell PRCC (also known as clear cell tubulopapillary carcinoma) is a renal epithelial neoplasm accounting for up to 5% of all resected renal tumors and arises sporadically in end-stage renal disease and VHL(von Hippel-Lindau) syndrome syndrome[52,53]; according to current knowledge, it has an indolent behavior.

Clear cell PRCC is composed of low-grade clear epithelial cells that in cell block preparations are arranged in tubules and papillae with a predominantly linear nuclear alignment away from the basement membrane, a feature that may be difficult to be appreciated in smears (**Fig. 7**).[54]

The tumor cells express CAIX in a distinctive pattern characterized by a positive staining limited to the cytoplasmic membrane along the basal and

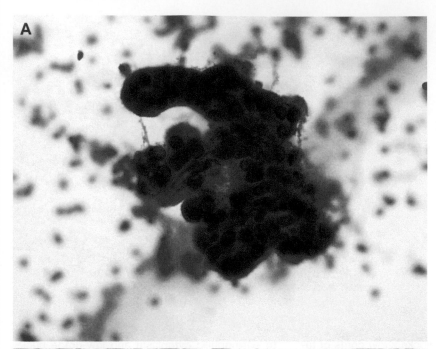

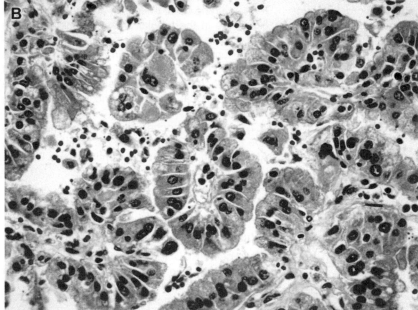

Fig. 5. PRCC. (*A*) Papillary structure with single layer of small bland cuboidal cells with uniform round nuclei (Papanicolaou-stained smear; original magnification ×60); (*B*) papillae covered by large eosinophilic cells with enlarged nuclei and prominent nucleoli (cell block; original magnification ×60).

lateral aspects of the cell, sparing the luminal border (cuplike staining).[53,55–57]

IHC may be helpful in differentiating Clear cell PRCC from CCRCC and PRCC (see **Tables 2** and **3**). Clear cell PRCC exhibit diffuse immunoreactivity for CK7 unlike CCRCC but they lack staining for AMACR, unlike the usual PRCC. Cytokeratin 34b E12 is positive but not generally useful. They are negative for TFE3-TBEB and cathepsin K. Unlike CCRCC, these tumors are

CD10 negative or they may express focal and weak staining.[53,58,59]

Hereditary Leiomyomatosis and Renal Cell Carcinoma Syndrome–Associated Renal Cell Carcinoma

Hereditary leiomyomatosis and RCC syndrome–associated RCC is an autosomal dominant disorder associated with increased risk of

Table 3
Differential diagnosis of tumors with a significant papillary component

Tumor Type	Carbonic Anhydrase IX	CK7	AMACR	Cathepsin K	34BE12	TFE3/TFEB
CCRCC with papillary growth	Positive, membranous	Negative	Negative	Negative	Negative	Negative
PRCC	Negative	Positive/Negative	Positive	Negative	Negative	Negative
Clear cell PRCC	Positive, cuplike	Positive, diffuse	Negative	Negative	Negative	Negative
MiTF-TFE tumors	Variable but focal	Negative	Positive	Positive (50%)	Negative	Positive

cutaneous and uterine leiomyomas as well as RCC, bearing a poor prognosis.[51] Hereditary leiomyomatosis and RCC syndrome–associated RCC demonstrate germline fumarate hydratase mutations.[60] The most striking characteristic is the presence of a prominent inclusion-like eosinophilic nucleolus surrounded by a perinucleolar halo, but this finding may not be uniformly present throughout the tumor. Loss of expression of fumarate hydratase is characteristic of this neoplasm.

Acquired Cystic Disease of Kidney–Associated Renal Cell Carcinoma

The RCC, acquired cystic disease of kidney–associated RCC, is associated with end-stage kidneys with acquired cystic disease and has an indolent behavior.[51] Characteristically is composed of large eosinophilic cells with prominent nucleoli, and intracellular spaces. Foci with clear or amphophilic cytoplasm also may be present. Calcium oxalate crystals are frequently seen. Most of the aggressive examples have sarcomatoid features.

IHC staining for AMACR and glutathione S–transferase alpha is diffusely and strongly positive; CK7 is typically negative in these neoplasms.[51]

MiTF Translocation–Associated Renal Cell Carcinoma

The neoplasm, MiTF translocation–associated RCC, is defined by translocations involving MiTF/TFE family genes (TFE3 and TFEB).[51] The TFE3 gene is localized to Xp11.2, and the result of these alterations is the overexpression of the TFE3 protein. Nuclear TFE3 expression can be identified by IHC and is a relatively specific diagnostic aid.[51] Tumor cells may vary in appearance, according to the specific mutation

in each case. Tumor cells commonly have abundant clear cell cytoplasm and high nuclear grade; alveolar or solid growth is commonly present in cell blocks (**Fig. 8**A). Granular eosinophilic cytoplasm also may be seen. Another relevant feature is the presence of psammomatous calcifications that may be abundant (**Fig. 8**B). Hyaline nodules also may be found. MiTF/TFE translocation–associated RCCs are commonly negative for all epithelial markers, although EMA may be focally positive. Some neoplasms may stain for HMB-45 or Melan-A (**Fig. 8**C).[51] TFE3 (in a nuclear distribution) (**Fig. 8**D) and cathepsin K are positive[51] (see **Tables 2** and **3**).

FISH probes for TFE3 and TFEB are increasingly used in daily practice[51] and cell blocks are suitable for testing (**Fig. 8**).

Collecting Duct Carcinoma

Collecting duct carcinoma (CDC) is a rare and aggressive tumor believed to arise from cells of collecting ducts.[50] This is predominantly a high-grade adenocarcinoma, with tendency for a prominent inflammatory reaction, including a neutrophilic infiltrate, within and around the tumor (**Fig. 9**A). A few reports of CDC in FNAC exist in the literature.[51]

The immunoprofile is usually characterized by positive PAX8 (**Fig. 9**B) and EMA and negative for p63 and GATA3.[51] Negativity for the latter 2 markers is helpful when distinguishing CDC from high-grade urothelial carcinoma of renal pelvis.

Renal Medullary Carcinoma

Renal neoplasm with poor prognosis that almost exclusive occurs in young patients with sickle cell trait or disease; therefore, sickled red blood cells are often found in the

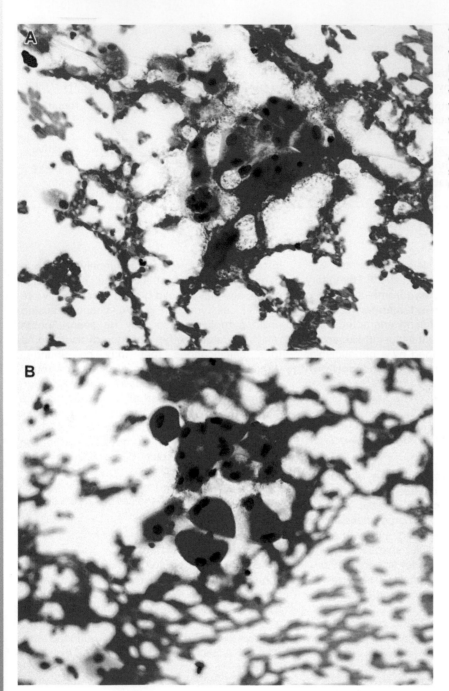

Fig. 6. Chromophobe RCC. (*A*) Polygonal cells with abundant cytoplasm and sharply defined cell borders with hyperchromatic wrinkled nuclei (Papanicolaou-stained smear; original magnification ×60); (*B*) binucleation is common (Papanicolaou-stained smear; original magnification ×60).

small vessels within and around the tumor. A neutrophil-dominant inflammatory infiltrate is commonly present. Tumor cells present high-grade cytology with a frequent finding of cytoplasmic mucin.

Immunocytochemical profile is characterized by the loss of nuclear expression of INI1 protein but cannot be considered a defining feature,

considering it has been reported in approximately 15% of CDC.[51]

Renal Cell Carcinoma Unclassified

Diagnosis of RCC unclassified should be reserved to those tumors that do not fit into one established histologic subtype in the current 2016 WHO

Table 4
Differential diagnosis of tumors with oncocytic features

Tumor Type	CD117	CK7	HMB-45	Cathepsin K	HNF1B	S100A1
Oncocytoma	Positive, membranous	Negative	Negative	Negative	Positive	Positive
Chromophobe RCC, eosinophilic	Positive, membranous	Positive but variable	Negative	Negative	Negative	Negative
Oncocytic PRCC	Negative	Positive but focal	Negative	Unknown	Positive	Negative but variable
Oncocytic AML	Negative	Negative	Positive, focal	Positive	Unknown	Positive

classification or that the morphology and immunocytochemical profile are noncompatible with any established RCC type.[35] The incorporation of molecular testing has been yielding the recognition of new entities that were previously classified as RCC unclassified. Ancillary studies should be performed to exclude distinct subtypes of RCC, AMLs, adrenal tumors, or metastatic neoplasms.

UNUSUAL MALIGNANT NEOPLASMS

Other solid renal cell tumors classified as independent entities in the 2016 WHO classification, such as succinate dehydrogenase–deficient RCC and tubulocystic RCC, are not discussed in this review due to rarity in routine cytologic practice.

The 2016 WHO classification includes rare neoplasms, such as mesenchymal tumors, neuroendocrine tumors, miscellaneous tumors, and metastasis.[35] Mesenchymal tumors include many of the ones seen in soft tissues, such as leiomyosarcoma, angiosarcoma, rhaddomyosarcoma, osteosarcoma, synovial sarcoma, Ewing sarcoma, solitary fibrous tumor, and benign mesenchymal neoplastic forms. Cytologic characteristics of these neoplasms are similar to the

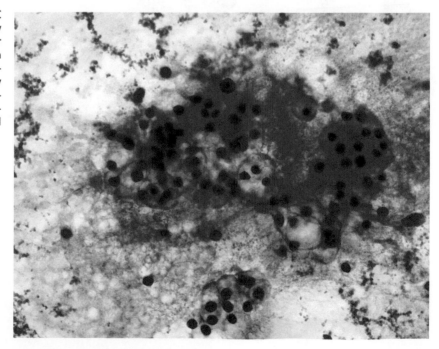

Fig. 7. Clear cell PRCC (clear cell tubulopapillary RCC). Low-grade clear epithelial cells with a predominantly linear nuclear alignment away from the basement membrane (Papanicolaou-stained smear; original magnification ×60).

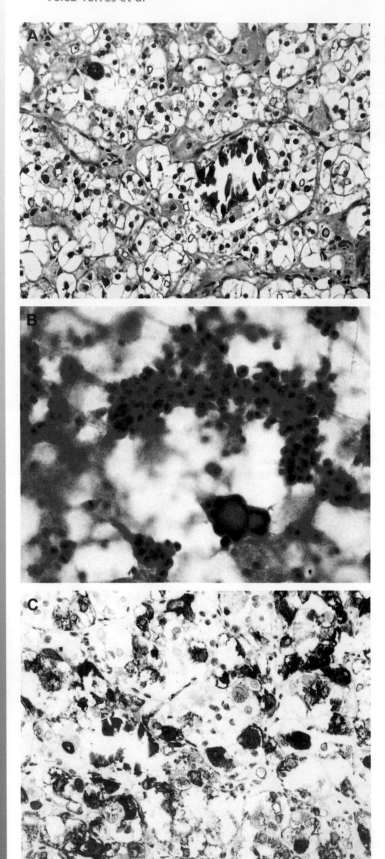

Fig. 8. TFE-3 translocation–associated RCC. (*A*) Tumor cells with abundant clear cell cytoplasm and high nuclear grade; alveolar or solid growth is commonly present in cell blocks (cell block; original magnification ×40). (*B*) Cells with granular eosinophilic cytoplasm and psammoma bodies (Papanicolaou-stained smear; original magnification ×60). (*C*) Melan-A positive (Melan-A immunostaining on cell block; original magnification ×60).

Fig. 8. (*continued*). (*D*) TFE3 positive (TFE-3 immunostaining. on cell block; original magnification ×60.) (*E*) TFE-3 FISH positive.

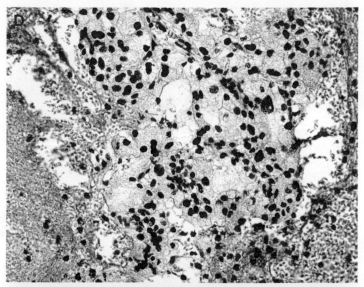

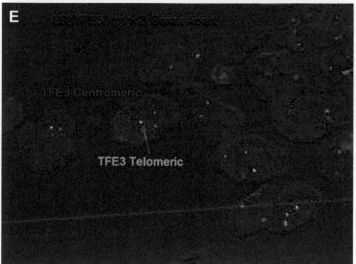

ones seen in other organs. Similarly, neuroendocrine neoplasms, including well-differentiated neuroendocrine tumor, large cell neuroendocrine carcinoma, small cell neuroendocrine carcinoma, and pheochromocytoma, show similar characteristics as the neuroendocrine neoplasm of other body parts.

GRADING RENAL CARCINOMA IN CYTOLOGIC SAMPLES

The 2012 ISUP grading system is currently in used. The ISUP grading classification for RCC is based on nucleolar prominence for grades 1 to 3,

whereas grade 4 is defined as tumors with highly pleomorphic tumor giant cells or the presence of sarcomatoid and/or rhabdoid morphology.[61] Overall grade is assigned based on the single high-power field showing the highest grade. There was also agreement that the presence of rhabdoid or sarcomatoid morphology within any of the morphologies of RCC represents dedifferentiation, showing similar prognosis of those presenting extreme nuclear pleomorphism or tumor giant cells.[62]

Correlation between the cytologic and histologic grades within the same tumor has been reported occur in more than 75% of cases.[63] For each

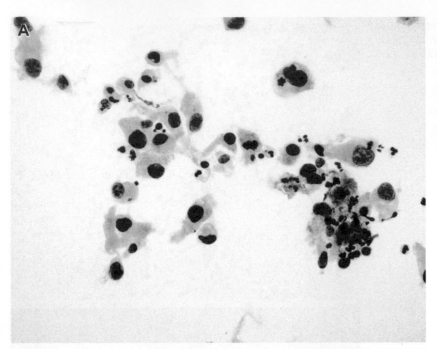

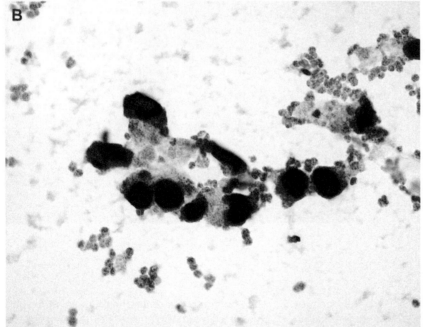

Fig. 9. CDC. (*A*) High-grade carcinoma with prominent inflammatory reaction, including a neutrophilic infiltrate, within and around the tumor (Papanicolaou-stained smear; original magnification ×60); (*B*) PAX-8 expression supports renal differentiation (PAX-8 immunostaining on smear; original magnification ×60).

discrepancy, the difference was no more than 1 grade. When grading as high grade or low grade was used, agreement was seen in 100% of the cases. The most reliable cytologic features distinguishing low from high-grade tumors were the nuclear/cytoplasmic ratio and the presence or absence of nucleoli. Pleomorphism, naked nuclei, and increased cellularity were less distinguishing features.

DIFFERENTIAL DIAGNOSIS BETWEEN RENAL NEOPLASM BASED IN CYTOLOGIC AND ARCHITECTURAL CHARACTERISTICS

Renal neoplasms can be grouped in several clusters, depending on the cytologic and architectural characteristic. This helps in using limited IHC panels, which is important especially in small samples, such as the ones obtained by FNAC. The main groups are defined in **Tables 2–4.**

Key Points
FNAC OF ADULT RENAL NEOPLASMS

- FNAC of renal masses, including SRMs, in comparison to CB, is relatively less invasive, cost effective, and amenable to immediate assessment.

- FNAC can separate benign from malignant renal neoplasms and it is helpful in subtyping RCC, especially if ancillary techniques, such as IHC and cytogenetics are used for the final interpretation.

- FNAC of renal tumors is highly valuable in the diagnosis of advanced stage disease, in patients with poor surgical status and/or with prior history of other malignancy, and in cases of discrepant clinical presentation and CT findings.

- Both FNAC and CB demonstrate excellent diagnostic accuracy when diagnosing malignancy demonstrating synergistic results.

Key Points
DIFFERENTIAL DIAGNOSIS OF ADULT RENAL NEOPLASMS

- Renal neoplasms can be grouped in several clusters, depending on the cytologic and architectural characteristic. This helps in using limited IHC panels, important especially in limited samples, such as the ones obtained by FNAC.
  - Tumors composed predominantly of clear cells
  - Tumors with a significant papillary component
  - Tumors with oncocytic features

REFERENCES

1. Bosniak MA. The current radiological approach to renal cysts. Radiology 1986;158(1):1–10.
2. Moreland WS, Zagoria RJ, Geisinger KR. Use of fine needle aspiration biopsy in radiofrequency ablation. Acta Cytol 2002;46(5):819–22.
3. Lew M, Foo WC, Roh MH. Diagnosis of metastatic renal cell carcinoma on fine-needle aspiration cytology. Arch Pathol Lab Med 2014;138(10):1278–85.
4. Alasker A, Williams SK, Ghavamian R. Small renal mass: to treat or not to treat. Curr Urol Rep 2013;14(1):13–8.
5. Volpe A, Cadeddu JA, Cestari A, et al. Contemporary management of small renal masses. Eur Urol 2011;60(3):501–15.
6. Farrell JJ, Brugge WR. EUS-guided fine-needle aspiration of a renal mass: an alternative method for diagnosis of malignancy. Gastrointest Endosc 2002;56(3):450–2.
7. Davis CJ Jr. Pathology of renal neoplasms. Semin Roentgenol 1987;22(4):233–40.
8. Lopes RI, Moura RN, Artifon E. Endoscopic ultrasound-guided fine-needle aspiration for the diagnosis of kidney lesions: a review. World J Gastrointest Endosc 2015;7(3):253–7.
9. Glassman D, Chawla SN, Waldman I, et al. Correlation of pathology with tumor size of renal masses. Can J Urol 2007;14(4):3616–20.
10. Ozen H, Colowick A, Freiha FS. Incidentally discovered solid renal masses: what are they? Br J Urol 1993;72(3):274–6.
11. Frank I, Blute ML, Cheville JC, et al. Solid renal tumors: an analysis of pathological features related to tumor size. J Urol 2003;170(6, Part 1):2217–20.
12. Jewett MAS, Mattar K, Basiuk J, et al. Active surveillance of small renal masses: progression patterns of early stage kidney cancer. Eur Urol 2011;60(1):39–44.
13. Rothman J, Egleston B, Wong YN, et al. Histopathological characteristics of localized renal cell carcinoma correlate with tumor size: a SEER analysis. J Urol 2009;181(1):29–34.
14. Lane BR, Samplaski MK, Herts BR, et al. Renal mass biopsy–a renaissance? J Urol 2008;179(1):20–7.
15. Sahni VA, Silverman SG. Biopsy of renal masses: when and why. Cancer Imaging 2009;9:44–55.
16. Volpe A, Finelli A, Gill IS, et al. Rationale for percutaneous biopsy and histologic characterisation of renal tumours. Eur Urol 2012;62(3):491–504.
17. Volpe A, Kachura JR, Geddie WR, et al. Techniques, safety and accuracy of sampling of renal tumors by fine needle aspiration and core biopsy. J Urol 2007;178(2):379–86.
18. Rioja J, de la Rosette JJ, Wijkstra H, et al. Advances in diagnosis and follow-up in kidney cancer. Curr Opin Urol 2008;18(5):447–54.
19. Laguna MP, Kummerlin I, Rioja J, et al. Biopsy of a renal mass: where are we now? Curr Opin Urol 2009;19(5):447–53.
20. Chow W, Devesa SS, Warren JL, et al. Rising incidence of renal cell cancer in the united states. JAMA 1999;281(17):1628–31.
21. Dragoescu EA, Liu L. Indications for renal fine needle aspiration biopsy in the era of modern imaging modalities. Cytojournal 2013;10:15.

22. Bardales R, Stelow EB, Mallery S, et al. Review of endoscopic ultrasound-guided fine needle aspiration cytology. Diagn Cytopathol 2006;34(2):140–75.

23. Truong LD, Todd TD, Dhurandhar B, et al. Fine-needle aspiration of renal masses in adults: analysis of results and diagnostic problems in 108 cases. Diagn Cytopathol 1999;20(6):339–49.

24. Silverman SG, Gan YU, Mortele KJ, et al. Renal masses in the adult patient: the role of percutaneous biopsy. Radiology 2006;240(1):6–22.

25. Renshaw AA, Granter SR, Cibas ES. Fine-needle aspiration of the adult kidney. Cancer 1997;81(2):71–88.

26. Caoili EM, Bude RO, Higgins EJ, et al. Evaluation of sonographically guided percutaneous core biopsy of renal masses. AJR Am J Roentgenol 2002;179(2):373–8.

27. Wood BJ, Khan MA, McGovern F, et al. Imaging guided biopsy of renal masses: indications, accuracy and impact on clinical management. J Urol 1999;161(5):1470–4.

28. Gattuso P, Ramzy I, Truong LD, et al. Utilization of fine-needle aspiration in the diagnosis of metastatic tumors to the kidney. Diagn Cytopathol 1999;21(1):35–8.

29. Lee CH, Chung SY, Moon KC, et al. A pilot study evaluating fine-needle aspiration cytology of clear-cell renal cell carcinoma: comparison of ancillary immunocytochemistry and cytomorphological characteristics of surepath liquid-based preparations with conventional smears. Acta Cytol 2015;59(3):239–47.

30. Yang CS, Choi E, Idrees MT, et al. Percutaneous biopsy of the renal mass: FNA or core needle biopsy? Cancer Cytopathol 2017;125(6):407–15.

31. Renshaw AA, Cibas ES. Kidney and adrenal gland, [Chapter 14]. In: Cytology. 3rd edition. Philadelphia: W.B. Saunders ELSEVIER; 2009. p. 403–31.

32. Renshaw AA, Lee KR, Madge R, et al. Accuracy of fine needle aspiration in distinguishing subtypes of renal cell carcinoma. Acta Cytol 1997;41(4):987–94.

33. Gowrishankar B, Cahill L, Arndt AE, et al. Subtyping of renal cortical neoplasms in fine needle aspiration biopsies using a decision tree based on genomic alterations detected by fluorescence in situ hybridization. BJU Int 2014;114(6):881–90.

34. Roh MH, Dal Cin P, Silverman SG, et al. The application of cytogenetics and fluorescence in situ hybridization to fine-needle aspiration in the diagnosis and subclassification of renal neoplasms. Cancer Cytopathol 2010;118(3):137–45.

35. Moch H, Cubilla AL, Humphrey PA, et al. The 2016 WHO classification of tumours of the urinary system and male genital organs-part a: renal, penile, and testicular tumours. Eur Urol 2016;70(1):93–105.

36. Lohse CM, Gupta S, Cheville JC. Outcome prediction for patients with renal cell carcinoma. Semin Diagn Pathol 2015;32(2):172–83.

37. Bostwick DG, Cheng L. Urologic surgical pathology. Philadelphia: Elsevier/Saunders; 2014.

38. Kryvenko ON, Jorda M, Argani P, et al. Diagnostic approach to eosinophilic renal neoplasms. Arch Pathol Lab Med 2014;138(11):1531–41.

39. Tickoo SK, Amin MB. Discriminant nuclear features of renal oncocytoma and chromophobe renal cell carcinoma. Analysis of their potential utility in the differential diagnosis. Am J Clin Pathol 1998;110(6):782–7.

40. Reuter VE, Argani P, Zhou M, et al. Best practices recommendations in the application of immunohistochemistry in the kidney tumors: report from the International Society of Urologic Pathology consensus conference. Am J Surg Pathol 2014;38(8):e35–49.

41. Conner JR, Hirsch MS, Jo VY. HNF1β and S100A1 are useful biomarkers for distinguishing renal oncocytoma and chromophobe renal cell carcinoma in FNA and core needle biopsies. Cancer Cytopathol 2015;123(5):298–305.

42. Yasir S, Herrera L, Gomez-Fernandez C, et al. CD10+ and CK7/RON- immunophenotype distinguishes renal cell carcinoma, conventional type with eosinophilic morphology from its mimickers. Appl Immunohistochem Mol Morphol 2012;20(5):454–61.

43. Barocas DA, Mathew S, DelPizzo JJ, et al. Renal cell carcinoma sub-typing by histopathology and fluorescence in situ hybridization on a needle-biopsy specimen. BJU Int 2007;99(2):290–5.

44. Chyhrai A, Sanjmyatav J, Gajda M, et al. Multi-colour FISH on preoperative renal tumour biopsies to confirm the diagnosis of uncertain renal masses. World J Urol 2010;28(3):269–74.

45. Receveur AO, Couturier J, Molinie V, et al. Characterization of quantitative chromosomal abnormalities in renal cell carcinomas by interphase four-color fluorescence in situ hybridization. Cancer Genet Cytogenet 2005;158(2):110–8.

46. Choueiri TK, Cheville J, Palescandolo E, et al. BRAF mutations in metanephric adenoma of the kidney. Eur Urol 2012;62(5):917–22.

47. Brunelli M, Eble JN, Zhang S, et al. Metanephric adenoma lacks the gains of chromosomes 7 and 17 and loss of Y that are typical of papillary renal cell carcinoma and papillary adenoma. Mod Pathol 2003;16(10):1060–3.

48. Doros LA, Rossi CT, Yang J, et al. DICER1 mutations in childhood cystic nephroma and its relationship to DICER1-renal sarcoma. Mod Pathol 2014;27:1267.

49. Reuter VE, Tickoo SK. Differential diagnosis of renal tumours with clear cell histology. Pathology 2010;42(4):374–83.

50. Al-Ahmadie HA, Alden D, Qin LX, et al. Carbonic anhydrase IX expression in clear cell renal cell carcinoma: an immunohistochemical study comparing 2 antibodies. Am J Surg Pathol 2008; 32(3):377–82.

51. Tickoo SK, Chen YB, Zynger DL. Biopsy interpretation of the kidney and adrenal gland. Philadelphia: Wolters Kluwer; 2015.

52. Zhou H, Zheng S, Truong LD, et al. Clear cell papillary renal cell carcinoma is the fourth most common histologic type of renal cell carcinoma in 290 consecutive nephrectomies for renal cell carcinoma. Hum Pathol 2014;45(1):59–64.

53. Rohan SM, Xiao Y, Liang Y, et al. Clear-cell papillary renal cell carcinoma: molecular and immunohistochemical analysis with emphasis on the von Hippel-Lindau gene and hypoxia-inducible factor pathway-related proteins. Mod Pathol 2011;24(9): 1207–20.

54. Tickoo SK, dePeralta-Venturina MN, Harik LR, et al. Spectrum of epithelial neoplasms in end-stage renal disease: an experience from 66 tumor-bearing kidneys with emphasis on histologic patterns distinct from those in sporadic adult renal neoplasia. Am J Surg Pathol 2006;30(2): 141–53.

55. Delahunt B, Sika-Paotonu D, Bethwaite PB, et al. Fuhrman grading is not appropriate for chromophobe renal cell carcinoma. Am J Surg Pathol 2007;31(6):957–60.

56. Delahunt B, Cheville JC, Martignoni G, et al. The International Society of Urological Pathology (ISUP) grading system for renal cell carcinoma and other prognostic parameters. Am J Surg Pathol 2013; 37(10):1490–504.

57. Hakimi AA, Tickoo SK, Jacobsen A, et al. TCEB1-mutated renal cell carcinoma: a distinct genomic and morphological subtype. Mod Pathol 2015;28: 845.

58. Tickoo SK, Reuter VE. Differential diagnosis of renal tumors with papillary architecture. Adv Anat Pathol 2011;18(2):120–32.

59. Williamson SR, Eble JN, Cheng L, et al. Clear cell papillary renal cell carcinoma: differential diagnosis and extended immunohistochemical profile. Mod Pathol 2013;26(5):697–708.

60. Tomlinson IP, Alam NA, Rowan AJ, et al, Multiple Leiomyoma Consortium. Germline mutations in FH predispose to dominantly inherited uterine fibroids, skin leiomyomata and papillary renal cell cancer. Nat Genet 2002;30: 406–10.

61. Samaratunga H, Gianduzzo T, Delahunt B. The ISUP system of staging, grading and classification of renal cell neoplasia. J Kidney Cancer VHL 2014; 1(3):26–39.

62. Chapman-Fredricks JR, Herrera L, Bracho J, et al. Adult renal cell carcinoma with rhabdoid morphology represents a neoplastic dedifferentiation analogous to sarcomatoid carcinoma. Ann Diagn Pathol 2011;15(5):333–7.

63. Nazer MA, Mourad WA. Succesful grading of renal cell carcinoma in fine-needle aspirates. Diagn Cytopathol 2000;22(4):223–6.

Applications of Ancillary Testing in the Cytologic Diagnosis of Soft Tissue Neoplasms

Vickie Y. Jo, MD

KEYWORDS

- Soft tissue • Sarcoma • Fine-needle aspiration • Immunohistochemistry
- Fluorescence in situ hybridization

Key points

- A pattern-based approach for soft tissue neoplasms provides a practical framework for formulating differential diagnoses and applying ancillary tests.

- Ancillary tests can identify characteristic immunophenotypes and molecular alterations, enabling accurate cytologic diagnoses for soft tissue neoplasms.

- Ancillary testing allows for efficient work-up of fine-needle aspiration material, and rapid on-site evaluation has the added benefit of allowing specimen triage for ancillary testing.

- The diagnostic utility of ancillary testing relies on correlation with clinical and morphologic features and judicious application and appropriate interpretation.

ABSTRACT

Soft tissue neoplasms are diagnostically challenging, although many advances in ancillary testing now enable accurate classification of fine-needle aspiration biopsies by detection of characteristic immunophenotypes (including protein correlates of molecular alterations) and molecular features. Although there are many useful diagnostic immunohistochemical markers and molecular assays, their diagnostic utility relies on correlation with clinical and morphologic features, judicious application, and appropriate interpretation because no single test is perfectly sensitive or specific. This review discusses applications of ancillary testing for commonly encountered soft tissue neoplasms in cytopathologic practice in the context of a pattern-based approach.

OVERVIEW

Soft tissue neoplasms frequently present diagnostic challenges in cytopathology, as tumors are rare and comprise numerous and diverse entities. The World Health Organization classification includes more than 100 distinct tumor types, which are categorized according to common histogenesis.[1] The rapid rate of molecular advances in soft tissue pathology has facilitated refinements in tumor classification, recognition of novel entities, and development of diagnostic tests. Definitive cytologic diagnosis is now feasible for many tumors sampled by fine-needle aspiration (FNA) with use of ancillary tests, which can detect specific immunophenotypes and molecular alterations as well as prognostic and predictive markers. Clinical management of patients with soft tissue tumors relies on accurate reporting of biologic behavior, and in this regard ancillary testing can help refine differential diagnoses even when precise classification is not possible. Ancillary testing is also useful for tumors presenting in unusual clinical contexts (such as unexpected patient age/gender or tumor site), and molecular testing is especially helpful for tumors showing uncharacteristic cytomorphologic features or inconclusive immunophenotypes.

Disclosures: The author has no disclosures.
Brigham and Women's Hospital, 75 Francis Street, Boston, MA 02115, USA
E-mail address: vjo@partners.org

Surgical Pathology 11 (2018) 633–656
https://doi.org/10.1016/j.path.2018.06.002

surgpath.theclinics.com

The traditional role of immunohistochemistry in identifying line of differentiation is now expanded to include lineage-specific markers, protein correlates of specific molecular alterations, and novel tumor-type specific markers identified by gene expression profiling. Molecular methods have largely replaced conventional karyotype analysis. Fluorescence in situ hybridization (FISH) is used to detect translocations and amplifications. Reverse transcriptase–polymerase chain reaction detects specific fusion genes, which can be more specific than FISH given the promiscuity of many molecular alterations (eg, *EWSR1* and *FUS* rearrangements[2]). Single-gene analysis is relevant for some tumors, such as *KIT* mutations in GIST. There have been many developments in next-generation sequencing (NGS) that have specific applications in soft tissue pathology,[3] and it is expected that NGS will have wider clinical implementation and replace low-throughput techniques in the future. Most immunohistochemical antibodies and molecular assays have been clinically validated on formalin-fixed, paraffin-embedded (FFPE) material, and FFPE cell blocks are the favored substrate for ancillary testing. All cytologic preparations, however, have proved reliable substrates for FISH and sequencing-based methods,[4–6] and testing of direct smears and liquid-based preparations should be considered if material is limited. Rapid on-site evaluation gives an opportunity for specimen triage for ancillary testing during FNA.

The diagnosis of soft tissue tumors requires integration of clinical data, cytomorphology, and ancillary tests. A pattern-based approach provides a practical framework for formulating differential diagnoses and applying ancillary tests, and most soft tissue tumors fall into one of the following morphologic patterns: adipocytic, myxoid, spindle, round cell, epithelioid, and pleomorphic.[7] This review discusses updates in ancillary tests for the more commonly encountered soft tissue neoplasms on FNA in the context of this pattern-based approach.

ADIPOCYTIC NEOPLASMS

Tumors that show prominent adipocytic, or fatty, features include benign and malignant adipocytic neoplasms and several nonadipocytic tumors that have fatty components. Some adipocytic neoplasms overlap with other morphologic patterns: for instance, spindle cell lipoma, myxoid liposarcoma, and lipoblastoma have myxoid features; and pleomorphic liposarcoma and dedifferentiated liposarcoma (DDLPS) are part of the differential for pleomorphic neoplasms.

The presence of a mature fatty component and absence of cytologic atypia allows for general classification as a benign lipomatous tumor, although definitive subclassification can be more challenging on cytology.[8] The most commonly encountered benign tumors are lipoma, hibernoma, and spindle cell lipoma. Most cases of lipoma and hibernoma are diagnostically straightforward, with the former appearing as predominantly mature fat and the latter showing an admixture of mature adipocytes and brown fat with multiple cytoplasmic vacuoles.[9] Lipomas showing fat necrosis and hibernomas may mimic atypical lipomatous tumor/well-differentiated liposarcoma (ALT/WDL) and require MDM2 testing to exclude ALT/WDL (discussed later).

Spindle cell/pleomorphic lipoma shows a broad morphologic spectrum, with variable proportions of its constituent features of myxoid or collagenous stroma, uniform short ovoid-to-spindle nuclei, long ropey collagen fibers, and mature fat[10]; some cases may show multinucleated floret-like cells or small lipoblasts. Immunohistochemistry can be helpful in the diagnosis of spindle cell lipoma, which is positive for CD34 and shows loss of expression of RB1 secondary to loss of heterozygosity of 13q10,[11,12] similarly to its related tumors mammary-type myofibroblastoma and cellular angiofibroma.[13,14] Some tumors may need MDM2 and CDK4 immunohistochemistry to exclude ALT/WDL and others with more myxoid stroma may require *DDIT3* FISH to exclude myxoid liposarcoma.

ALT/WDL and DDLPS is characterized by amplification of chromosome 12q13-15. This region includes the *MDM2, CDK4,* and *HMGA2* genes, and amplification can be detected by FISH for the *MDM2* locus or immunohistochemistry for MDM2 and CDK4 (and HGMA2)[15] (**Fig. 1**). ALT/WDL shows atypical hyperchromatic stromal cells and variably sized adipocytes. These features are often subtle, and cases of lipoma-like ALT/WDL are especially challenging. Lipoblasts are rarely present and are not required for diagnosis. Fat necrosis may appear worrisome for ALT/WDL, and histiocytes can show MDM2 positivity.[16] Accurate diagnosis of ALT/WDL is important given its risk for recurrence and dedifferentiation to DDLPS. Nuclear expression of MDM2 and CDK4 is sufficiently diagnostic in many scenarios, although *MDM2* FISH has higher sensitivity for ALT/WDL in small biopsies[17] and should be considered for challenging cases. Testing for MDM2 amplification should always be performed for large (>10.0-cm) deep-seated extremity masses, tumors within body cavities (retroperitoneum and mediastinum), recurrent lesions, and tumors with equivocal atypia, because these scenarios favor ALT/WDL over lipoma.[18,19]

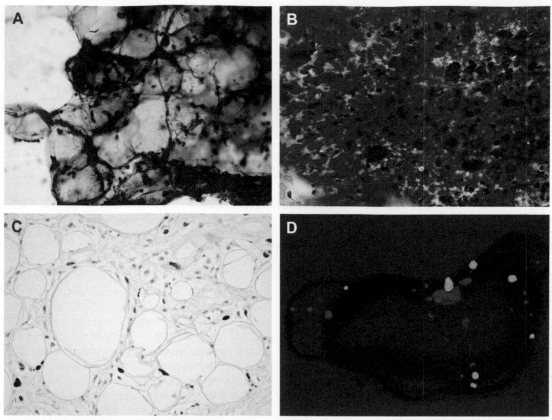

Fig. 1. ALT/WDL and DDLPS are characterized by amplification of chromosome 12q13-15, which includes the *MDM2* locus. ALT/WDL shows subtle features of variation in adipocyte size and scattered atypical stromal cells ([*A*] Diff-Quik stain, ×400). DDLPS often appears as an indistinct nonlipogenic pleomorphic sarcoma ([*B*] Diff-Quik stained, ×400). Immunohistochemistry for MDM2 ([*C*] ALT/WDL, ×400) and CDK4 serves as a surrogate for 12q13-15 amplification; *MDM2* FISH is confirmatory ([*D*] *MDM2* probe [*red*]; centromeric probe *CEP12* [*green*]).

DDLPS shows a broad morphologic spectrum, for which MDM2/CDK4 immunohistochemistry and/or *MDM2* FISH are necessary for definitive diagnosis.[20–23] Most tumors show a wide spectrum of nonlipogenic morphologies and may be considered in the differential diagnosis of spindle, myxoid, and pleomorphic patterns. A subset is lipogenic with numerous large atypical lipoblasts (so-called homologous dedifferentiation) and resembles pleomorphic liposarcoma.[24–26] DDLPS is the chief consideration when encountering any nonlipogenic neoplasm in the retroperitoneum.

Pleomorphic liposarcoma has no specific immunohistochemical features and harbors a complex karyotype. Tumors have high-grade spindle, pleomorphic, or epithelioid tumor cells and characteristic pleomorphic, multivacuolated lipoblasts, which can be abundant or more sparsely present.[25,27] The presence of lipoblasts is the key diagnostic feature; pleomorphic liposarcoma is otherwise indistinguishable from other high-grade pleomorphic sarcomas, such as high-grade myxofibrosarcoma, and definitive diagnosis is often deferred to surgical resection. Tumors can be distinguished from DDLPS by negativity for MDM2 and CDK4.

Myxoid liposarcoma, which harbors *FUS-DDIT3* fusion,[28] has the characteristic features of myxoid stroma, delicate branching capillaries, and small lipoblasts that are often univaculoted or bivacuolated. Tumors have a uniform ovoid, spindle, and round cell population that shows increased cellularity with higher grade; high-grade myxoid liposarcoma can appear as a round cell sarcoma. Most cases are recognizable according to these characteristic morphologic features, although many cases undergo molecular confirmation. FISH for *DDIT3* FISH is commonly used because it is more specific for myxoid liposarcoma than *FUS* FISH and also detects the small subset that harbor *EWSR1-DDIT3* fusion[29,30] (**Fig. 2**).

Lipoblastomas are benign but resemble myxoid liposarcoma by having abundant myxoid matrix,

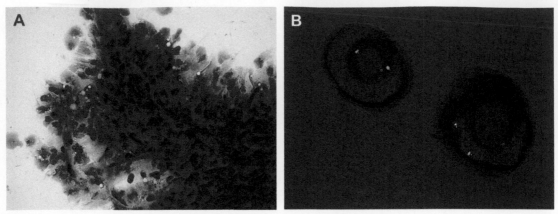

Fig. 2. Myxoid liposarcoma. This high-grade example is hypercellular but still shows the characteristic features of delicate branching vessels and small lipoblasts ([A] Diff-Quik stain, ×400). *DDIT3* rearrangement is confirmed by FISH with separate green telomeric *DDIT3* and red centromeric *DDIT3* signals (*B*).

thin branching capillaries, uniform spindle cells, and varying bland lipoblasts and mature fat.[31] Lipoblastoma is distinct, however, in that tumors typically arise during infancy and lacks nuclear atypia. Tumors are characterized by *PLAG1* rearrangements that can be detected by *PLAG1* FISH or PLAG1 immunohistochemsitry.[31,32]

Several nonlipomatous tumors may show prominent fat, and immunohistochemistry is helpful in characterizing their respective cellular components: PEComa (SMA, desmin, HMB-45, and MelanA), fat-forming solitary fibrous tumor (SFT) (CD34 and STAT6), myolipoma (desmin and SMA), and mammary-type myofibroblastoma and cellular angiofibroma (CD34, desmin, and Rb loss). Myelolipoma may be a mimic for ALT, but megakaryocytes within the trilineage hematopoiesis are negative for MDM2/CDK4.

Key Features
ADIPOCYTIC NEOPLASMS

Tumor	Cytomorphologic Pattern(s)	Immunohistochemical Features	Molecular Features
Lipoma	Adipocytic/lipogenic	—	12q rearrangement; 6p21 rearrangement; or 13q deletion
Hibernoma	Adipocytic/lipogenic	—	11q alterations
Spindle cell lipoma	Adipocytic/lipogenic Myxoid	CD34, Rb-loss	Loss of 13q or 16q
Lipoblastoma	Adipocytic/lipogenic Myxoid	PLAG1	*PLAG1* rearrangement
ALT/WDL	Adipocytic/lipogenic	MDM2, CDK4	12q13-15 amplification
Myxoid liposarcoma	Adipocytic/lipogenic Myxoid	—	*FUS-DDIT3;* rare *EWSR1-DDIT3*
Pleomorphic liposarcoma	Adipocytic/lipogenic Spindle Epithelioid Pleomorphic	—	Complex karyotype
DDLPS	Adipocytic/lipogenic Myxoid Spindle Pleomorphic	MDM2, CDK4	12q13-15 amplification

MYXOID NEOPLASMS

Myxoid neoplasms encompass a wide spectrum of tumor types that includes benign tumors and sarcomas with spindle or epithelioid morphology. Several adipocytic neoplasms (spindle cell lipoma, myxoid liposarcoma, and lipoblastoma) can show a prominent extracellular myxoid matrix (discussed earlier). Tumors with abundant myxoid matrix can yield hypocellular smears that appear deceptively bland, which are challenging to classify and especially misleading for tumors with unsampled high grade areas.

Smears showing hypocellular low-grade myxoid neoplasms with relatively bland spindle or ovoid cells are diagnostically challenging, and ancillary studies are primarily helpful in excluding malignant neoplasms after which a diagnosis of "benign myxoid spindle cell neoplasm" is appropriate.[33] The main diagnostic considerations in somatic sites are the benign entities, intramusclar/cellular myxoma and soft tissue perineurioma, and low-grade fibromyxoid sarcoma (LGFMS). Soft tissue perineurioma is typically positive for CD34, EMA, and Claudin-1; however, expression of these markers is variable, and EMA is positive in subsets of both LGFMS and myxoma.[33] Myxoma has no specific immunohistochemical features but is characterized by *GNAS1* mutations,[34] which can be detected by molecular testing.

Aspirate smears of LGFMS show deceptively bland spindle and ovoid cells embedded in a myxoid matrix.[35] Definitive diagnosis is feasible if cell block material is available for immunohistochemistry, and cytoplasmic MUC4 expression is a highly sensitive and marker for LGFMS[36] (**Fig. 3**). LGFMS is characterized by *FUS* rearrangements, most commonly with fusion partners *CREB3L2* or *CREB3L1*.[37,38] *FUS* FISH is diagnostic in most cases; *EWSR1* FISH may be needed to identify rare cases of variant *EWSR1* fusions. Tumors with hybrid features of LGFMS and sclerosing epithelioid fibrosarcoma occur; sclerosing epithelioid fibrosarcoma seems genetically related and a subset harbors *FUS-CREB3L1* and MUC4 expression.[39–41]

Myxofibrosarcoma lacks specific immunohistochemical features and has a complex

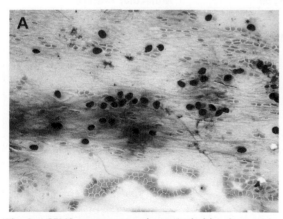
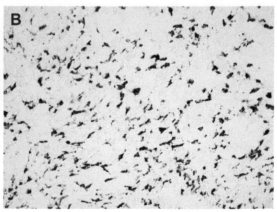

Fig. 3. LGFMS appears as a deceptively bland myxoid neoplasm with mildly atypical ovoid nuclei ([*A*] Diff-Quik stain, 400×). LGFMS shows diffuse cytoplasmic staining for MUC4, which distinguishes LGFMS from its cytomorphologic mimics (*B*, 100×).

karyotype. All smears show some degree of cytologic atypia and characteristic curvilinear vessels; low-grade tumors show lower cellularity (and may resemble cellular myxoma) and high-grade tumors often show areas of solid growth of spindle, pleomorphic, or even epithelioid cells (discussed later).[42–44] High-grade myxofibrosarcoma can closely resemble pleomorphic liposarcoma and may even show pseudolipoblasts; distinction between the two is typically deferred to surgical resection because their respective characteristic features may not be represented. Immunohistochemistry is helpful to exclude DDLPS.

For myxoid neoplasms showing a uniform ovoid and epithelioid morphology arranged in cords and nests within a myxoid stroma, extraskeletal myxoid chondrosarcoma (EMC), myoepithelial neoplasms of soft tissue, and ossifying fibromyxoid tumor (OFMT) should be considered in the differential diagnosis. Tumor cells of EMC often have tapered cytoplasmic processes.[45] Tumors express S100 in 50% of cases.[46] EMC harbors NR4A3 rearrangements with either EWSR1 or TAF15 partners[47,48]; FISH for NR4A3 is a common diagnostic approach and is more specific than EWSR1 FISH.[49] Myoepithelial neoplasms of soft tissue show more cytomorphologic heterogeneity with a spectrum of ovoid, spindle, epithelioid, and occasionally plasmacytoid or rhabdoid morphology. Tumors show variable expression of keratin, EMA, S100, GFAP, and p63,[50] and a subset shows loss of INI1 expression.[51] Myoepithelial carcinomas have frequent EWSR1 fusions involving various partners as well as rare variant FUS fusions[52–56]; SMARCB1 deletions are present in a subset.[57] In pediatric patients, myoepithelial carcinomas can show epithelioid or round cell morphology.[51] OFMT also shows uniform epithelioid cells embedded in a fibromyxoid stroma[58,59]; its characteristic peripheral shell of bone is unlikely to be sampled. OFMT is positive for S100 and desmin and has PHF1 rearrangements.[60,61]

Key Features
COMMON NEOPLASMS WITH MYXOID PATTERNS

Tumor Type	Immunophenotype	Molecular Features
Myxoma	—	GNAS1 mutation
Soft tissue perineurioma	EMA, Claudin-1	—
LGFMS	MUC4	FUS-CREB3L2, FUS-CREB3L1
Spindle cell lipoma	CD34, Rb-loss	Loss of 13q or 16q
Myxoid liposarcoma	—	FUS-DDIT3; rare EWSR1-DDIT3
Lipoblastoma	PLAG1	PLAG1 rearrangement
EMC	S100 (50%)	EWSR1-NR4A3; TAF15-NR4A3
Myoepithelial neoplasms of soft tissue	Keratin, EMA, S100, SOX10, p63 (50%), INI1-loss	EWSR1 rearrangement (various partners: PBX1, PBX3, POU5F1, ATF1, KLF17, ZNF44)
OFMT	S100, desmin	PHF1 rearrangement
Myxofibrosarcoma	—	Complex karyotype
Pleomorphic liposarcoma	—	Complex karyotype
DDLPS	MDM2, CDK4	12q15-13 amplification

SPINDLE CELL NEOPLASMS

Spindle cell neoplasms may be challenging to classify given the significant overlap between benign tumors, intermediate-grade neoplasms, and sarcomas, and ancillary testing has a central role in the diagnostic work-up. The diagnostic approach should focus on accurate assignment of biologic grade to guide appropriate management; if definitive classification is not possible, descriptive cytologic diagnoses, such as low-grade spindle cell neoplasm, atypical spindle cell neoplasm, and high-grade sarcoma, are appropriate.

Among benign spindle cell neoplasms, schwannomas and soft tissue leiomyomas are common. Schwannomas yield smears with large cohesive syncytial fragments of spindle cells having wavy or bent nuclei with tapered ends and fibrillary cytoplasm; tumors may show nuclear pseudoinclusions and degenerative nuclear changes. Cellular schwannomas are fascicular, which can be worrisome for low-grade sarcomas. Diffuse nuclear S100 staining is characteristic of schwannoma. Leiomyomas show fascicular fragments of bland spindle cells having plump ovoid nuclei and eosinophilic cytoplasm; severe atypia, significant mitotic activity, and necrosis are absent. SMA, desmin, and caldesmon support smooth muscle differentiation.

Nodular fasciitis, now known to be a transient benign neoplasm that harbors USP6-MYH9 fusion,[62] follows a pathognomonic self-limited clinical course of rapid growth of a tender subcutaneous nodule followed by spontaneous regression. Smears are cellular with unipolar or bipolar spindle and stellate cells in loose clusters and fascicles, an inflammatory infiltrate, and myxoid or collagenous stroma.[63–65] Most diagnoses are based on the characteristic clinical picture, but diagnostic confirmation by USP6 FISH is feasible on FNA material.[66]

Desmoid fibromatosis presents as extra-abdominal, intra-abdominal, and abdominal wall tumors and can arise during pregnancy and post-cesarean section. Tumors are locally aggressive with frequent recurrences. Long fascicular fragments of bland bipolar spindle cells within a collagenous stroma is typical.[67,68] Sporadic tumors have CTNNB1 mutations[69] and tumors associated with familial adenomatous polyposis harbor APC mutations.[70] These mutations result in nuclear accumulation of β-catenin, which can be detected by immunohistochemistry in up to 80% of cases.[71] SMA is variable. Sequencing is helpful in certain circumstances.

Inflammatory myofibroblastic tumor (IMT) shows cellular smears of plump, mildly atypical myofibroblastic cells singly dispersed and arranged in loosely cohesive groups and an inflammatory infiltrate of lymphocytes, plasma cells, and histiocytes.[72] IMT is positive for SMA and variably positive for desmin and keratin; up to 50% of cases show ALK expression secondary to ALK rearrangements involving a heterogeneous group of partners. ALK expression is typically diffusely cytoplasmic, and the pattern seems to reflect the function of the involved fusion partner; for instance, TPM3 and TPM4 are cytoplasmic proteins.[73,74] IMT is characterized by repeated recurrences and small risk for metastasis.

Gastrointestinal stromal tumor (GIST) is the most common mesenchymal neoplasm in the gastrointestinal tract (but are rare in the esophagus and rectum), and tumors range in biologic behavior from essentially benign to highly aggressive. Although immunohistochemistry enables the cytologic diagnosis of GIST, risk stratification using the National Comprehensive Cancer Network scheme[75] is not possible and is deferred to surgical resection. The spindle cells of GIST are uniform with wispy cytoplasm and frequent cytoplasmic extensions and are arranged in clusters, with frequent isolated cells and bare nuclei.[76–79] Some extent of epithelioid morphology is seen in up to 30% of cases. Most GISTs (80%) harbor KIT mutations. PDGFRA mutations are second most common (10%–15%)[80]; the remaining KIT wild-type GISTs include BRAF V600E, association with neurofibromatosis type 1, and succinate dehydrogenase (SDH)-deficient GISTs (discussed later). KIT immunohistochemistry is positive in most (95%) GISTs, regardless of KIT mutation status. DOG1 is also a useful marker and stains up to 30% of KIT-negative GISTs[81,82] and is more robust stain than KIT in cytologic samples processed in methanol-based fixatives.[83] KIT exon 11 mutations are most common in GIST (80%) and render sensitivity to the tyrosine kinase inhibitor imatinib, the first-line therapy for GIST. Mutational analysis is sometimes necessary to identify mutations that render poor or no response to imatinib, such as KIT exon 9 mutations and PDGFRA D842V. Sequencing is also diagnostically helpful to identify GISTs that show treatment-related histologic responses and the subset (2%) that is negative for both KIT and DOG1.

Aspirates of SFT are composed of uniform spindle cells variably arranged in anastomosing fascicles and singly dispersed, often with cytoplasmic processes.[84,85] CD34 has long been used for the diagnosis of SFT but is not sensitive or specific. SFT harbors *NAB2-STAT6* fusion, secondary to an intrachromosomal rearrangement on 12q13[86,87] that cannot be detected by karyotype or FISH due to the close proximity of the involved genes. Immunohistochemistry, however, can detect resultant nuclear overexpression of STAT6, which is highly sensitive and specific for SFT[88,89] and has diagnostic utility in FNA samples.[90]

Dermatofibrosarcoma protuberans (DFSP) can resemble SFT and is also positive for CD34 but negative for STAT6. The characteristic storiform growth pattern is a helpful feature.[91,92] The diagnosis can be confirmed by *PDGFB* FISH to detect the characteristic *COL1A1-PDGFB* fusion[93]; molecular testing may be particularly helpful for cases of high-grade fibrosarcomatous transformation, which appear as an indistinct spindle cell sarcomas.

Spindle cell neoplasms of intermediate biologic potential (such as SFT) can often be difficult to distinguish from spindle cell sarcomas on cytomorphologic grounds. Most spindle cell sarcomas show cellular smears with frequent singly dispersed nuclei; if present, the features of cytologic atypia, mitotic activity, and necrosis are helpful in determining malignancy. The differential diagnosis commonly includes synovial sarcoma, MPNST, leiomyosarcoma, spindle cell rhabdomyosarcoma (RMS), and DDLPS. Leiomyosarcomas are positive for SMA, desmin, and caldesmon. Spindle cell/sclerosing RMS shows diffuse desmin positivity, and most cases show diffuse nuclear expression of MyoD1 secondary to *MyoD1* L122R mutations.[94,95] MDM2 and CDK4 identify DDLPS.

Nearly all cases of synovial sarcoma show cellular smears of spindle cells in clusters intermixed with singly disperse nuclei. Transgressing delicate vessels are commonly present, and epithelial structures are present for biphasic tumors. The spindle cell component expresses at least focal EMA and/or keratin in most cases. TLE1 has been shown highly sensitive but more modestly specific for synovial sarcoma (**Fig. 4**); most tumors show diffuse nuclear staining but TLE1 expression may be seen in multiple mimics, including MPNST and SFT.[96–98] *SS18-SSX* fusions are characteristic of synovial sarcoma,[99] which can be detected by *SS18* FISH or sequencing. Ancillary testing may be especially helpful in recognizing the 10% of cases that are poorly differentiated and show round cell or epithelioid morphology.[100]

There are numerous diagnostic challenges for MPNST. The diagnosis can be favored in certain clinical contexts, such as neurofibromatosis type I, origin from a peripheral nerve or neurofibroma, or postradiation. Smears are composed of spindle cells arranged in clusters and singly dispersed, and tumors show greater atypia and pleomorphism, necrosis, and mitotic activity with increased histologic grade.[101,102] Tumors show limited, if any, expression of S100, SOX10, and GFAP. Desmin may be focally positive, even in the absence of heterologous rhabdomyoblastic differentiation. Inactivation of the polycomb repressor complex 2 (PRC2) via mutations of coding genes for its subunits SUZ12 or EED1 is present in a subset of MPNST[103,104];

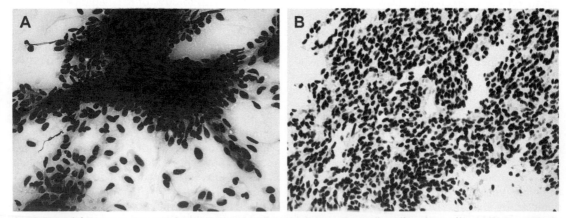

Fig. 4. Synovial sarcoma. Smears show clustered and singly dispersed spindle cells, often with traversing delicate vessels ([A] Diff-Quik stain). Synovial sarcoma shows diffuse nuclear expression of TLE1 (B), although specificity is imperfect and may require confirmatory molecular testing for *SS18* rearrangement.

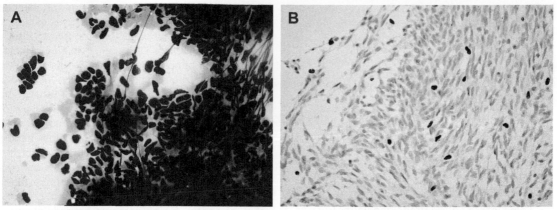

Fig. 5. MPNST is difficult to distinguish from other spindle cell sarcomas ([*A*] Diff-Quik stain, ×400). Immunohistochemical loss of H3K27me3 is a useful marker for high-grade MPNST (*B*, ×400), although overall sensitivity and specificity is imperfect.

PRC2 inactivation leads to loss of histone H3 trimethylation at lysine 27, which can be detected by immunohistochemistry (H3K27me3).[105–108] Loss of H3K27me is most frequent in high-grade tumors (**Fig. 5**) and thus is not entirely sensitive for MPNST. H3K27me3 loss should be interpreted with an inclusive panel given its moderate specificity, because loss occurs in several mimics including synovial sarcoma and DDLPS.[108,109]

Key Features
SELECTED SPINDLE CELL NEOPLASMS

Tumor Type	Immunophenotype	Molecular Features
Benign tumors		
Schwannoma	S100, SOX10	—
Leiomyoma	SMA, desmin, caldesmon	—
Nodular fasciitis	SMA	*MYH9-USP6*
Tumors with intermediate biologic potential		
Desmoid fibromatosis	β-catenin, SMA±	*CTNNB1* or *APC* mutations
IMT	SMA±, ALK (50%)	*ALK* rearrangements (partners include *TPM3*, *TPM4*, *CLTC*, *RANBP2*)
GIST	KIT, DOG1	*KIT* mutations (80%) Also: *PDGFRA* mutations, *BRAF* V600E, association with NF-1
SFT	CD34, STAT6	*NAB2-STAT6*
DFSP	CD34	*COL1A1-PDGFB*
Sarcomas		
Synovial sarcoma	EMA, keratin, TLE1	*SS18-SSX1*, *SS18-SSX2*
MPNST	±S100, ±SOX10, ±GFAP, H3K27me3-loss (in higher-grade tumors)	*NF1*, *CDKN2A*, *SUZ12*, *EED1* mutations
Leiomyosarcoma	SMA, desmin, caldesmon	Complex karyotype
Spindle cell RMS	Desmin, MyoD1	*MyoD1* L122R
DDLPS	MDM2, CDK4	12q13-15 amplification

Abbreviation: NF, neurofibromatosis.

ROUND CELL NEOPLASMS

Accurate classification of round cell neoplasms requires ancillary testing, and many tumors in this group have specific treatment regiments, such as Ewing sarcoma and alveolar RMS. The initial immunohistochemical panel should ideally include CD99 for Ewing sarcoma, desmin for alveolar RMS, keratin for carcinoma, S100 for melanoma, and TdT for lymphoblastic lymphoma. Pitfalls include nonspecific CD99 staining in many mimics of Ewing sarcoma and aberrant expression of keratin and neuroendocrine markers in numerous round cell sarcomas, a pitfall in older adults who are more likely to have carcinoma.

Ewing sarcoma was the first sarcoma identified to harbor a recurrent translocation. Most tumors harbor *EWSR1-FLI* fusion[110]; a small subset has alternate fusions involving *EWSR1* with partners from other members of the *ETS* transcription factor family,[111–114] with *ERG* the second most common (5% of cases). Ewing sarcoma typically shows a uniform tumor cell population with round nuclei having slightly irregular contours, small or inconspicuous nucleoli, and frequently vacuolated cytoplasm due to increased glycogen[115–117]; nuclear molding is frequent. Smears may show naked nuclei in a background of glycogen-rich cytoplasmic fragments (which may appear tigroid) and a second population of hyperchromatic, degenerating cells. Immunohistochemistry is helpful to identify cases for confirmatory molecular testing, either by *EWSR1* FISH or sequencing (**Fig. 6**).

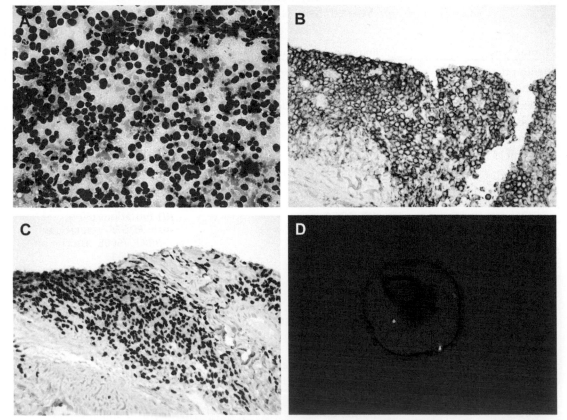

Fig. 6. Ewing sarcoma is a round cell sarcoma that has a uniform appearance; a tigroid background is common ([*A*] Diff-Quik stain, ×400). Tumors show a characteristic diffuse membranous staining pattern for CD99 (*B*, ×400). Nuclear NKX2.2 is highly sensitive, but less specific, for Ewing sarcoma (*C*, ×400). FISH confirms *EWSR1* rearrangement ([*D*] telomeric *EWSR1* [*green*] and centromeric *EWSR1* [*red*]).

Ewing sarcoma shows a characteristic membranous staining pattern for CD99, although CD99 staining should be evaluated carefully given that numerous other round cell sarcomas and nonmesenchymal mimics (such as well-differentiated neuroendocrine tumors) can show nonspecific CD99 expression. FLI1 is positive in up to 70% of cases, and ERG is positive in tumors with EWSR1-ERG.[118] NKX2.2 has been shown to have high sensitivity for Ewing sarcoma but more modest specificity.[119] Aberrant expression of keratin, synaptophysin, and chromogranin occurs in up to 30% of cases, and pitfalls of misclassification as a neuroendocrine tumor is well known.[120] If EWSR1 rearrangement is not detected, testing for FUS fusions should be considered.[121]

Alveolar RMS has the cytomorphologic appearance of atypical round cells with large, irregular hyperchromatic nuclei, and occasional wreath-like giant cells.[122] Tumors show desmin and myogenin positivity, similarly to all other RMS subtypes (embryonal, spindle cell/sclerosing, and pleomorphic), however nuclear expression of myogenin is specific for alveolar RMS and a useful diagnostic feature.[123] Alveolar RMS may show positivity for keratin, synaptophysin, and chromogranin,[124] which could be mistaken for neuroendocrine carcinoma, especially in adult patients. PAX3-FOXO1 and PAX7-FOXO1 fusions are characteristic,[125,126] and FOXO1 FISH is a common diagnostic approach.

Smears of desmoplastic small round cell tumor (DSRCT) show round cells arranged in irregularly shaped groups with nuclear molding at the periphery, and desmoplastic stroma may be present.[127] Most tumors arise as intra-abdominal masses in young male patients. DSRCT shows expression of keratin, EMA, and NSE; dotlike positivity for desmin; and reactivity to antibodies to the C-terminus of WT1. DSRCT harbors EWSR1-WT1[128]; EWSR1 rearrangements detected by FISH alone should be interpreted with caution, especially because DSRCT can show variable positivity for CD99, synaptophysin, and chromogranin. Identification of the specific fusion gene by sequencing facilitates definitive diagnosis.

Other round cell sarcomas show CD99 expression, including poorly differentiated synovial sarcoma, high-grade myxoid liposarcoma, myoepithelial carcinomas of soft tissue with round cell morphology, and mesenchymal chondrosarcoma. TLE1 immunohistochemistry and SS18 FISH is helpful for synovial sarcoma. High-grade myxoid liposarcoma may only have focal areas of its characteristic features; molecular testing for FUS-DDIT3 is confirmatory. Soft tissue myoepithelial carcinomas show expression of keratin, EMA, S100, and GFAP; tumors have EWSR1 rearrangements and sequencing may be helpful to identify the specific fusion partners. Mesenchymal chondrosarcoma is a biphasic tumor and shows a round cell population admixed with a well-differentiated cartilaginous component and harbors HEY1-NCOA2 fusion.[129]

Rare molecular subsets have been identified among undifferentiated round cell sarcomas and should be considered after exclusion of Ewing sarcoma and other round cell sarcomas. CIC-rearranged sarcoma[130–134] and BCOR-CCNB3 sarcoma[135–139] are newly described entities that show variable (often negative) CD99 expression and differ from Ewing sarcoma by showing increased cytologic atypia, prominent nucleoli, increased cytoplasm, spindle morphology, myxoid stroma, and necrosis. Diagnosis requires molecular confirmation due to their novelty and rarity. Identification of their respective immunophenotypes is helpful to identify cases for molecular testing. CIC-rearranged sarcoma shows nuclear expression of WT1 and ETV4[140–142]; most cases have CIC-DUX4 fusion, which can be detected by CIC FISH. CCNB3 is sensitive and specific for BCOR-CCNB3 sarcoma[143]; tumors also express of BCOR, TLE1, and SATB2,[139] which have more limited sensitivity and specificity.

Key Points

PRACTICAL CONSIDERATIONS FOR ROUND CELL SARCOMAS

- Careful assessment of the CD99 staining pattern is necessary; if staining pattern is variable staining, consider alternative diagnoses to Ewing sarcoma.

- Nonmesenchymal neoplasms (lymphoid, epithelial, and melanoma) should always be considered in the differential diagnosis.

- An initial immunohistochemical panel should ideally include CD99, desmin, keratin, S100, and TdT.

- EWSR1 and FUS rearrangements are features of various round cell neoplasms and molecular testing results should be interpreted in conjunction with clinical, morphologic, and immunohistochemical features.

<table>
<tr><th colspan="4" align="center">**Differential Diagnosis**
ROUND CELL SARCOMAS</th></tr>
<tr><th>Tumor Type</th><th>Immunophenotype</th><th>Molecular Features</th><th>Other</th></tr>
<tr>
<td>Ewing sarcoma</td>
<td>CD99+++, NKX2.2, FLI-1</td>
<td>*EWSR1-FLI1*</td>
<td>Rare variant fusions of *EWSR1* with other ETS family members (*ERG, ETV1, ETV4* [*EIAF*], and *FEV*)
ERG positive in tumors with *EWSR1-ERG*
Rare variant *FUS* fusions</td>
</tr>
<tr>
<td>Alveolar RMS</td>
<td>Desmin, myogenin</td>
<td>*PAX3-FOXO1, PAX7-FOXO1*</td>
<td>Rare *PAX3-NCOA1* or *PAX3-NCOA2*</td>
</tr>
<tr>
<td>DSRCT</td>
<td>EMA, NSE, desmin, WT1 (C-terminus Ab)</td>
<td>*EWSR1-WT1*</td>
<td>May show variable CD99 staining
Negative for N-terminus WT1 Ab</td>
</tr>
<tr>
<td>Synovial sarcoma, poorly differentiated</td>
<td>EMA, keratin, TLE1</td>
<td>*SS18-SSX1, SS18-SSX2*</td>
<td>May show variable CD99 staining</td>
</tr>
<tr>
<td>Myxoid liposarcoma, high grade</td>
<td>*FUS-DDIT3*</td>
<td>Rare *EWSR1-DDIT3*</td>
<td>Morphologic features: myxoid stroma, delicate branching vessels, small lipoblasts
Subset with *EWSR1-DDIT3*</td>
</tr>
<tr>
<td>Myoepithelial carcinoma</td>
<td>Keratin, EMA, S100, SOX10, p63 (50%), INI1-loss</td>
<td>*EWSR1* rearrangement with various partners (*PBX1, PBX3, POU5F1, ATF1, KLF17,* and *ZNF44*)</td>
<td>Rare variant *FUS* fusions</td>
</tr>
<tr>
<td>Mesenchymal chondrosarcoma</td>
<td>CD99, SOX9</td>
<td>*HEY1-NCOA2*</td>
<td>Biphasic tumor, also has a cartilaginous component</td>
</tr>
<tr>
<td>*CIC*-rearranged sarcoma</td>
<td>CD99±, WT1, ETV4</td>
<td>*CIC-DUX4*</td>
<td>Rare *CIC-FOXO4*</td>
</tr>
<tr>
<td>*BCOR-CCNB3* sarcoma</td>
<td>CD99f±, CCNB3, BCOR, SATB2, TLE1</td>
<td>*BCOR-CCNB3*</td>
<td>Most tumors in bone
Rare *BCOR-MAML3* and *ZC3H7B-BCOR*</td>
</tr>
</table>

EPITHELIOID NEOPLASMS

Soft tissue tumors with epithelioid morphology are diverse and include a few benign entities, many neoplasms of intermediate and malignant potential, and epithelioid variants of specific tumor types. Although many epithelioid neoplasms have characteristic histopathologic features, these are often subtle or absent in smears. Carcinoma and melanoma should always be considered in the differential diagnosis. Inclusive immunohistochemical panels are necessary, however, because many epithelioid soft tissue tumors are positive for keratin, EMA, or S100.

The benign neoplasm granular cell tumor shows tumor cells with abundant granular cytoplasm; nuclei are typically small and round but occasionally show enlargement and mild atypia, which may appear worrisome for malignancy. Granular cell tumors are positive for S100 and SOX10 and the less specific markers NKI-C3 and NSE; TFE3 expression has been reported though tumors lack *TFE3* rearrangements.[144,145] Malignant granular cell tumors are rare, and diagnostic criteria are often not discernible on cytology.[146]

Epithelioid sarcoma has the distinct immunophenotype of EMA and keratin positivity, frequent CD34 expression (50%), and consistent loss of expression of INI1 (**Fig. 7**). Smears show epithelioid and polygonal cells with round nuclei having prominent nucleoli and frequent binucleation and multinucleation; the cytoplasm is dense with

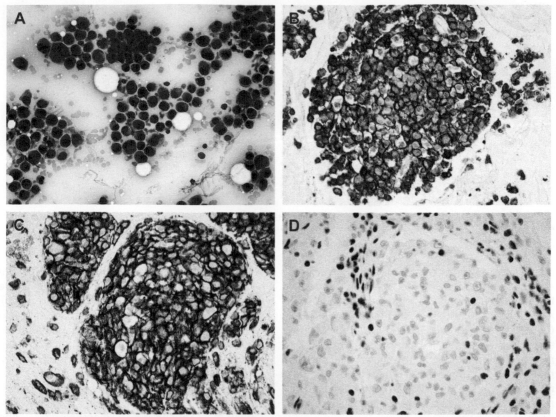

Fig. 7. Proximal-type epithelioid sarcoma shows atypical but uniform epithelioid cells with round nuclei (some binucleated), prominent nucleoli, and dense cytoplasm ([A] Diff-Quik stain, ×400) and has a distinct immunophenotype. Tumors show expression of EMA (B, ×400) and keratin and frequent (50%) CD34 positivity (C, ×400). Loss of INI1 expression occurs secondary to *SMARCB1* alterations (D).

distinct borders and occasional vacuoles and perinuclear zones.[147,148] The conventional (distal) subtype typically arises in distal extremities and also shows spindle cells and granulomata-type structures. Proximal-type epithelioid sarcoma commonly arises in proximal/truncal sites and is composed solely of epithelioid cells with occasional rhabdoid morphology.[149] Loss of INI1 expression occurs secondary to alterations of *SMARCB1* on 22q11.2.[57,150–152] Several pitfalls should be considered. Keratin and EMA expression alone may be misinterpreted as carcinoma, especially considering that epithelioid sarcoma commonly metastasizes to lung and lymph nodes. ERG positivity is seen in a subset when using antibodies to the N-terminus,[153,154] which may be mistaken for vascular differentiation. Loss of INI1 expression also occurs in other neoplasms, including malignant rhabdoid tumor, renal medullary carcinoma, epithelioid MPNST, and neoplasms with *EWSR1* rearrangement[155,156]; correlation with clinical data and an inclusive immunohistochemical panel are necessary.

Epithelioid hemangioendothelioma (EHE) also has the cytomorphologic appearance of dispersed round and polygonal epithelioid cells with mildly atypical nuclei, frequent binucleation, and dense cytoplasm. The characteristic intracytoplasmic vacuoles is a helpful feature if present; some cases show myxoid and fibrous stroma. EHE shows positivity for endothelial markers ERG, CD31, and CD34, and 30% of cases express keratin and EMA. EHE is characterized by *CAMTA1-WWTR1* fusion.[157] CAMTA1 is a highly sensitive and specific marker for EHE[158] (**Fig. 8**) and is especially helpful in excluding cytomorphologic mimics of epithelioid sarcoma and epithelioid angiosarcoma. A subset of EHE that is often vasoformative has *YAP1-TFE3* fusions and is positive for TFE3 immunohistochemistry.[159]

Clear cell sarcoma shows melanocytic differentiation and is positive for S100, SOX10, and melanocytic markers HMB-45 and MiTF. Tumor cells have nuclei with large prominent nucleoli and intranuclear pseudoinclusions and vacuolated cytoplasm with wispy ends and wreath-like

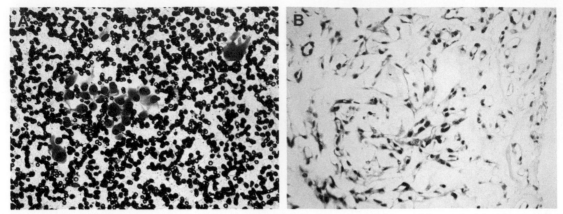

Fig. 8. EHE shows epithelioid and polygonal cells with abundant cytoplasm and frequent binucleation ([*A*] Diff-Quik stain, ×400). Tumors have *WWTR1-CAMTA1* fusion, and CAMTA1 is a highly sensitive and specific marker (*B*, ×400).

multinucleated giant cells.[160] Malignant melanoma should be excluded in older patients. Molecular testing can identify the characteristic *EWSR1-ATF1* fusion gene (or, less commonly, *EWSR1-CREB1*).[161] *EWSR1-ATF1* and *EWSR1-CREB1* fusions are also present in clear cell sarcoma-like tumor of the gastrointestinal tract (also known as malignant gastrointestinal neuroectodermal tumor), which are positive for S100 but negative for melanocytic markers, and are aggressive neoplasms.[162,163]

The epithelioid cells of alveolar soft part sarcoma (ASPS) have abundant fragile granular cytoplasm, and smears often show naked nuclei and granular cytoplasmic contents.[164] Rhomboid crystals (which are periodic acid-Schiff [PAS] positive and diastase resistant) are a distinctive feature but rare in cytologic samples.[165] ASPS harbors *ASPSCR1-TFE3* fusion, which can be detected by *TFE3* FISH; immunohistochemistry can detect resultant nuclear TFE3 expression. TFE3 expression is also seen in rare subsets of EHE and PEComa that have *TFE3* fusions,[166,167] as well as granular cell tumor, which lacks *TFE3* rearrangement.

Many specific tumor types have epithelioid variants, and have distinctive clinicopathologic features. The epithelioid variant of IMT is an aggressive subtype that is characterized by *ALK-RANBP2* and shows a distinctive nuclear membranous ALK staining pattern.[168] Tumors commonly present as intra-abdominal masses in young men and may also show CD30 and desmin expression. Smears show large atypical epithelioid cells associated with myxoid stroma, neutrophils, and delicate vessels.[169] The epithelioid variant of MPNST has distinctive clinicopathologic features, including consistent diffuse S100 expression and loss of INI1 expression in up to 67% of cases.[156] Smears show epithelioid tumor cells with round

vesicular nuclei, prominent nucleoli, and frequent cytoplasmic vacuolization.[170] Tumors are negative for melanocytic markers (HMB-45 and MelanA0), allowing distinction from melanoma. Epithelioid variants of myxofibrosarcoma and pleomorphic liposarcoma should be considered in the limbs of older patients, which may be recognizable by their respective characteristic features.

SDH-deficient GIST has specific clinicopathologic features (exclusively gastric location, predominant epithelioid morphology, and multinodular growth pattern) and important management implications. SDH deficiency refers to dysfunction of the SDH complex, a tetrameric mitochondrial membrane protein, which is caused by mutations in any of the 4 subunit encoding genes (*SDHA, SDHB, SDHC,* and *SDHD*) or other epigenetic mechanisms. Immunohistochemical loss of SDHB expression occurs in all tumors with SDH deficiency regardless of mechanism of dysfunction.[171,172] Immunohistochemical loss of SDHA correlates, however, with *SDHA* mutations.[173] Despite being wild-type for *KIT*, SDH-deficient GISTs are positive for KIT and DOG1. SDH-deficient GISTs include pediatric cases and sporadic adult wild-type tumors,[172,174] and a subset has syndromic associations. Patients are referred for genetic testing and counseling given that tumors may arise as part of Carney-Stratakis syndrome (GIST and paragangliomas; germline *SDH* mutations)[175] and the nonhereditary Carney triad syndrome (GIST, paragangliomas, and pulmonary chondroma; *SDHC* promoter hypermethylation[176]). Unlike conventional GISTs, SDH-deficient GISTs frequently show nodal and distant metastases but overall follow an indolent course; tumors are imatinib resistant and their biologic behavior cannot be predicted by conventional risk stratification.[177]

⚠️ Differential Diagnosis
EPITHELIOID NEOPLASMS

Tumor Type	Immunophenotype	Molecular Features	Other Features
Granular cell tumor	S100, Sox10, NKI-C3, NSE	—	TFE positive but lacks *TFE3* rearrangement
Epithelioid sarcoma	EMA, keratin, CD34 (50%) Loss of INI1	*SMARCB1* alterations	Distal type also shows spindle cells and granulomatous structures Subset positive for ERG (N-terminus Ab)
EHE	CAMTA1, ERG, CD31, CD34	*CAMTA1-WWTR1*	Keratin + 30% Subset with *YAP1-TFE3* (TFE3 positive)
CCS of soft tissue	S100, HMB-45	*EWSR1-ATF1, EWSR1-CREB1*	Wreath-like giant cells
CCS-like tumor of the GI tract	S100	*EWSR1-CREB1; EWSR1-ATF1*	Negative for HMB-45
ASPS	TFE3	*ASPSCR1-TFE3*	PAS, diastase-resistant rhomboid crystals
Epithelioid IMT	ALK, CD30, desmin	*ALK-RANBP2*	Myxoid stroma, delicate vessels, neutrophils
Epithelioid MPNST	S100, INI1-loss	—	Negative for HMB-45, MelanA
Epithelioid variant of myxofibrosarcoma	No specific immunophenotype	Complex karyotype	Morphologic features: curvilinear thin-walled vessels and myxoid stroma
Epithelioid variant of pleomorphic liposarcoma	No specific immunophenotype	Complex karyotype	Morphologic features: large atypical lipoblasts
SDH-deficient GIST	KIT, DOG1 Loss of SDHB (all tumors) SDHA loss if *SDHA* mutant	Mutations in *SDHA, SDHB, SDHC, SDHD*; or epigenetic mechanisms	—

Abbreviations: CCS, clear cell sarcoma; GI, gastrointestinal.

PLEOMORPHIC NEOPLASMS

A majority of neoplasms showing high-grade pleomorphic morphology are aggressive sarcomas with complex cytogenetic features; the presence of severe cytologic atypia, necrosis, and frequent mitotic activity with atypical forms allows classification as a high-grade sarcoma for management purposes. The differential diagnosis typically includes myxofibrosarcoma, pleomorphic liposarcoma, pleomorphic RMS, DDLPS, and unclassified pleomorphic sarcoma. Many cases of myxofibrosarcoma show at least focal characteristic areas of curvilinear vessels and myxoid stroma, and careful search of large atypical lipoblasts is useful for the diagnosis of pleomorphic liposarcoma. In older patients, carcinoma and melanoma should be excluded.

Pleomorphic RMS is strongly positive for desmin, and skeletal muscle differentiation can be confirmed by myogenin immunohistochemistry (**Fig. 9**). Several high-grade malignancies, however, can show heterologous rhabdomyoblastic differentiation and should be excluded: carcinosarcoma (epithelial component positive for keratin and PAX8), MPNST (S100, SOX10, GFAP,

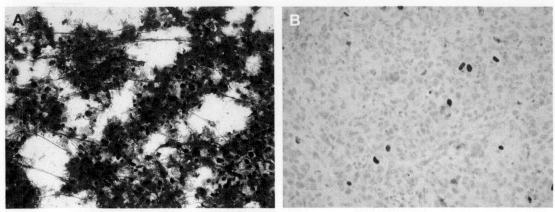

Fig. 9. Pleomorphic RMS appears as a high-grade pleomorphic neoplasia ([A] Diff-Quik stain, ×400). Skeletal muscle differentiation can be identified by immunohistochemistry for desmin and nuclear myogenin expression (B, ×400).

and H3K27me3), and DDLPS (MDM2 and CDK4, or *MDM2* FISH).

DDLPS should always be considered in the differential diagnosis of any pleomorphic sarcoma and is the most likely diagnosis in retroperitoneal sites. Most tumors are nonlipogenic and show a wide range of morphologic appearances[24–26] (see **Fig. 1**B). Some smears may include areas of the precursor ALT/WDL. Diagnosis of DDLPS is confirmed by identification of 12q13-15 amplification.[15] Coexpression of MDM2 and CDK4 is sufficiently diagnostic in many cases; however, *MDM2* FISH is helpful when the immunohistochemical results are not straightforward.[15,178] MDM2 expression may be seen in other sarcomas, including myxofibrosarcoma and MPNST[15];

however, these mimics rarely show coexpression of CDK4. *MDM2* gene amplification also is a feature of intimal sarcoma[179,180] as well as parosteal osteosarcoma and central low-grade osteosarcoma[181–183]; clinical and radiologic correlation may be required in some scenarios.

Undifferentiated pleomorphic sarcoma is a diagnosis of exclusion, and requires exclusion of all specific pleomorphic tumor types, which typically requires a broad immunohistochemical panel and thorough histologic sampling. Definitive diagnosis may not be possible on FNA even if cases are negative for MDM2/CDK4 and myogenic markers, and a cytologic diagnosis of high-grade pleomorphic sarcoma with a differential diagnosis is appropriate.

Key Points
PRACTICAL CONSIDERATIONS FOR
PLEOMORPHIC NEOPLASMS

- DDLPS is in the differential diagnosis for all pleomorphic neoplasms and is the chief consideration in the retroperitoneum; MDM2/CDK4 immunohistochemistry should always be performed.

- Carcinoma and melanoma should always be excluded.

- Pleomorphic RMS is positive for desmin and myogenin; however, diagnosis requires exclusion of heterologous rhabdomyoblastic differentiation in other malignancies (eg, carcinosarcoma, MPNST, and DDLPS).

- Myxofibrosarcoma, pleomorphic liposarcoma, and unclassified pleomorphic sarcoma lack specific immunophenotypes and have complex karyotypes; definitive diagnosis is typically deferred to resection.

- Myxofibrosarcoma is favored when there are curvilinear thin-walled vessels and myxoid stroma.

- Pleomorphic liposarcoma is supported by the presence of large atypical lipoblasts.

- Unclassified pleomorphic sarcoma is a diagnosis of exclusion and typically primary diagnosis is not made on cytology.

SUMMARY

A pattern-based approach in soft tissue cytology offers a practical framework to guide differential diagnoses and ancillary testing. The numerous advances in ancillary tests now enable accurate classification for many tumor types on cytologic specimens. Immunohistochemistry is central to the diagnostic work-up and is helpful for identifying line of differentiation and tumor-specific immunophenotypes. FISH and sequencing-based methods, such as reverse transcriptase–polymerase chain reaction, are useful for detecting molecular alterations, and rapidly developing NGS technologies have many potential future applications. Despite the many advances in ancillary testing, diagnostic pitfalls remain in soft tissue cytology, including limited evaluation of architectural features, overlapping protein expression patterns between tumor types, aberrant expression of keratin and neuroendocrine markers in many mesenchymal neoplasms, and shared molecular alterations (such as *EWSR1* rearrangement), among numerous entities. Appropriate use of ancillary tests requires an understanding of the advantages and limitations of these tests, and diagnostic practice requires integration of these diagnostic markers with clinical and cytomorphologic data.

REFERENCES

1. Fletcher CDM, Bridge JA, Hogendoorn PCW, et al. WHO classification of tumours of soft tissue and bone. Pathology and genetics of tumours of soft tissue and bone. 4th edition. Lyon (France): IARC Press; 2013.

2. Antonescu CR, Dal Cin P. Promiscuous genes involved in recurrent chromosomal translocations in soft tissue tumours. Pathology 2014;46(2): 105–12.

3. Marino-Enriquez A. Advances in the molecular analysis of soft tissue tumors and clinical implications. Surg Pathol Clin 2015;8(3):525–37.

4. Abati A, Sanford JS, Fetsch P, et al. Fluorescence in situ hybridization (FISH): a user's guide to optimal preparation of cytologic specimens. Diagn Cytopathol 1995;13(5):486–92.

5. Hwang DH, Garcia EP, Ducar MD, et al. Next-generation sequencing of cytologic preparations: an analysis of quality metrics. Cancer Cytopathol 2017;125(10):786–94.

6. Roy-Chowdhuri S, Chen H, Singh RR, et al. Concurrent fine needle aspirations and core needle biopsies: a comparative study of substrates for next-generation sequencing in solid organ malignancies. Mod Pathol 2017;30(4):499–508.

7. Qian X. Soft tissue. In: Cibas ES, editor. Cytology: diagnostic principles and clinical correlates. 4th edition. Philadelphia: Elsevier; 2014. p. 471–518.

8. Kapila K, Ghosal N, Gill SS, et al. Cytomorphology of lipomatous tumors of soft tissue. Acta Cytol 2003;47(4):555–62.

9. Lemos MM, Kindblom LG, Meis-Kindblom JM, et al. Fine-needle aspiration characteristics of hibernoma. Cancer 2001;93(3):206–10.

10. Domanski HA, Carlen B, Jonsson K, et al. Distinct cytologic features of spindle cell lipoma. A cytologic-histologic study with clinical, radiologic, electron microscopic, and cytogenetic correlations. Cancer 2001;93(6):381–9.

11. Chen BJ, Marino-Enriquez A, Fletcher CD, et al. Loss of retinoblastoma protein expression in spindle cell/pleomorphic lipomas and cytogenetically related tumors: an immunohistochemical study with diagnostic implications. Am J Surg Pathol 2012;36(8):1119–28.

12. Bartuma H, Nord KH, Macchia G, et al. Gene expression and single nucleotide polymorphism array analyses of spindle cell lipomas and conventional lipomas with 13q14 deletion. Genes Chromosomes Cancer 2011;50(8):619–32.

13. Maggiani F, Debiec-Rychter M, Vanbockrijck M, et al. Cellular angiofibroma: another mesenchymal tumour with 13q14 involvement, suggesting a link with spindle cell lipoma and (extra)-mammary myofibroblastoma. Histopathology 2007;51(3):410–2.

14. Pauwels P, Sciot R, Croiset F, et al. Myofibroblastoma of the breast: genetic link with spindle cell lipoma. J Pathol 2000;191(3):282–5.

15. Binh MB, Sastre-Garau X, Guillou L, et al. MDM2 and CDK4 immunostainings are useful adjuncts in diagnosing well-differentiated and dedifferentiated liposarcoma subtypes: a comparative analysis of 559 soft tissue neoplasms with genetic data. Am J Surg Pathol 2005;29(10):1340–7.

16. Weaver J, Goldblum JR, Turner S, et al. Detection of MDM2 gene amplification or protein expression distinguishes sclerosing mesenteritis and retroperitoneal fibrosis from inflammatory well-differentiated liposarcoma. Mod Pathol 2009;22(1):66–70.

17. Weaver J, Rao P, Goldblum JR, et al. Can MDM2 analytical tests performed on core needle biopsy be relied upon to diagnose well-differentiated liposarcoma? Mod Pathol 2010;23(10):1301–6.

18. Zhang H, Erickson-Johnson M, Wang X, et al. Molecular testing for lipomatous tumors: critical analysis and test recommendations based on the analysis of 405 extremity-based tumors. Am J Surg Pathol 2010;34(9):1304–11.

19. Clay MR, Martinez AP, Weiss SW, et al. MDM2 amplification in problematic lipomatous tumors: analysis of FISH testing criteria. Am J Surg Pathol 2015;39(10):1433–9.

20. Sandberg AA. Updates on the cytogenetics and molecular genetics of bone and soft tissue tumors: liposarcoma. Cancer Genet Cytogenet 2004; 155(1):1–24.

21. Dei Tos AP, Doglioni C, Piccinin S, et al. Molecular abnormalities of the p53 pathway in dedifferentiated liposarcoma. J Pathol 1997;181(1):8–13.

22. Mertens F, Fletcher CD, Dal Cin P, et al. Cytogenetic analysis of 46 pleomorphic soft tissue sarcomas and correlation with morphologic and clinical features: a report of the CHAMP Study Group. Chromosomes and MorPhology. Genes Chromosomes Cancer 1998;22(1):16–25.

23. Meis-Kindblom JM, Sjogren H, Kindblom LG, et al. Cytogenetic and molecular genetic analyses of liposarcoma and its soft tissue simulators: recognition of new variants and differential diagnosis. Virchows Arch 2001;439(2):141–51.

24. Marino-Enriquez A, Fletcher CD, Dal Cin P, et al. Dedifferentiated liposarcoma with "homologous" lipoblastic (pleomorphic liposarcoma-like) differentiation: clinicopathologic and molecular analysis of a series suggesting revised diagnostic criteria. Am J Surg Pathol 2010;34(8):1122–31.

25. Marino-Enriquez A, Hornick JL, Dal Cin P, et al. Dedifferentiated liposarcoma and pleomorphic liposarcoma: a comparative study of cytomorphology and MDM2/CDK4 expression on fine-needle aspiration. Cancer Cytopathol 2014;122(2):128–37.

26. Liau JY, Lee JC, Wu CT, et al. Dedifferentiated liposarcoma with homologous lipoblastic differentiation: expanding the spectrum to include low-grade tumours. Histopathology 2013;62(5):702–10.

27. Klijanienko J, Caillaud JM, Lagace R. Fine-needle aspiration in liposarcoma: cytohistologic correlative study including well-differentiated, myxoid, and pleomorphic variants. Diagn Cytopathol 2004; 30(5):307–12.

28. Aman P, Ron D, Mandahl N, et al. Rearrangement of the transcription factor gene CHOP in myxoid liposarcomas with t(12;16)(q13;p11). Genes Chromosomes Cancer 1992;5(4):278–85.

29. Dal Cin P, Sciot R, Panagopoulos I, et al. Additional evidence of a variant translocation t(12;22) with EWS/CHOP fusion in myxoid liposarcoma: clinicopathological features. J Pathol 1997;182(4):437–41.

30. Panagopoulos I, Hoglund M, Mertens F, et al. Fusion of the EWS and CHOP genes in myxoid liposarcoma. Oncogene 1996;12(3):489–94.

31. Ferreira J, Esteves G, Fonseca R, et al. Fine-needle aspiration of lipoblastoma: cytological, molecular, and clinical features. Cancer Cytopathol 2017; 125(12):934–9.

32. Yoshida H, Miyachi M, Ouohi K, et al. Identification of COL3A1 and RAB2A as novel translocation partner genes of PLAG1 in lipoblastoma. Genes Chromosomes Cancer 2014;53(7):606–11.

33. Yang EJ, Hornick JL, Qian X. Fine-needle aspiration of soft tissue perineurioma: a comparative analysis of cytomorphology and immunohistochemistry with benign and malignant mimics. Cancer Cytopathol 2016;124(9):651–8.

34. Delaney D, Diss TC, Presneau N, et al. GNAS1 mutations occur more commonly than previously thought in intramuscular myxoma. Mod Pathol 2009;22(5):718–24.

35. Domanski HA, Mertens F, Panagopoulos I, et al. Low-grade fibromyxoid sarcoma is difficult to diagnose by fine needle aspiration cytology: a cytomorphological study of eight cases. Cytopathology 2009;20(5):304–14.

36. Doyle LA, Moller E, Dal Cin P, et al. MUC4 is a highly sensitive and specific marker for low-grade fibromyxoid sarcoma. Am J Surg Pathol 2011;35(5): 733–41.

37. Panagopoulos I, Storlazzi CT, Fletcher CD, et al. The chimeric FUS/CREB3l2 gene is specific for low-grade fibromyxoid sarcoma. Genes Chromosomes Cancer 2004;40(3):218–28.

38. Mertens F, Fletcher CD, Antonescu CR, et al. Clinicopathologic and molecular genetic characterization of low-grade fibromyxoid sarcoma, and cloning of a novel FUS/CREB3L1 fusion gene. Lab Invest 2005;85(3):408–15.

39. Guillou L, Benhattar J, Gengler C, et al. Translocation-positive low-grade fibromyxoid sarcoma: clinicopathologic and molecular analysis of a series expanding the morphologic spectrum and suggesting potential relationship to sclerosing epithelioid fibrosarcoma: a study from the French Sarcoma Group. Am J Surg Pathol 2007;31(9): 1387–402.

40. Doyle LA, Wang WL, Dal Cin P, et al. MUC4 is a sensitive and extremely useful marker for sclerosing epithelioid fibrosarcoma: association with FUS gene rearrangement. Am J Surg Pathol 2012;36(10):1444–51.

41. Arbajian E, Puls F, Magnusson L, et al. Recurrent EWSR1-CREB3L1 gene fusions in sclerosing epithelioid fibrosarcoma. Am J Surg Pathol 2014; 38(6):801–8.

42. Colin P, Lagace R, Caillaud JM, et al. Fine-needle aspiration in myxofibrosarcoma: experience of Institut Curie. Diagn Cytopathol 2010;38(5):343–6.

43. Kilpatrick SE, Ward WG, Bos GD. The value of fine-needle aspiration biopsy in the differential diagnosis of adult myxoid sarcoma. Cancer 2000; 90(3):167–77.

44. Olson MT, Ali SZ. Myxofibrosarcoma: cytomorphologic findings and differential diagnosis on fine needle aspiration. Acta Cytol 2012;56(1):15–24.

45. Jakowski JD, Wakely PE Jr. Cytopathology of extraskeletal myxoid chondrosarcoma: report of 8 cases. Cancer 2007;111(5):298–305.

46. Okamoto S, Hisaoka M, Ishida T, et al. Extraskeletal myxoid chondrosarcoma: a clinicopathologic, immunohistochemical, and molecular analysis of 18 cases. Hum Pathol 2001;32(10):1116–24.

47. Attwooll C, Tariq M, Harris M, et al. Identification of a novel fusion gene involving hTAFII68 and CHN from a t(9;17)(q22;q11.2) translocation in an extraskeletal myxoid chondrosarcoma. Oncogene 1999; 18(52):7599–601.

48. Panagopoulos I, Mertens F, Isaksson M, et al. Molecular genetic characterization of the EWS/CHN and RBP56/CHN fusion genes in extraskeletal myxoid chondrosarcoma. Genes Chromosomes Cancer 2002;35(4):340–52.

49. Flucke U, Tops BB, Verdijk MA, et al. NR4A3 rearrangement reliably distinguishes between the clinicopathologically overlapping entities myoepithelial carcinoma of soft tissue and cellular extraskeletal myxoid chondrosarcoma. Virchows Arch 2012; 460(6):621–8.

50. Hornick JL, Fletcher CD. Myoepithelial tumors of soft tissue: a clinicopathologic and immunohistochemical study of 101 cases with evaluation of prognostic parameters. Am J Surg Pathol 2003; 27(9):1183–96.

51. Gleason BC, Fletcher CD. Myoepithelial carcinoma of soft tissue in children: an aggressive neoplasm analyzed in a series of 29 cases. Am J Surg Pathol 2007;31(12):1813–24.

52. Brandal P, Panagopoulos I, Bjerkehagen B, et al. Detection of a t(1;22)(q23;q12) translocation leading to an EWSR1-PBX1 fusion gene in a myoepithelioma. Genes Chromosomes Cancer 2008;47(7):558–64.

53. Brandal P, Panagopoulos I, Bjerkehagen B, et al. t(19;22)(q13;q12) Translocation leading to the novel fusion gene EWSR1-ZNF444 in soft tissue myoepithelial carcinoma. Genes Chromosomes Cancer 2009;48(12):1051–6.

54. Antonescu CR, Zhang L, Chang NE, et al. EWSR1-POU5F1 fusion in soft tissue myoepithelial tumors. A molecular analysis of sixty-six cases, including soft tissue, bone, and visceral lesions, showing common involvement of the EWSR1 gene. Genes Chromosomes Cancer 2010;49(12):1114–24.

55. Agaram NP, Chen HW, Zhang L, et al. EWSR1-PBX3: a novel gene fusion in myoepithelial tumors. Genes Chromosomes Cancer 2015;54(2):63–71.

56. Huang SC, Chen HW, Zhang L, et al. Novel FUS-KLF17 and EWSR1-KLF17 fusions in myoepithelial tumors. Genes Chromosomes Cancer 2015;54(5): 267–75.

57. Le Loarer F, Zhang L, Fletcher CD, et al. Consistent SMARCB1 homozygous deletions in epithelioid sarcoma and in a subset of myoepithelial carcinomas can be reliably detected by FISH in archival material. Genes Chromosomes Cancer 2014;53(6): 475–86.

58. Ahmed OI, Qasem SA, Salih ZT. Ossifying fibromyxoid tumor: report of a case with cytomorphologic description. Diagn Cytopathol 2015;43(8): 646–9.

59. Alvarez-Rodriguez F, Jimenez-Heffernan J, Salas C, et al. Cytological features of ossifying fibromyxoid tumor of soft parts. J Cytol 2012;29(3): 205–7.

60. Gebre-Medhin S, Nord KH, Moller E, et al. Recurrent rearrangement of the PHF1 gene in ossifying fibromyxoid tumors. Am J Pathol 2012;181(3): 1069–77.

61. Graham RP, Weiss SW, Sukov WR, et al. PHF1 rearrangements in ossifying fibromyxoid tumors of soft parts: a fluorescence in situ hybridization study of 41 cases with emphasis on the malignant variant. Am J Surg Pathol 2013;37(11):1751–5.

62. Erickson-Johnson MR, Chou MM, Evers BR, et al. Nodular fasciitis: a novel model of transient neoplasia induced by MYH9-USP6 gene fusion. Lab Invest 2011;91(10):1427–33.

63. Plaza JA, Mayerson J, Wakely PE Jr. Nodular fasciitis of the hand: a potential diagnostic pitfall in fine-needle aspiration cytopathology. Am J Clin Pathol 2005;123(3):388–93.

64. Sakuma T, Matsuo K, Koike S, et al. Fine needle aspiration cytology of nodular fasciitis of the breast. Diagn Cytopathol 2015;43(3):222–9.

65. Wong NL, Di F. Pseudosarcomatous fasciitis and myositis: diagnosis by fine-needle aspiration cytology. Am J Clin Pathol 2009;132(6):857–65.

66. Kang A, Kumar JB, Thomas A, et al. A spontaneously resolving breast lesion: imaging and cytological findings of nodular fasciitis of the breast with FISH showing USP6 gene rearrangement. BMJ Case Rep 2015;2015, [pii:bcr2015213076].

67. Owens CL, Sharma R, Ali SZ. Deep fibromatosis (desmoid tumor): cytopathologic characteristics, clinicoradiologic features, and immunohistochemical findings on fine-needle aspiration. Cancer 2007;111(3):166–72.

68. Rege TA, Madan R, Qian X. Long fascicular tissue fragments in desmoid fibromatosis by fine needle aspiration: a new cytologic feature. Diagn Cytopathol 2012;40(1):45–7.

69. Lazar AJ, Tuvin D, Hajibashi S, et al. Specific mutations in the beta-catenin gene (CTNNB1) correlate with local recurrence in sporadic desmoid tumors. Am J Pathol 2008;173(5):1518–27.

70. Miyaki M, Konishi M, Kikuchi-Yanoshita R, et al. Coexistence of somatic and germ-line mutations of APC gene in desmoid tumors from patients with familial adenomatous polyposis. Cancer Res 1993;53(21):5079–82.

71. Bhattacharya B, Dilworth HP, Iacobuzio-Donahue C, et al. Nuclear beta-catenin expression distinguishes deep fibromatosis from other benign

and malignant fibroblastic and myofibroblastic lesions. Am J Surg Pathol 2005;29(5):653–9.

72. Stoll LM, Li QK. Cytology of fine-needle aspiration of inflammatory myofibroblastic tumor. Diagn Cytopathol 2011;39(9):663–72.

73. Cook JR, Dehner LP, Collins MH, et al. Anaplastic lymphoma kinase (ALK) expression in the inflammatory myofibroblastic tumor: a comparative immunohistochemical study. Am J Surg Pathol 2001;25(11):1364–71.

74. Bridge JA, Kanamori M, Ma Z, et al. Fusion of the ALK gene to the clathrin heavy chain gene, CLTC, in inflammatory myofibroblastic tumor. Am J Pathol 2001;159(2):411–5.

75. Demetri GD, von Mehren M, Antonescu CR, et al. NCCN Task Force report: update on the management of patients with gastrointestinal stromal tumors. J Natl Compr Canc Netw 2010;8(Suppl 2): S1–41, [quiz: S2–4].

76. Stelow EB, Stanley MW, Mallery S, et al. Endoscopic ultrasound-guided fine-needle aspiration findings of gastrointestinal leiomyomas and gastrointestinal stromal tumors. Am J Clin Pathol 2003; 119(5):703–8.

77. Dodd LG, Nelson RC, Mooney EE, et al. Fine-needle aspiration of gastrointestinal stromal tumors. Am J Clin Pathol 1998;109(4):439–43.

78. Wieczorek TJ, Faquin WC, Rubin BP, et al. Cytologic diagnosis of gastrointestinal stromal tumor with emphasis on the differential diagnosis with leiomyosarcoma. Cancer 2001;93(4):276–87.

79. Rader AE, Avery A, Wait CL, et al. Fine-needle aspiration biopsy diagnosis of gastrointestinal stromal tumors using morphology, immunocytochemistry, and mutational analysis of c-kit. Cancer 2001;93(4):269–75.

80. Rubin BP, Heinrich MC, Corless CL. Gastrointestinal stromal tumour. Lancet 2007;369(9574):1731–41.

81. West RB, Corless CL, Chen X, et al. The novel marker, DOG1, is expressed ubiquitously in gastrointestinal stromal tumors irrespective of KIT or PDGFRA mutation status. Am J Pathol 2004; 165(1):107–13.

82. Espinosa I, Lee CH, Kim MK, et al. A novel monoclonal antibody against DOG1 is a sensitive and specific marker for gastrointestinal stromal tumors. Am J Surg Pathol 2008;32(2):210–8.

83. Hwang DG, Qian X, Hornick JL. DOG1 antibody is a highly sensitive and specific marker for gastrointestinal stromal tumors in cytology cell blocks. Am J Clin Pathol 2011;135(3):448–53.

84. Bishop JA, Rekhtman N, Chun J, et al. Malignant solitary fibrous tumor: cytopathologic findings and differential diagnosis. Cancer Cytopathol 2010; 118(2):83–9.

85. Clayton AC, Salomao DR, Keeney GL, et al. Solitary fibrous tumor: a study of cytologic features of six cases diagnosed by fine-needle aspiration. Diagn Cytopathol 2001;25(3):172–6.

86. Robinson DR, Wu YM, Kalyana-Sundaram S, et al. Identification of recurrent NAB2-STAT6 gene fusions in solitary fibrous tumor by integrative sequencing. Nat Genet 2013;45(2):180–5.

87. Chmielecki J, Crago AM, Rosenberg M, et al. Whole-exome sequencing identifies a recurrent NAB2-STAT6 fusion in solitary fibrous tumors. Nat Genet 2013;45(2):131–2.

88. Doyle LA, Vivero M, Fletcher CD, et al. Nuclear expression of STAT6 distinguishes solitary fibrous tumor from histologic mimics. Mod Pathol 2014; 27(3):390–5.

89. Yoshida A, Tsuta K, Ohno M, et al. STAT6 immunohistochemistry is helpful in the diagnosis of solitary fibrous tumors. Am J Surg Pathol 2014;38(4): 552–9.

90. Tani E, Wejde J, Astrom K, et al. FNA cytology of solitary fibrous tumors and the diagnostic value of STAT6 immunocytochemistry. Cancer Cytopathol 2018;126(1):36–43.

91. Domanski HA, Gustafson P. Cytologic features of primary, recurrent, and metastatic dermatofibrosarcoma protuberans. Cancer 2002;96(6):351–61.

92. Klijanienko J, Caillaud JM, Lagace R. Fine-needle aspiration of primary and recurrent dermatofibrosarcoma protuberans. Diagn Cytopathol 2004; 30(4):261–5.

93. Patel KU, Szabo SS, Hernandez VS, et al. Dermatofibrosarcoma protuberans COL1A1-PDGFB fusion is identified in virtually all dermatofibrosarcoma protuberans cases when investigated by newly developed multiplex reverse transcription polymerase chain reaction and fluorescence in situ hybridization assays. Hum Pathol 2008;39(2):184–93.

94. Agaram NP, Chen CL, Zhang L, et al. Recurrent MYOD1 mutations in pediatric and adult sclerosing and spindle cell rhabdomyosarcomas: evidence for a common pathogenesis. Genes Chromosomes Cancer 2014;53(9):779–87.

95. Szuhai K, de Jong D, Leung WY, et al. Transactivating mutation of the MYOD1 gene is a frequent event in adult spindle cell rhabdomyosarcoma. J Pathol 2014;232(3):300–7.

96. Jagdis A, Rubin BP, Tubbs RR, et al. Prospective evaluation of TLE1 as a diagnostic immunohistochemical marker in synovial sarcoma. Am J Surg Pathol 2009;33(12):1743–51.

97. Foo WC, Cruise MW, Wick MR, et al. Immunohistochemical staining for TLE1 distinguishes synovial sarcoma from histologic mimics. Am J Clin Pathol 2011;135(6):839–44.

98. Kosemehmetoglu K, Vrana JA, Folpe AL. TLE1 expression is not specific for synovial sarcoma: a whole section study of 163 soft tissue and bone neoplasms. Mod Pathol 2009;22(7):872–8.

99. Crew AJ, Clark J, Fisher C, et al. Fusion of SYT to two genes, SSX1 and SSX2, encoding proteins with homology to the Kruppel-associated box in human synovial sarcoma. EMBO J 1995;14(10):2333–40.

100. Folpe AL, Schmidt RA, Chapman D, et al. Poorly differentiated synovial sarcoma: immunohistochemical distinction from primitive neuroectodermal tumors and high-grade malignant peripheral nerve sheath tumors. Am J Surg Pathol 1998; 22(6):673–82.

101. Klijanienko J, Caillaud JM, Lagace R, et al. Cytohistologic correlations of 24 malignant peripheral nerve sheath tumor (MPNST) in 17 patients: the Institut Curie experience. Diagn Cytopathol 2002; 27(2):103–8.

102. Wakely PE Jr, Ali SZ, Bishop JA. The cytopathology of malignant peripheral nerve sheath tumor: a report of 55 fine-needle aspiration cases. Cancer Cytopathol 2012;120(5):334–41.

103. Lee W, Teckie S, Wiesner T, et al. PRC2 is recurrently inactivated through EED or SUZ12 loss in malignant peripheral nerve sheath tumors. Nat Genet 2014;46(11):1227–32.

104. Zhang M, Wang Y, Jones S, et al. Somatic mutations of SUZ12 in malignant peripheral nerve sheath tumors. Nat Genet 2014;46(11):1170–2.

105. Cleven AH, Sannaa GA, Briaire-de Bruijn I, et al. Loss of H3K27 tri-methylation is a diagnostic marker for malignant peripheral nerve sheath tumors and an indicator for an inferior survival. Mod Pathol 2016;29(6):582–90.

106. Prieto-Granada CN, Wiesner T, Messina JL, et al. Loss of H3K27me3 expression is a highly sensitive marker for sporadic and radiation-induced MPNST. Am J Surg Pathol 2016;40(4):479–89.

107. Schaefer IM, Fletcher CD, Hornick JL. Loss of H3K27 trimethylation distinguishes malignant peripheral nerve sheath tumors from histologic mimics. Mod Pathol 2016;29(1):4–13.

108. Mito JK, Qian X, Doyle LA, et al. Role of histone H3K27 trimethylation loss as a marker for malignant peripheral nerve sheath tumor in fine-needle aspiration and small biopsy specimens. Am J Clin Pathol 2017;148(2):179–89.

109. Le Guellec S, Macagno N, Velasco V, et al. Loss of H3K27 trimethylation is not suitable for distinguishing malignant peripheral nerve sheath tumor from melanoma: a study of 387 cases including mimicking lesions. Mod Pathol 2017;30(12):1677–87.

110. Delattre O, Zucman J, Melot T, et al. The Ewing family of tumors–a subgroup of small-round-cell tumors defined by specific chimeric transcripts. N Engl J Med 1994;331(5):294–9.

111. Ginsberg JP, de Alava E, Ladanyi M, et al. EWS-FLI1 and EWS-ERG gene fusions are associated with similar clinical phenotypes in Ewing's sarcoma. J Clin Oncol 1999;17(6):1809–14.

112. Jeon IS, Davis JN, Braun BS, et al. A variant Ewing's sarcoma translocation (7;22) fuses the EWS gene to the ETS gene ETV1. Oncogene 1995; 10(6):1229–34.

113. Kaneko Y, Yoshida K, Handa M, et al. Fusion of an ETS-family gene, EIAF, to EWS by t(17;22)(q12;q12) chromosome translocation in an undifferentiated sarcoma of infancy. Genes Chromosomes Cancer 1996; 15(2):115–21.

114. Peter M, Couturier J, Pacquement H, et al. A new member of the ETS family fused to EWS in Ewing tumors. Oncogene 1997;14(10):1159–64.

115. Bakhos R, Andrey J, Bhoopalam N, et al. Fine-needle aspiration cytology of extraskeletal Ewing's sarcoma. Diagn Cytopathol 1998;18(2):137–40.

116. Klijanienko J, Couturier J, Bourdeaut F, et al. Fine-needle aspiration as a diagnostic technique in 50 cases of primary Ewing sarcoma/peripheral neuroectodermal tumor. Institut Curie's experience. Diagn Cytopathol 2012;40(1):19–25.

117. Silverman JF, Joshi VV. FNA biopsy of small round cell tumors of childhood: cytomorphologic features and the role of ancillary studies. Diagn Cytopathol 1994;10(3):245–55.

118. Wang WL, Patel NR, Caragea M, et al. Expression of ERG, an Ets family transcription factor, identifies ERG-rearranged Ewing sarcoma. Mod Pathol 2012;25(10):1378–83.

119. Hung YP, Fletcher CD, Hornick JL. Evaluation of NKX2-2 expression in round cell sarcomas and other tumors with EWSR1 rearrangement: imperfect specificity for Ewing sarcoma. Mod Pathol 2016;29(4):370–80.

120. Doyle LA, Wong KK, Bueno R, et al. Ewing sarcoma mimicking atypical carcinoid tumor: detection of unexpected genomic alterations demonstrates the use of next generation sequencing as a diagnostic tool. Cancer Genet 2014;207(7–8):335–9.

121. Shing DC, McMullan DJ, Roberts P, et al. FUS/ERG gene fusions in Ewing's tumors. Cancer Res 2003; 63(15):4568–76.

122. Klijanienko J, Caillaud JM, Orbach D, et al. Cytohistological correlations in primary, recurrent and metastatic rhabdomyosarcoma: the institut Curie's experience. Diagn Cytopathol 2007;35(8): 482–7.

123. Dias P, Chen B, Dilday B, et al. Strong immunostaining for myogenin in rhabdomyosarcoma is significantly associated with tumors of the alveolar subclass. Am J Pathol 2000;156(2):399–408.

124. Bahrami A, Gown AM, Baird GS, et al. Aberrant expression of epithelial and neuroendocrine markers in alveolar rhabdomyosarcoma: a potentially serious diagnostic pitfall. Mod Pathol 2008;21(7):795–806.

125. Barr FG. Gene fusions involving PAX and FOX family members in alveolar rhabdomyosarcoma. Oncogene 2001;20(40):5736–46.

126. Sorensen PH, Lynch JC, Qualman SJ, et al. PAX3-FKHR and PAX7-FKHR gene fusions are prognostic indicators in alveolar rhabdomyosarcoma: a report from the children's oncology group. J Clin Oncol 2002;20(11):2672–9.

127. Klijanienko J, Colin P, Couturier J, et al. Fine-needle aspiration in desmoplastic small round cell tumor: a report of 10 new tumors in 8 patients with clinicopathological and molecular correlations with review of the literature. Cancer Cytopathol 2014;122(5):386–93.

128. Ladanyi M, Gerald W. Fusion of the EWS and WT1 genes in the desmoplastic small round cell tumor. Cancer Res 1994;54(11):2837–40.

129. Wang L, Motoi T, Khanin R, et al. Identification of a novel, recurrent HEY1-NCOA2 fusion in mesenchymal chondrosarcoma based on a genome-wide screen of exon-level expression data. Genes Chromosomes Cancer 2012;51(2):127–39.

130. Yoshimoto M, Graham C, Chilton-MacNeill S, et al. Detailed cytogenetic and array analysis of pediatric primitive sarcomas reveals a recurrent CIC-DUX4 fusion gene event. Cancer Genet Cytogenet 2009;195(1):1–11.

131. Graham C, Chilton-MacNeill S, Zielenska M, et al. The CIC-DUX4 fusion transcript is present in a subgroup of pediatric primitive round cell sarcomas. Hum Pathol 2012;43(2):180–9.

132. Italiano A, Sung YS, Zhang L, et al. High prevalence of CIC fusion with double-homeobox (DUX4) transcription factors in EWSR1-negative undifferentiated small blue round cell sarcomas. Genes Chromosomes Cancer 2012;51(3):207–18.

133. Choi EY, Thomas DG, McHugh JB, et al. Undifferentiated small round cell sarcoma with t(4;19)(q35;q13.1) CIC-DUX4 fusion: a novel highly aggressive soft tissue tumor with distinctive histopathology. Am J Surg Pathol 2013;37(9):1379–86.

134. Chebib I, Jo VY. Round cell sarcoma with CIC-DUX4 gene fusion: discussion of the distinctive cytomorphologic, immunohistochemical, and molecular features in the differential diagnosis of round cell tumors. Cancer Cytopathol 2016;124(5):350–61.

135. Pierron G, Tirode F, Lucchesi C, et al. A new subtype of bone sarcoma defined by BCOR-CCNB3 gene fusion. Nat Genet 2012;44(4):461–6.

136. Cohen-Gogo S, Cellier C, Coindre JM, et al. Ewing-like sarcomas with BCOR-CCNB3 fusion transcript: a clinical, radiological and pathological retrospective study from the Societe Francaise des Cancers de L'Enfant. Pediatr Blood Cancer 2014;61(12):2191–8.

137. Puls F, Niblett A, Marland G, et al. BCOR-CCNB3 (Ewing-like) sarcoma: a clinicopathologic analysis of 10 cases, in comparison with conventional Ewing sarcoma. Am J Surg Pathol 2014;38(10):1307–18.

138. Peters TL, Kumar V, Polikepahad S, et al. BCOR-CCNB3 fusions are frequent in undifferentiated sarcomas of male children. Mod Pathol 2015;28(4):575–86.

139. Kao YC, Owosho AA, Sung YS, et al. BCOR-CCNB3 fusion positive sarcomas: a clinicopathologic and molecular analysis of 36 cases with comparison to morphologic spectrum and clinical behavior of other round cell sarcomas. Am J Surg Pathol 2018;42(5):604–15.

140. Specht K, Sung YS, Zhang L, et al. Distinct transcriptional signature and immunoprofile of CIC-DUX4 fusion-positive round cell tumors compared to EWSR1-rearranged Ewing sarcomas: further evidence toward distinct pathologic entities. Genes Chromosomes Cancer 2014;53(7):622–33.

141. Hung YP, Fletcher CD, Hornick JL. Evaluation of ETV4 and WT1 expression in CIC-rearranged sarcomas and histologic mimics. Mod Pathol 2016;29(11):1324–34.

142. Le Guellec S, Velasco V, Perot G, et al. ETV4 is a useful marker for the diagnosis of CIC-rearranged undifferentiated round-cell sarcomas: a study of 127 cases including mimicking lesions. Mod Pathol 2016;29(12):1523–31.

143. Shibayama T, Okamoto T, Nakashima Y, et al. Screening of BCOR-CCNB3 sarcoma using immunohistochemistry for CCNB3: a clinicopathological report of three pediatric cases. Pathol Int 2015;65(8):410–4.

144. Chamberlain BK, McClain CM, Gonzalez RS, et al. Alveolar soft part sarcoma and granular cell tumor: an immunohistochemical comparison study. Hum Pathol 2014;45(5):1039–44.

145. Schoolmeester JK, Lastra RR. Granular cell tumors overexpress TFE3 without corollary gene rearrangement. Hum Pathol 2015;46(8):1242–3.

146. Wieczorek TJ, Krane JF, Domanski HA, et al. Cytologic findings in granular cell tumors, with emphasis on the diagnosis of malignant granular cell tumor by fine-needle aspiration biopsy. Cancer 2001;93(6):398–408.

147. Rekhi B, Singh N. Spectrum of cytopathologic features of epithelioid sarcoma in a series of 7 uncommon cases with immunohistochemical results, including loss of INI1/SMARCB1 in two test cases. Diagn Cytopathol 2016;44(7):636–42.

148. Cardillo M, Zakowski MF, Lin O. Fine-needle aspiration of epithelioid sarcoma: cytology findings in nine cases. Cancer 2001;93(4):246–51.

149. Pendse AA, Dodd LG. Fine-needle-aspiration cytology of a proximal type epithelioid sarcoma: a case report. Diagn Cytopathol 2015;43(10):859–62.

150. Hornick JL, Dal Cin P, Fletcher CD. Loss of INI1 expression is characteristic of both conventional and proximal-type epithelioid sarcoma. Am J Surg Pathol 2009;33(4):542–50.

151. Flucke U, Slootweg PJ, Mentzel T, et al. Re: infrequent SMARCB1/INI1 gene alteration in epithelioid sarcoma: a useful tool in distinguishing epithelioid sarcoma from malignant rhabdoid tumor: direct evidence of mutational inactivation of SMARCB1/INI1 in epithelioid sarcoma. Hum Pathol 2009;40(9): 1361–2, [author reply: 2–4].

152. Sullivan LM, Folpe AL, Pawel BR, et al. Epithelioid sarcoma is associated with a high percentage of SMARCB1 deletions. Mod Pathol 2013;26(3): 385–92.

153. Stockman DL, Hornick JL, Deavers MT, et al. ERG and FLI1 protein expression in epithelioid sarcoma. Mod Pathol 2014;27(4):496–501.

154. Miettinen M, Wang Z, Sarlomo-Rikala M, et al. ERG expression in epithelioid sarcoma: a diagnostic pitfall. Am J Surg Pathol 2013;37(10):1580–5.

155. Hollmann TJ, Hornick JL. INI1-deficient tumors: diagnostic features and molecular genetics. Am J Surg Pathol 2011;35(10):e47–63.

156. Jo VY, Fletcher CD. Epithelioid malignant peripheral nerve sheath tumor: clinicopathologic analysis of 63 cases. Am J Surg Pathol 2015;39(5):673–82.

157. Errani C, Zhang L, Sung YS, et al. A novel WWTR1-CAMTA1 gene fusion is a consistent abnormality in epithelioid hemangioendothelioma of different anatomic sites. Genes Chromosomes Cancer 2011;50(8):644–53.

158. Doyle LA, Fletcher CD, Hornick JL. Nuclear expression of CAMTA1 distinguishes epithelioid hemangioendothelioma from histologic mimics. Am J Surg Pathol 2016;40(1):94–102.

159. Antonescu CR, Le Loarer F, Mosquera JM, et al. Novel YAP1-TFE3 fusion defines a distinct subset of epithelioid hemangioendothelioma. Genes Chromosomes Cancer 2013;52(8):775–84.

160. Creager AJ, Pitman MB, Geisinger KR. Cytologic features of clear cell sarcoma (malignant melanoma) of soft parts: a study of fine-needle aspirates and exfoliative specimens. Am J Clin Pathol 2002; 117(2):217–24.

161. Wang WL, Mayordomo E, Zhang W, et al. Detection and characterization of EWSR1/ATF1 and EWSR1/CREB1 chimeric transcripts in clear cell sarcoma (melanoma of soft parts). Mod Pathol 2009;22(9): 1201–9.

162. Antonescu CR, Nafa K, Segal NH, et al. EWS-CREB1: a recurrent variant fusion in clear cell sarcoma–association with gastrointestinal location and absence of melanocytic differentiation. Clin Cancer Res 2006;12(18):5356–62.

163. Stockman DL, Miettinen M, Suster S, et al. Malignant gastrointestinal neuroectodermal tumor: clinicopathologic, immunohistochemical, ultrastructural, and molecular analysis of 16 cases with a reappraisal of clear cell sarcoma-like tumors of the gastrointestinal tract. Am J Surg Pathol 2012;36(6):857–68.

164. Wakely PE Jr, McDermott JE, Ali SZ. Cytopathology of alveolar soft part sarcoma: a report of 10 cases. Cancer 2009;117(6):500–7.

165. Machhi J, Kouzova M, Komorowski DJ, et al. Crystals of alveolar soft part sarcoma in a fine needle aspiration biopsy cytology smear. A case report. Acta Cytol 2002;46(5):904–8.

166. Folpe AL, Mentzel T, Lehr HA, et al. Perivascular epithelioid cell neoplasms of soft tissue and gynecologic origin: a clinicopathologic study of 26 cases and review of the literature. Am J Surg Pathol 2005;29(12):1558–75.

167. Argani P, Aulmann S, Illei PB, et al. A distinctive subset of PEComas harbors TFE3 gene fusions. Am J Surg Pathol 2010;34(10):1395–406.

168. Marino-Enriquez A, Wang WL, Roy A, et al. Epithelioid inflammatory myofibroblastic sarcoma: an aggressive intra-abdominal variant of inflammatory myofibroblastic tumor with nuclear membrane or perinuclear ALK. Am J Surg Pathol 2011;35(1): 135–44.

169. Lee JC, Wu JM, Liau JY, et al. Cytopathologic features of epithelioid inflammatory myofibroblastic sarcoma with correlation of histopathology, immunohistochemistry, and molecular cytogenetic analysis. Cancer Cytopathol 2015;123(8):495–504.

170. Jiwani S, Gokden M, Lindberg M, et al. Fine-needle aspiration cytology of epithelioid malignant peripheral nerve sheath tumor: a case report and review of the literature. Diagn Cytopathol 2016;44(3): 226–31.

171. Doyle LA, Nelson D, Heinrich MC, et al. Loss of succinate dehydrogenase subunit B (SDHB) expression is limited to a distinctive subset of gastric wild-type gastrointestinal stromal tumours: a comprehensive genotype-phenotype correlation study. Histopathology 2012;61(5):801–9.

172. Miettinen M, Wang ZF, Sarlomo-Rikala M, et al. Succinate dehydrogenase-deficient GISTs: a clinicopathologic, immunohistochemical, and molecular genetic study of 66 gastric GISTs with predilection to young age. Am J Surg Pathol 2011;35(11):1712–21.

173. Wagner AJ, Remillard SP, Zhang YX, et al. Loss of expression of SDHA predicts SDHA mutations in gastrointestinal stromal tumors. Mod Pathol 2013; 26(2):289–94.

174. Gill AJ, Chou A, Vilain RE, et al. "Pediatric-type" gastrointestinal stromal tumors are SDHB negative ("type 2") GISTs. Am J Surg Pathol 2011;35(8): 1245–7, [author reply: 7–8].

175. Pasini B, McWhinney SR, Bei T, et al. Clinical and molecular genetics of patients with the Carney-Stratakis syndrome and germline mutations of the genes coding for the succinate dehydrogenase subunits SDHB, SDHC, and SDHD. Eur J Hum Genet 2008;16(1):79–88.

176. Haller F, Moskalev EA, Faucz FR, et al. Aberrant DNA hypermethylation of SDHC: a novel mechanism of tumor development in Carney triad. Endocr Relat Cancer 2014;21(4):567–77.

177. Mason EF, Hornick JL. Conventional risk stratification fails to predict progression of succinate dehydrogenase-deficient gastrointestinal stromal tumors: a clinicopathologic study of 76 cases. Am J Surg Pathol 2016;40(12):1616–21.

178. Sirvent N, Coindre JM, Maire G, et al. Detection of MDM2-CDK4 amplification by fluorescence in situ hybridization in 200 paraffin-embedded tumor samples: utility in diagnosing adipocytic lesions and comparison with immunohistochemistry and real-time PCR. Am J Surg Pathol 2007;31(10): 1476–89.

179. Bode-Lesniewska B, Zhao J, Speel EJ, et al. Gains of 12q13-14 and overexpression of mdm2 are frequent findings in intimal sarcomas of the pulmonary artery. Virchows Arch 2001;438(1):57–65.

180. Zhang H, Macdonald WD, Erickson-Johnson M, et al. Cytogenetic and molecular cytogenetic findings of intimal sarcoma. Cancer Genet Cytogenet 2007;179(2):146–9.

181. Mejia-Guerrero S, Quejada M, Gokgoz N, et al. Characterization of the 12q15 MDM2 and 12q13-14 CDK4 amplicons and clinical correlations in osteosarcoma. Genes Chromosomes Cancer 2010;49(6):518–25.

182. Tarkkanen M, Bohling T, Gamberi G, et al. Comparative genomic hybridization of low-grade central osteosarcoma. Mod Pathol 1998;11(5):421–6.

183. Duhamel LA, Ye H, Halai D, et al. Frequency of Mouse Double Minute 2 (MDM2) and Mouse Double Minute 4 (MDM4) amplification in parosteal and conventional osteosarcoma subtypes. Histopathology 2012;60(2):357–9.

Updates in Primary Bone Tumors
Current Challenges and New Opportunities in Cytopathology

Xiaohua Qian, MD, PhD

KEYWORDS

- Aneurysmal bone cyst • Chondroblastoma • Chondrosarcoma • Giant cell–rich
- Giant cell tumor of bone • Notochordal tumors • Chordoma • Fine-needle aspiration

Key points

- Collaboration within a multidisciplinary team is still the fundamental approach to establishing a correct and/or clinically relevant diagnosis of primary bone tumors.

- The identification of histone 3.3 mutations in giant cell tumor of bone and chondroblastoma has led to the development of diagnostically useful mutation-specific markers, H3G34W and H3K36M, which can improve the diagnostic accuracy among giant cell–rich neoplasms, especially in needle biopsy samples.

- Recurrent molecular alterations have been found, including *IDH1/2* mutations in both benign and malignant cartilaginous tumors and *HEY1-NCOA2* fusion in mesenchymal chondrosarcoma. Molecular studies may help in some but not all difficult differential diagnoses of chondrosarcomas on needle biopsy samples.

- Bimorphic bone tumors, such as mesenchymal chondrosarcoma, dedifferentiated chondrosarcoma, and dedifferentiated chordoma, pose significant diagnostic pitfalls in fine-needle aspiration biopsies due to potential sampling errors.

- An additional advantage of fine-needle aspiration over surgical biopsy for bone tumors is the ability to obtain samples with high-quality DNA and RNA for molecular/genetic testing without the damage of decalcification.

ABSTRACT

The review summarizes the current diagnostic challenges in fine-needle aspiration of primary bone tumors, with focus on the application of new molecular and immunohistochemical techniques in the diagnosis of giant cell–rich neoplasms, chondrosarcomas, and notochordal tumors.

OVERVIEW

Evaluation of primary bone tumors by minimally invasive biopsy techniques, such as fine-needle aspiration (FNA) and core needle biopsy (CNB), remains one of the most challenging areas in surgical pathology, particularly in cytopathology.[1,2] The practice has been limited to a few large tertiary centers because of the uneasiness of general cytopathologists with primary bone tumors, which are uncommon and require a high level of collaboration within a multidisciplinary team to make a correct diagnosis.[3] Recent advances in understanding the underlying molecular genetics in certain bone tumors not only have increased knowledge of their pathogenesis but also led to the development of novel molecular and surrogate immunohistochemical (IHC) diagnostic tools. A new era of using FNA material for the judicious application of ancillary

Department of Pathology, Brigham and Women's Hospital, 75 Francis Street, Boston, MA 02115, USA
E-mail address: xqian@bwh.harvard.edu

Surgical Pathology 11 (2018) 657–668
https://doi.org/10.1016/j.path.2018.06.004

studies to supplement the traditional approach of integration of clinical and imaging characteristics for the diagnosis of primary bone tumors is expected to emerge in the horizon. General discussion of cytologic diagnosis of bone tumors is beyond of scope of this focused review, and readers are directed to prior excellent reviews[1,2] and book chapters.[3,4] In this review, entities with recent molecular advances and their respective opportunities for cytopathologic practice are selected for discussion. Relevant updates in the current 2013 World Health Organization (WHO) classification of tumors of soft tissue and bone are included.[5]

GIANT CELL–RICH TUMORS

Giant cell–rich tumors represent a broad group of tumors and tumor-like lesions, which are characterized morphologically by the presence of numerous osteoclasts or osteoclast-like giant cells. A summary of differential diagnosis of giant cell–rich tumors is provided in **Table 1**.

GIANT CELL TUMOR OF BONE

Giant cell tumor (GCT) of bone is a locally aggressive neoplasm that has a predilection for young adults with a mature skeleton and usually arises in the epiphyseal-metaphyseal region of long bones around the knee. GCT of bone represents approximately 5% of primary bone tumors and 20% of benign bone tumors. The treatment options include surgical curettage and receptor activator of nuclear factor κB (RANK) ligand (RANKL) inhibitors, such as denosumab.[6] Up to one-third of patients recur after treatment by curettage, and fewer than 5% of cases show malignant transformation, either occurring de novo or developing during recurrence. Classically, GCT of bone on image studies shows an eccentric, large, and pure lytic intramedullary lesion with sharp borders in the epiphyseal-metaphyseal region of distal femur. Aspirates are typically cellular and characterized by a dual cell population: mononuclear spindled or ovoid cells and admixed with numerous large osteoclast-like giant cells containing 20 to 50 (or more) nuclei (**Fig. 1**). In the presence of these characteristic radiographic and cytologic features, the diagnosis of GCT by FNA can be straightforward. Significant clinical, radiologic, and morphologic overlap exists, however, among many benign and malignant giant cell–rich neoplasms, posing considerable diagnostic challenges, especially in FNA/CNB samples.[2,7]

The main diagnostic challenges of GCT of bone include (1) separating from other giant cell–rich benign neoplasms/lesions, such as solid aneurysmal bone cyst (ABC), chondroblastoma, chondromyxoid fibroma, GCT of Paget disease, nonossifying fibroma, giant cell lesion of the small bones (GCLSB) (giant cell reparative granuloma), and brown tumor of hyperparathyroidism; (2) distinguishing giant cell–rich osteosarcoma from GCT of bone with atypical features (cytologic atypia, necrosis, and mitosis); and finally (3) recognizing denosumab-treated GCT of bone, which shows markedly diminished osteoclast-like giant cells and increased fibrosis and hyalinization.[6,8]

> ### Main Diagnostic Challenges of GCT of Bone
> - To separate GCT of bone from other giant cell–rich benign neoplasms/lesions
> - To distinguish giant cell–rich osteosarcoma from GCT of bone with atypical features
> - To recognize denosumab-treated GCT of bone

One of the updates in the 2013 WHO classification was separating GCT of bone from GCLSB.[5,9] GCLSB, along with similar lesions arising in jaw bones, is also called giant cell reparative granuloma in practice. Giant cells clustering around the areas of hemorrhage, a key histologic feature in GCLSB, is usually absent in FNA cytology preparations.[10] In fact, the cytomorphologic features of GCT of bone, GCLSB, GCT of Paget disease, and brown tumor of hyperparathyroidism are usually indistinguishable.[2,3,10,11] The presence of benign fibrous histocytoma-like areas in GCT of bone mimics nonossifying fibroma. The cyst formation in GCT of bone makes distinguishing it from primary ABC difficult.[7,12] Considering the differences in recurrence rates, prognoses, and treatment strategies, it is important to distinguish GCT of bone from its benign giant cell–rich mimics. Definitive distinction, however, is not always possible, even with correlation of clinical and radiologic findings, especially when a tumor arises at unusual anatomic sites and/or shows atypical morphologic features (**Fig. 2**). In such settings, traditionally, a descriptive diagnosis, such as "giant cell–rich neoplasm" is often given with a list of differential diagnoses.

The recent discovery of recurrent somatic driver mutations in *H3F3A* (located at 1q42.12) and *H3F3B* (located at 17q25.1) in the majority GCTs of bone and chondroblastomas, respectively,[13] has forever reshaped the diagnostic field of giant cell–rich neoplasms. *H3F3A* and *H3F3B* have different DNA sequences but both encode replication-independent histone proteins (H3.3) of identical amino acid sequences. The most

Table 1
Differential diagnoses of common giant cell rich neoplasms of bone

Diagnosis	Age (y), Male:Female	Common Location	Imaging Features	Cytomorphology	Ancillary Tests
ABC	<20; 1:1	Metaphysis of long bones; lumbar and cervical vertebrae	Cystic, expansile, multiloculated lesion with soft tissue septa and fluid-fluid levels	Hypocellular bloody smears, spindle cells, and scattered GCs; intratumoral reactive bone on CNB	FISH for *USP6* rearrangement
Chondro-blastoma	10–25 2:1	Epiphysis of long bones	Well-defined, scalloped borders, sclerotic rim, and internal mineralization	Cellular smears with matrix, chondroblasts with nuclear grooves, and scattered GCs	Mutation-specific IHC K36M DOG1, SOX9
GCT	20–40; 2:1	Epiphyseal-metaphyseal region of long bones; sacrum	Large, pure lytic intramedullary lesion with sharp borders, no matrix mineralization	Hypercellular smears with a dual cell population: mononuclear spindled or ovoid cells and multinucleated GCs; absence of matrix	Mutation-specific IHC G36W/L/V/R
Osteoblastoma	10–30 2:1	Metadiaphyseal region of tubular bones; spine; sacrum	Expansile, well-defined mixed lytic and blastic lesion, 2–5 cm	Mononucleated and binucleated osteoblasts, dispersed or in small clusters; scattered GCs and scant stroma	N/A
Osteosarcoma, giant cell–rich	10–20 and >50 1.3:1	Metaphysis of long bones	Destructive and ill-defined, soft tissue component with matrix mineralization	Variably cellular smears with epithelioid to pleomorphic cells, both tumor GCs and benign osteoclast-like GCs, necrosis, mitoses, and strands of osteoid matrix	N/A
Nonossifying fibroma[a]	10–15; 2:1	Metaphysis of long bones in lower extremities	Lytic and lobulated lesion with a sclerotic rim	Spindled fibroblasts, scattered GCs, and foam cells; peripheral reactive bone on CNB	N/A

[a] Radiologic features are often diagnostic and a biopsy is not necessary in most cases.

Abbreviations: ABC, aneurysmal bone cyst; FISH, fluorescence in situ hybridization; GCs, giant cells; IHC, immunohisto-chemistry; N/A, not applicable.

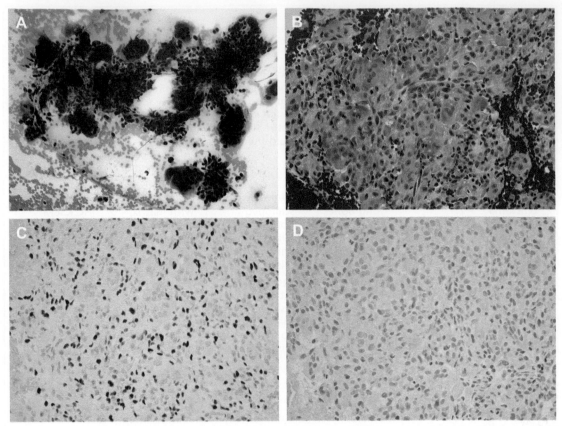

Fig. 1. GCT of bone. Aspirates demonstrating clusters of oval to spindled mononucleated cells admixed with numerous multinucleated giant cells are characteristic (Diff-Quik stain [A]; cell block hematoxylin-eosin stain [B]). IHC for H3G34W (C) is positive in the mononuclear stromal cells, the true neoplastic cells in GCT of bone. The multinucleated giant cells and their precursors, non-neoplastic bystanders, are negative for H3G34W. IHC for H3K36M (D), a mutation-specific marker for chondroblastoma, is negative in GCT of bone. ([A–D], original magnification ×400)

common mutation in GCT of bone is *H3F3A* G34W and accounts for 85% to 95% cases, but alternate G34V, G34R, and G34L mutations have been reported in a subset of cases.[13–17] The *H3F3A* mutations and the resulting mutant H3.3G34W protein or its variants are restricted to the mononuclear stromal cells, the true neoplastic cells in GCT of bone (see **Fig. 1**C). The multinucleated giant cells and their precursors are non-neoplastic bystanders, making GCT of bone a true misnomer. Mutation analysis of *H3F3A* has been shown to effectively distinguish GCT of bone from many aforementioned giant cell–rich neoplasms, because *H3F3A* mutations are absent in these mimics.[14–16,18] Most recently, mutation-specific IHC using monoclonal antibodies directed against the mutant H3.3 G34W and its variant proteins has been shown highly specific and sensitive for the diagnosis of GCT of bone.[17,19,20] It is particularly exciting that these mutation-specific antibodies have been validated to work well on FNA and CNB samples and help clarify the diagnosis in morphologically ambiguous cases[11] (see **Fig. 2**).

GCT of bone can exhibit atypical features including cytologic atypia (nuclear hyperchromasia and enlargement in mononuclear cells),[21] mitotic activity, and even necrosis and/or hemorrhage due to infarction. These features could be alarming for malignancy and lead to the confusion with giant cell–rich osteosarcoma or malignant transformation in GCT of bone. Traditionally, the infiltrative growth pattern and diffuse marked atypia in mononuclear cells would favor giant cell–rich osteosarcoma. Now, the detection of *H3F3A* mutations by either sequencing or mutation-specific IHC can distinguish conventional GCT of bone with atypia from giant cell–rich osteosarcoma but not from malignant GCT of bone, which also harbors *H3F3A* mutations.[19]

Denosumab, a fully humanized monoclonal antibody directed against the RANKL, has been used to control unresectable or metastatic GCT of bone since 2010.[22,23] Denosumab suppresses the RANK-RANKL interaction, a key mechanism of osteoclast activity, thereby resulting in marked diminishing of osteoclast-like giant cells, reduction

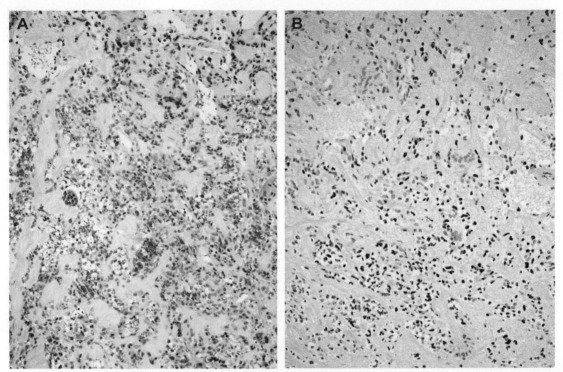

Fig. 2. A giant-cell rich neoplasm arising in distal femur in an 83-year-old female. The core needle biopsy showing mononuclear cell proliferation with extensive fibrosis, hyalinization, and a rich vasculature. There are only a few osteoclast-like giant cells, unrecognizable as giant cell tumor of bone (*A*, H&E stain). Immunohistochemistry for H3G34W is positive in mononucleated cells (*B*), confirming the diagnosis of GCT of bone with unusual morphology. [*A, B* original magnification ×200].

of bone destruction, and increased production of fibro-osseous tissue. Therefore, denosumab-treated GCTs of bone can morphologically mimic other fibro-osseous lesions, such as fibrous dysplasia, nonossifying fibroma, osteoblastoma, and low-grade osteosarcoma.[6,8,24,25] The neoplastic stromal cells, however, survive the denosumab treatment and their *H3F3A* mutations usually remain unchanged. In diagnostically challenging post-denosumab treatment cases, detection of *H3F3A* by mutation analysis and/or mutation specific H3G34W IHC has proven helpful.[11,25]

CHONDROBLASTOMA

Chondroblastoma is a rare benign, cartilage-producing tumor composed of chondroblasts, which occurs in children and adolescents with an immature skeleton. It accounts for less than 1% of primary bone tumors and less than 3% of benign bone tumors. The most common site is the epiphysis of long bones, such as distal and proximal femur, but tumors may arise in the small tubular bones in hands and feet and flat bones, such as talus, calcaneus, and patella. Chondroblastoma tends to be a painful, solitary lesion. The typical

radiograph shows a small (3–6 cm), well-defined, intramedullary lytic lesion with a sclerotic rim and internal mineralization. The FNA smears usually have the diagnostic features of a mixture of mononuclear chondroblasts and multinucleated osteoclast-like giant cell, in clusters and single cells (**Fig. 3**A, B). Fragments of chondroid matrix with calcifications, if present, are a helpful clue.[26–28]

In cases with classic imaging and cytomorphologic features, diagnosis of chondroblastoma is usually straightforward. Several mimics, however, enter the differential diagnosis of chondroblastoma, which include other giant cell–rich tumors, such as GCT of bone and ABC, chondromyxoid fibroma, clear cell chondrosarcoma, and chondroblastoma-like osteosarcoma.[27,29]

Although a few makers, such as S100 protein, SOX9, and DOG1, have been shown positive in chondroblastoma and other neoplasms with cartilaginous differentiation,[29–32] truly sensitive and specific markers for the difficult differential diagnoses of chondroblastoma were not available until recently. In 2013, Behjati and colleagues[13] identified mutations in either *H3F3B* (majority) or *H3F3A* at codon K36M in 95% of chondroblastoma, along with *H3F3A* mutations in 92% of GCT of bone. This

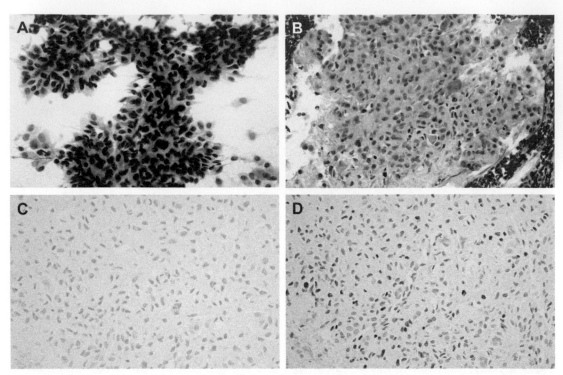

Fig. 3. Chondroblastoma. Aspirates are hypercellular with mononuclear chondroblasts with characteristic nuclear grooves and scattered multinucleated osteoclast-like giant cell (Papanicolaou stain [*A*]). The mononucleated cells are typically embedded in a chondroid matrix (cell block hematoxylin-eosin stain [*B*]); IHC for H3K36M is positive in chondroblasts and not in osteoclast-like giant cells (*D*). IHC for H3G34W (*C*), a mutation-specific marker for giant cell tumor of bone, is negative in chondroblastoma [*A–D*, original magnification ×400].

breakthrough discovery was further confirmed by others.[14] Subsequently, Amary and colleagues[33] demonstrated mutation-specific H3K36M IHC to be highly sensitive and specific for the diagnosis of chondroblastoma among giant cell–rich tumors. Like in GCT of bone, *H3F3B* mutations and the resulting mutant H3.3K36M protein are present in chondroblasts and not in osteoclast-like giant cells (**Fig.** 3C, D). The H3K36M antibody (clone RM193) seems to achieve higher sensitivity in FNA samples than in decalcified resection sections.[11] This highly sensitive and specific mutation-specific IHC is extremely helpful in small biopsy samples to distinguish chondroblastoma from its malignant mimics, such as clear cell chondrosarcoma and chondroblastoma-like osteosarcoma.

ANEURYSMAL BONE CYST

ABC is a benign but locally destructive multicystic bone lesion with blood-filled spaces. It may occur as a primary bone lesion (primary ABC) or be associated with a preexisting bone lesion (secondary ABC). Primary ABC usually affects patients in their first 2 decades with a slight female predominance. The common sites of involvement include the metaphysis of long bones, posterior elements of vertebra, and small bones of hands and feet. Image findings are characteristic and show a cystic, expansile, multiloculated lesion with soft tissue septa and fluid-fluid levels.[5,7] Histologically, it is characterized by blood-filled spaces surrounded by septa of bland spindle cells, foamy macrophages, and osteoclastic-like giant cells.[7] Diagnosing ABC on FNA is extremely difficult due to a high insufficient rate and nonspecific cytomorphology with a broad differential diagnosis ranging from benign giant cell–rich neoplasms to highly malignant telangiectatic osteosarcoma.[34] The solid variant of ABC is particularly problematic not only because of the absence of characteristic blood-filled cystic spaces, but also because of the presence of hypercellular, even mitotically active myofibroblasts with reactive woven bone fragments.

It is well known now that approximately 70% of primary but not secondary ABCs harbor a t (16;17) translation,[35] resulting in a fusion transcript *CDH11-USP6*. The fusion gene does not result in a fusion protein but instead leads to constitutive activation of *USP6* under the control of the *CDH11* promoter.[36] Many other fusion partners (*OMD, COL1A1, ZNF9,* and *TRAP*) identified so far function in a similar manner.[37] Fluorescence in situ hybridization (FISH) with break-apart probes for *USP6* can detect all fusion variants in ABCs, which may be helpful in distinguishing primary ABC from secondary ABC, other giant cell–rich neoplasms, and telangiectatic osteosarcoma. *USP6* rearrangement is only present in neoplastic stromal cells, the fraction of which in ABCs ranges from 8% to 82%; as a result, a false-negative FISH result may occur, which not necessarily excludes the diagnosis of ABC.[38]

CHONDROSARCOMA AND ITS VARIANTS

Cartilage-forming tumors form a clinical and histologic spectrum ranging from benign, such as enchondroma; to intermediate, such as chondrosarcoma grade 1; to malignant, such as conventional chondrosarcoma, grades 2 to 3.[5,39] In recent years, there have been both remarkable advances in molecular alterations and noticeable updates in the 2013 WHO classification regarding chondrosarcoma, which is thereby the focus of discussion.

Chondrosarcomas are a heterogeneous group of malignant cartilaginous tumors, which include conventional chondrosarcoma (primary and secondary, central and periosteal), dedifferentiated chondrosarcoma, clear cell chondrosarcoma, and mesenchymal chondrosarcoma. Primary central chondrosarcoma accounts for approximately 85% of all chondrosarcomas. It is the third most common primary malignant bone tumor after plasma cell myeloma and osteosarcoma in adults. Chondrosarcoma can develop at any age but affects mainly older patients in the fifth to seventh decades of life. It can arise in any bone derived from enchondral ossification but originates mostly in bones of the trunk (pelvis, ribs, and scapula) and in bones around hip and shoulder girdles.[5] On imaging studies, low-grade tumors exhibit a lytic erosion with intratumoral mineralization, endosteal scalloping, and cortex thickening; high-grade ones show cortical destruction and soft tissue extension.[40]

One of the major updates of chondrogenic tumors in the 2013 WHO classification was to give chondrosarcoma two *International Classification of Disease* (ICD) codes to reflect the different prognosis of chondrosarcoma based on grade.[5] Grade 1 chondrosarcoma was separated from grade 2 and grade 3 chondrosarcomas and given the synonym "atypical cartilaginous tumor" to reflect its relatively indolent clinical course.[9] Patients with atypical cartilaginous tumor/grade 1 chondrosarcoma in the long bones now tend be treated with curettage and local adjuvants and have a 10% recurrence rate and an 83% 5-year survival rate. In contrast, patients with grades 2 to 3 chondrosarcoma are treated with wide surgical resection and have a 5-year survival rate at 53%.[9,39,41]

Despite its clinical importance, preoperative diagnosis and grading chondrosarcoma remains one of most challenging dilemmas in bone pathology, even among experienced subspecialists.[42] The main diagnostic challenges include (1) distinguishing atypical cartilaginous tumor/grade 1 chondrosarcoma from benign cartilage-forming tumors, such as enchondroma and chondromyxoid fibroma; (2) separating atypical cartilaginous tumor/grade 1 chondrosarcoma from high-grade (grades 2–3) chondrosarcoma; (3) distinguishing chondrosarcoma from other malignant mimics, such as chondroblastic osteosarcoma and chordoma; and finally, (4) recognizing rare variants of chondrosarcoma, such as dedifferentiated chondrosarcoma, clear cell chondrosarcoma, and mesenchymal chondrosarcoma.

Main Diagnostic Challenges of Chondrosarcoma

- To distinguish atypical cartilaginous tumor/grade 1 chondrosarcoma from benign cartilage-forming tumors, such as enchondroma and chondromyxoid fibroma

- To separate atypical cartilaginous tumor/grade 1 chondrosarcoma from high-grade (grades 2–3) chondrosarcoma

- To distinguish chondrosarcoma from other malignant mimics, such as chondroblastic osteosarcoma and chordoma

- To recognize rare variants of chondrosarcoma, such as dedifferentiated chondrosarcoma, clear cell chondrosarcoma, and mesenchymal chondrosarcoma.

One of most significant genetic findings of bone tumors in recent years is the identification of point mutations in *isocitrate dehydrogenase* (*IDH1/2*) genes in a variety of benign and malignant cartilage-forming tumors. *IDH1/2* genes encode for the metabolic enzymes IDH1 and IDH2; these gain of function mutations have been linked to the pathogenesis of cartilage-forming tumors.[43] The prevalence of *IDH1/2* mutations is extremely variable: enchondroma (approximately 40% in solitary lesions and 87% in syndromic multiple lesions), conventional central chondrosarcomas, grades 1 to 3 (38%–70%), secondary central chondrosarcoma (86%), periosteal chondrosarcoma (100%), and dedifferentiated chondrosarcoma (50%–60%).[44] Mutational analysis is of little value for chondrosarcoma grading and for distinguishing atypical cartilaginous tumor/grade 1 chondrosarcoma from benign cartilage-forming tumors. In addition, only approximately 20% of the *IDH1* mutations can be detected by the mutation-specific IHC using the IDH R132H antibody.[44] A multidisciplinary approach with close historadiologic correlation is still indispensable for establishing a clinically relevant diagnosis in such difficult settings.[39]

Although cytomorphologic features of chondrosarcomas have been well described,[3,45–47] the fact that it is cytologically indistinguishable between atypical cartilaginous tumor/grade 1 chondrosarcoma (Fig. 4) and benign enchondroma cannot be overemphasized.[2] The infiltrative growth pattern, a diagnostic feature for low-grade chondrosarcoma, is absent in FNA samples. Therefore, the recommendation of a CNB, especially of the tumor-normal bone interface, should be discussed during the rapid on-site evaluation when a low-grade cartilaginous neoplasm is suspected. It is not uncommon that the radiologic and clinical worrisome features trump the benign morphology on biopsy. When it is impossible to distinguish the two based on both morphology and radiology, a diagnosis of "low-grade cartilaginous neoplasm" is still helpful for clinical management by confirming the cartilaginous and low-grade nature of the lesion.[2,48,49] In fact, many low-grade cartilaginous neoplasms in long bones are treated with curettage based on clinical and imaging features without a preoperative needle biopsy.[41] Chondrosarcoma grading on small biopsies, however, remains problematic, especially for tumors arising in the pelvic bones.[49,50]

Most high-grade chondrosarcomas are convenient targets for FNA due to the presence of cortical destruction and soft tissue extension. Aspirates often yield hypercellular smears with single

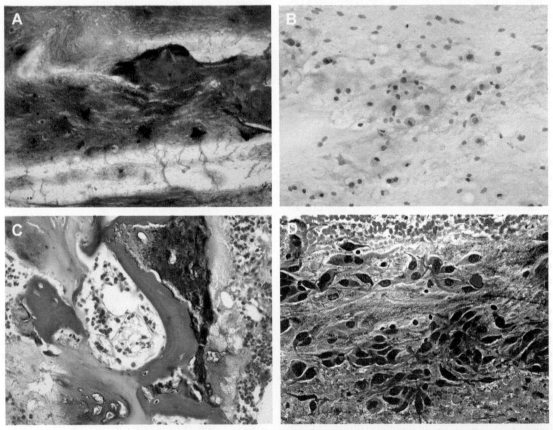

Fig. 4. Chondrosarcoma. Aspirates are usually hypocellular and composed of scattered epithelioid cells in an abundant chondromyxoid matrix, which is rich magenta on Diff-Quik stained smears (*A*) and pale grayish on Papanicolaou stained smears (*B*). The cytology of chondrosarcoma grade 1 is deceptively bland and the infiltrative pattern is best appreciated on core needle biopsies (hematoxylin-eosin stain [*C*]). Dedifferentiated chondrosarcoma is characterized by a bimorphic pattern with a chondrosarcoma grade 1 component juxtaposed with a high-grade noncartilaginous sarcomatous component (Diff-Quik stained smear [*D*]). Sampling only one of the components is a common pitfall in FNA samples. (original magnification: ABCD: 400×).

tumor cells, cartilaginous tissue fragments, and a myxoid background. The cellular and nuclear pleomorphism is conspicuous, as are the mitoses. The important differential diagnosis in this setting includes chondroblastic osteosarcoma and chordoma. In addition to careful clinical and radiology correlation, ancillary studies, including IHC (brachyury for chordoma [discussed later]) and mutational analysis to detect IDH1/2 mutations in chondrosarcoma, can aid the distinction between chondrosarcoma and its malignant mimics because both chordoma and chondroblastic osteosarcoma lack IDH1/2 mutations.[44,51,52]

Dedifferentiated chondrosarcoma occurs in approximately 10% to 15% of chondrosarcomas and carries a poor prognosis. It is characterized by two histologic components in variable proportions: a chondrosarcoma grade 1 component juxtaposed with a high-grade noncartilaginous sarcomatous component. Sampling only one of the components is a common pitfall in the FNA samples.[53]

Clear cell chondrosarcoma, a rare variant of chondrosarcoma often seen in femoral head, is characterized by sheets of clear cells with areas of conventional low-grade chondrosarcoma.[54] Cytomorphologic features of clear cell chondrosarcoma, described in a few case reports,[55,56] include cellular smears with dispersed large epithelioid tumor cells with abundant finely vacuolated cytoplasm, a central to slightly eccentric round nucleus, and prominent nucleoli. Fragments of chondromyxoid matrix and scattered osteoclast-like giant cells also are present.

Mesenchymal chondrosarcoma is a rare high-grade malignant tumor with a distinct bimorphic pattern composed of islands of low-grade hyaline cartilage and areas of primitive small round cells.[54] The cytologic features of mesenchymal chondrosarcoma in FNA smears have been reported in a few case reports.[57–59] Like other bimorphic sarcomas, sampling only one of components is a pitfall in small needle biopsies. The primitive round cell component can mimic Ewing sarcoma, small cell osteosarcoma, lymphomas, and even recently defined round cell sarcomas with CIC rearrangement or BCOR-CCNB3 rearrangement[60]; the low-grade cartilaginous component can be easily mistaken for more common entities, such as low-grade chondrosarcoma and chondroblastic osteosarcoma. The recent identification of HEY1-NCOA2 fusion can facilitate definitive diagnosis of mesenchymal chondrosarcoma in difficult cases by application of either FISH using HEY1 or NCOA2 probes or reverse transcriptase–polymerase chain reaction (TR-PCR) to detect the fusion transcripts.[61]

Mutational analysis to detect IDH1/2 mutations is also helpful in distinguishing dedifferentiated chondrosarcoma from other pleomorphic/spindle cell sarcomas[62] and low-grade chondrosarcoma from clear cell and mesenchymal variants of chondrosarcoma.[44]

NOTOCHORDAL TUMORS

Chordoma is a primary malignant bone tumor of notochordal differentiation. Although virtually restricted to axial skeleton, it can rarely occur at extra-axial skeletal locations. A destructive, lytic sacral mass with anterior soft tissue extension is a typical finding on image studies.[63] Brachyury (gene product of T) is an important transcription factor in notochord differentiation[64] and the antibody against brachyury is a sensitive and specific marker of notochordal tumors, even in small biopsies.[65] The FNA cytologic features in most cases are distinct: physaliferous (bubbles in Greek) cells within an abundant chondromyxoid matrix (deep magenta color on air-dried Diff-Quik–stained smears), making a diagnosis of chordoma often straightforward.[2,66–68] The main diagnostic challenges are (1) to separate well-differentiated chordoma from its benign counterpart, benign notochordal cell tumor (BNCT); (2) to distinguish it from morphologic mimics, such as conventional chondrosarcoma; and (3) to recognize dedifferentiated chordoma, a higher-grade tumor with a sarcoma-like appearance.

> ### Main Diagnostic Challenges of Chordoma
> - To separate well-differentiated chordoma from its benign counterpart, BNCT
> - To distinguish chordoma from morphologic mimics such as conventional chondrosarcoma
> - To recognize dedifferentiated chordoma, a higher-grade tumor with a sarcoma-like appearance.

BNCT was first described by Yamaguchi and colleagues[69] in 2002, and introduced as a new entity in the 2013 WHO classification.[5] BNCT may be considered a precursor lesion for chordoma.[70] It is sometimes a daunting task to distinguish chordoma from BNCT, especially in needle biopsies, because they share a morphologic spectrum and both express brachyury.[63,71,72] It is, therefore, important to acquire the radiologic evidence of a destructive mass before rendering the diagnosis of chordoma. In addition, chordoma needs to be distinguished from chondrosarcoma, myoepithelial neoplasms, chordoid meningioma, and even metastatic carcinomas, namely mucinous adenocarcinoma and clear cell renal cell carcinoma.[65,73] The demonstration of brachyury negativity in these morphologic mimics in addition to characteristics of each individual entity, such as *EWSR1* rearrangement in myoepithelial neoplasms, is essential to these differential diagnoses.[63]

Like dedifferentiated chondrosarcoma, dedifferentiation occurs either de novo or postradiation in a subset cases of chordoma, which shows a bimorphic pattern: a classic chordoma component juxtaposed with a high-grade sarcomatous component without notochordal differentiation.[74,75] The nonspecific morphology and lack of brachyury expression in the dedifferentiated component pose significant diagnostic challenges in small needle biopsies.[76,77] Finally, a subset of pediatric chordoma cases with a poorly differentiated histology has been described. These tumors have deletions at the *SMARCB1/INI-1* locus, with associated loss of SMARCB1/INI1 nuclear expression in addition to brachyury expression.[78,79]

SUMMARY

The many advances in the discovery of genetic alterations of bone tumors in recent years not only have broadened understanding of the pathogenesis of certain bone tumors but also facilitated the development of many useful ancillary molecular and IHC tests. These techniques have proved valuable on FNA and/or CNB samples to increase the diagnostic accuracy. Integration of morphologic, clinical, and radiographic features is still essential for establishing a clinical relevant diagnosis of bone tumors. FNA of bone lesions will become more and more acceptable as one of the actionable initial diagnostic tools for primary bone tumors.

REFERENCES

1. Layfield LJ. Cytologic diagnosis of osseous lesions: a review with emphasis on the diagnosis of primary neoplasms of bone. Diagn Cytopathol 2009;37:299–310.
2. Cardona DM, Dodd LG. Bone cytology: a realistic approach for clinical use. Surg Pathol Clin 2012;5:79–100.
3. Domanski HA, Qian X, Stanley DE. Chapter 16: bone. In: Domanski HA, editor. Atlas of fine needle aspiration cytology. 2nd edition. London: Springer; 2018.
4. Kilpatrick S. Diagnostic musculoskeletal surgical pathology. Philadelphia: Saunders; 2003.
5. Fletcher C, Bridge JA, Hogendoorn PCW, et al. WHO classification of tumours of soft tissue and bone. Lyon (France): IARC Press; 2013.
6. Girolami I, Mancini I, Simoni A, et al. Denosumab treated giant cell tumour of bone: a morphological, immunohistochemical and molecular analysis of a series. J Clin Pathol 2016;69:240–7.
7. Orosz Z, Athanasou NA. Giant cell-containing tumors of bone. Surg Pathol Clin 2017;10:553–73.
8. Roitman PD, Jauk F, Farfalli GL, et al. Denosumab-treated giant cell tumor of bone. Its histologic spectrum and potential diagnostic pitfalls. Hum Pathol 2017;63:89–97.
9. Doyle LA. Sarcoma classification: an update based on the 2013 world health organization classification of tumors of soft tissue and bone. Cancer 2014;120:1763–74.
10. Akerman M, Domanski HA, Jonsson K. Cytological features of bone tumours in FNA smears V: giant-cell lesions. Monogr Clin Cytol 2010;19:55–61.
11. Schaefer IM, Fletcher JA, Nielsen GP, et al. Immunohistochemistry for histone H3G34W and H3K36M is highly specific for giant cell tumor of bone and chondroblastoma, respectively, in FNA and core needle biopsy. Cancer Cytopathol 2018. https://doi.org/10.1002/cncy.22000.
12. Al-Ibraheemi A, Inwards CY, Zreik RT, et al. Histologic spectrum of giant cell tumor (GCT) of bone in patients 18 years of age and below: a study of 63 patients. Am J Surg Pathol 2016;40:1702–12.
13. Behjati S, Tarpey PS, Presneau N, et al. Distinct H3F3A and H3F3B driver mutations define chondroblastoma and giant cell tumor of bone. Nat Genet 2013;45:1479–82.
14. Cleven AH, Hocker S, Briaire-de Bruijn I, et al. Mutation analysis of H3F3A and H3F3B as a diagnostic tool for giant cell tumor of bone and chondroblastoma. Am J Surg Pathol 2015;39:1576–83.
15. Kervarrec T, Collin C, Larousserie F, et al. H3F3 mutation status of giant cell tumors of the bone, chondroblastomas and their mimics: a combined high resolution melting and pyrosequencing approach. Mod Pathol 2017;30:393–406.
16. Nohr E, Lee LH, Cates JM, et al. Diagnostic value of histone 3 mutations in osteoclast-rich bone tumors. Hum Pathol 2017;68:119–27.
17. Yamamoto H, Iwasaki T, Yamada Y, et al. Diagnostic utility of histone H3.3 G34W, G34R, and G34V mutant-specific antibodies for giant cell tumors of bone. Hum Pathol 2018;73:41–50.
18. Gomes CC, Diniz MG, Amaral FR, et al. The highly prevalent H3F3A mutation in giant cell tumours of bone is not shared by sporadic central giant cell lesion of the jaws. Oral Surg Oral Med Oral Pathol Oral Radiol 2014;118:583–5.
19. Amary F, Berisha F, Ye H, et al. H3F3A (Histone 3.3) G34W immunohistochemistry: a reliable marker defining benign and malignant giant cell tumor of bone. Am J Surg Pathol 2017;41:1059–68.

20. Luke J, von Baer A, Schreiber J, et al. H3F3A mutation in giant cell tumour of the bone is detected by immunohistochemistry using a monoclonal antibody against the G34W mutated site of the histone H3.3 variant. Histopathology 2017;71:125–33.

21. Sarungbam J, Agaram N, Hwang S, et al. Symplastic/pseudoanaplastic giant cell tumor of the bone. Skeletal Radiol 2016;45:929–35.

22. Thomas D, Henshaw R, Skubitz K, et al. Denosumab in patients with giant-cell tumour of bone: an open-label, phase 2 study. Lancet Oncol 2010;11:275–80.

23. van der Heijden L, Dijkstra PDS, Blay JY, et al. Giant cell tumour of bone in the denosumab era. Eur J Cancer 2017;77:75–83.

24. Wojcik J, Rosenberg AE, Bredella MA, et al. Denosumab-treated giant cell tumor of bone exhibits morphologic overlap with malignant giant cell tumor of bone. Am J Surg Pathol 2016;40:72–80.

25. Kato I, Furuya M, Matsuo K, et al. Giant cell tumours of bone treated with denosumab: histological, immunohistochemical and H3F3A mutation analyses. Histopathology 2018;72:914–22.

26. Fanning CV, Sneige NS, Carrasco CH, et al. Fine needle aspiration cytology of chondroblastoma of bone. Cancer 1990;65:1847–63.

27. Kilpatrick SE, Pike EJ, Geisinger KR, et al. Chondroblastoma of bone: use of fine-needle aspiration biopsy and potential diagnostic pitfalls. Diagn Cytopathol 1997;16:65–71.

28. Cabrera RA, Almeida M, Mendonca ME, et al. Diagnostic pitfalls in fine-needle aspiration cytology of temporomandibular chondroblastoma: report of two cases. Diagn Cytopathol 2006;34:424–9.

29. Chen W, DiFrancesco LM. Chondroblastoma: an update. Arch Pathol Lab Med 2017;141:867–71.

30. Akpalo H, Lange C, Zustin J. Discovered on gastrointestinal stromal tumour 1 (DOG1): a useful immunohistochemical marker for diagnosing chondroblastoma. Histopathology 2012;60:1099–106.

31. Konishi E, Nakashima Y, Iwasa Y, et al. Immunohistochemical analysis for Sox9 reveals the cartilaginous character of chondroblastoma and chondromyxoid fibroma of the bone. Hum Pathol 2010;41:208–13.

32. Cleven AH, Briaire-de Bruijn I, Szuhai K, et al. DOG1 expression in giant-cell-containing bone tumours. Histopathology 2016;68:942–5.

33. Amary MF, Berisha F, Mozela R, et al. The H3F3 K36M mutant antibody is a sensitive and specific marker for the diagnosis of chondroblastoma. Histopathology 2016;69:121–7.

34. Creager AJ, Madden CR, Bergman S, et al. Aneurysmal bone cyst: fine-needle aspiration findings in 23 patients with clinical and radiologic correlation. Am J Clin Pathol 2007;128:740–5.

35. Panoutsakopoulos G, Pandis N, Kyriazoglou I, et al. Recurrent t(16;17)(q22;p13) in aneurysmal bone cysts. Genes Chromosomes Cancer 1999;26:265–6.

36. Oliveira AM, Perez-Atayde AR, Inwards CY, et al. USP6 and CDH11 oncogenes identify the neoplastic cell in primary aneurysmal bone cysts and are absent in so-called secondary aneurysmal bone cysts. Am J Pathol 2004;165:1773–80.

37. Oliveira AM, Perez-Atayde AR, Dal Cin P, et al. Aneurysmal bone cyst variant translocations upregulate USP6 transcription by promoter swapping with the ZNF9, COL1A1, TRAP150, and OMD genes. Oncogene 2005;24:3419–26.

38. Oliveira AM, Chou MM. USP6-induced neoplasms: the biologic spectrum of aneurysmal bone cyst and nodular fasciitis. Hum Pathol 2014;45:1–11.

39. de Andrea CE, San-Julian M, Bovee J. Integrating morphology and genetics in the diagnosis of cartilage tumors. Surg Pathol Clin 2017;10:537–52.

40. Douis H, Singh L, Saifuddin A. MRI differentiation of low-grade from high-grade appendicular chondrosarcoma. Eur Radiol 2014;24:232–40.

41. Brown MT, Gikas PD, Bhamra JS, et al. How safe is curettage of low-grade cartilaginous neoplasms diagnosed by imaging with or without preoperative needle biopsy? Bone Joint J 2014;96-B:1098–105.

42. Eefting D, Schrage YM, Geirnaerdt MJ, et al. Assessment of interobserver variability and histologic parameters to improve reliability in classification and grading of central cartilaginous tumors. Am J Surg Pathol 2009;33:50–7.

43. Lu C, Venneti S, Akalin A, et al. Induction of sarcomas by mutant IDH2. Genes Dev 2013;27:1986–98.

44. Amary MF, Bacsi K, Maggiani F, et al. IDH1 and IDH2 mutations are frequent events in central chondrosarcoma and central and periosteal chondromas but not in other mesenchymal tumours. J Pathol 2011;224:334–43.

45. Olszewski W, Woyke S, Musiatowicz B. Fine needle aspiration biopsy cytology of chondrosarcoma. Acta Cytol 1983;27:345–9.

46. Dodd LG. Fine-needle aspiration of chondrosarcoma. Diagn Cytopathol 2006;34:413–8.

47. Agarwal S, Agarwal T, Agarwal R, et al. Fine needle aspiration of bone tumors. Cancer Detect Prev 2000;24:602–9.

48. Crim J, Schmidt R, Layfield L, et al. Can imaging criteria distinguish enchondroma from grade 1 chondrosarcoma? Eur J Radiol 2015;84:2222–30.

49. Rozeman LB, Hogendoorn PC, Bovee JV. Diagnosis and prognosis of chondrosarcoma of bone. Expert Rev Mol Diagn 2002;2:461–72.

50. Roitman PD, Farfalli GL, Ayerza MA, et al. Is needle biopsy clinically useful in preoperative grading of central chondrosarcoma of the pelvis and long bones? Clin Orthop Relat Res 2017;475:808–14.

51. Kerr DA, Lopez HU, Deshpande V, et al. Molecular distinction of chondrosarcoma from chondroblastic

osteosarcoma through IDH1/2 mutations. Am J Surg Pathol 2013;37:787–95.

52. Arai M, Nobusawa S, Ikota H, et al. Frequent IDH1/2 mutations in intracranial chondrosarcoma: a possible diagnostic clue for its differentiation from chordoma. Brain Tumor Pathol 2012;29: 201–6.

53. Rinas AC, Ward WG, Kilpatrick SE. Potential sampling error in fine needle aspiration biopsy of dedifferentiated chondrosarcoma: a report of 4 cases. Acta Cytol 2005;49:554–9.

54. Kilpatrick SE. Chondrosarcoma variants. Surg Pathol Clin 2012;5:163–81.

55. Jiang XS, Pantanowitz L, Bui MM, et al. Clear cell chondrosarcoma: cytologic findings in six cases. Diagn Cytopathol 2014;42:784–91.

56. McHugh KE, Emory CL, Parks GE, et al. Fine needle aspiration biopsy diagnosis of primary clear cell chondrosarcoma: a case report. Diagn Cytopathol 2018;46:165–9.

57. Trembath DG, Dash R, Major NM, et al. Cytopathology of mesenchymal chondrosarcomas: a report and comparison of four patients. Cancer 2003;99: 211–6.

58. Gonzalez-Campora R, Otal Salaverri C, Gomez Pascual A, et al. Mesenchymal chondrosarcoma of the retroperitoneum. Report of a case diagnosed by fine needle aspiration biopsy with immunohistochemical, electron microscopic demonstration of S-100 protein in undifferentiated cells. Acta Cytol 1995;39:1237–43.

59. Doria MI Jr, Wang HH, Chinoy MJ. Retroperitoneal mesenchymal chondrosarcoma. Report of a case diagnosed by fine needle aspiration cytology. Acta Cytol 1990;34:529–32.

60. Le Loarer F, Pissaloux D, Coindre JM, et al. Update on families of round cell sarcomas other than classical ewing sarcomas. Surg Pathol Clin 2017;10: 587–620.

61. Wang L, Motoi T, Khanin R, et al. Identification of a novel, recurrent HEY1-NCOA2 fusion in mesenchymal chondrosarcoma based on a genome-wide screen of exon-level expression data. Genes Chromosomes Cancer 2012;51:127–39.

62. Chen S, Fritchie K, Wei S, et al. Diagnostic utility of IDH1/2 mutations to distinguish dedifferentiated chondrosarcoma from undifferentiated pleomorphic sarcoma of bone. Hum Pathol 2017;65: 239–46.

63. Yamaguchi T, Imada H, Iida S, et al. Notochordal tumors: an update on molecular pathology with therapeutic implications. Surg Pathol Clin 2017;10: 637–56.

64. Vujovic S, Henderson S, Presneau N, et al. Brachyury, a crucial regulator of notochordal development, is a novel biomarker for chordomas. J Pathol 2006;209:157–65.

65. Jo VY, Hornick JL, Qian X. Utility of brachyury in distinction of chordoma from cytomorphologic mimics in fine-needle aspiration and core needle biopsy. Diagn Cytopathol 2014;42:647–52.

66. Qian X. Soft tissue. In: Cibas ES, editor. Cytology: diagnostic principles and clinical correlates. Philadelphia: Elsevier; 2014. p. 471–518.

67. Kay PA, Nascimento AG, Unni KK, et al. Chordoma. Cytomorphologic findings in 14 cases diagnosed by fine needle aspiration. Acta Cytol 2003; 47:202–8.

68. Walaas L, Kindblom LG. Fine-needle aspiration biopsy in the preoperative diagnosis of chordoma: a study of 17 cases with application of electron microscopic, histochemical, and immunocytochemical examination. Hum Pathol 1991;22:22–8.

69. Yamaguchi T, Yamato M, Saotome K. First histologically confirmed case of a classic chordoma arising in a precursor benign notochordal lesion: differential diagnosis of benign and malignant notochordal lesions. Skeletal Radiol 2002;31:413–8.

70. Deshpande V, Nielsen GP, Rosenthal DI, et al. Intraosseous benign notochord cell tumors (BNCT): further evidence supporting a relationship to chordoma. Am J Surg Pathol 2007;31:1573–7.

71. Kreshak J, Larousserie F, Picci P, et al. Difficulty distinguishing benign notochordal cell tumor from chordoma further suggests a link between them. Cancer Imaging 2014;14:4.

72. Tateda S, Hashimoto K, Aizawa T, et al. Diagnosis of benign notochordal cell tumor of the spine: is a biopsy necessary? Clin Case Rep 2018;6:63–7.

73. Layfield LJ. Cytologic differential diagnosis of myxoid and mucinous neoplasms of the sacrum and parasacral soft tissues. Diagn Cytopathol 2003;28:264–71.

74. Hanna SA, Tirabosco R, Amin A, et al. Dedifferentiated chordoma: a report of four cases arising 'de novo'. J Bone Joint Surg Br 2008;90:652–6.

75. Meis JM, Raymond AK, Evans HL, et al. "Dedifferentiated" chordoma. A clinicopathologic and immunohistochemical study of three cases. Am J Surg Pathol 1987;11:516–25.

76. Layfield LJ, Liu K, Dodd LG, et al. "Dedifferentiated" chordoma: a case report of the cytomorphologic findings on fine-needle aspiration. Diagn Cytopathol 1998;19:378–81.

77. Masood Q, Bilal M, Tariq A, et al. Dedifferentiated chordoma with a sarcomatous component: an overlooked diagnosis. J Ayub Med Coll Abbottabad 2009;21:164–5.

78. Mobley BC, McKenney JK, Bangs CD, et al. Loss of SMARCB1/INI1 expression in poorly differentiated chordomas. Acta Neuropathol 2010;120:745–53.

79. Antonelli M, Raso A, Mascelli S, et al. SMARCB1/INI1 involvement in pediatric chordoma: a mutational and immunohistochemical analysis. Am J Surg Pathol 2017;41:56–61.

Advances in Molecular Testing Techniques in Cytologic Specimens

Sinchita Roy-Chowdhuri, MD, PhD

KEYWORDS

• Molecular testing • Cytopathology • Precision medicine • ROSE

ABSTRACT

There has been a paradigm shift in the practice of cytopathology with the advent of highly sensitive molecular tests using small amounts of tissue that can provide diagnostic, prognostic, and predictive information for clinical management. The cytopathologist plays a key role in providing a timely and accurate diagnosis as well as ensuring appropriate processing and handling of the specimen and judicious triaging of the tissue for molecular testing that guide therapeutic decisions. As the era of "precision medicine" continues to evolve and expand, cytopathology remains a dynamic field with advances in the practice of molecular cytopathology providing new paradigms in clinical care.

OVERVIEW

In recent years, molecular cytopathology has developed into a rapidly evolving field, with the increasing use of cytopathology specimens for molecular testing. This paradigm shift in the practice of cytopathology from a strictly morphologic role to one that incorporates molecular testing for predictive and prognostic information guiding therapeutic decisions is largely due to (1) advances in molecular techniques with adaptation of highly sensitive molecular testing platforms that have minimal nucleic acid requirements and (2) the growing recognition of molecular-friendly cytologic substrates as an alternative to conventional formalin-fixed paraffin-embedded (FFPE) tissue blocks.

In a large fraction of patients with solid organ malignancies diagnosed with advanced-stage disease, the cytology sample may be the only tissue available for molecular testing. Therefore, the role of the cytopathologist has become increasingly critical in not only providing a timely and accurate diagnosis but also processing the specimens appropriately and triaging the tissue judiciously for molecular testing.[1–3] With the increasing use of cytologic specimens, there is also a growing recognition of the myriad preanalytical variables that play a role in determining the quality of a tissue sample.[4–9] Several factors can affect the quality and integrity of a specimen from the moment it is procured, through multiple steps of specimen fixation and processing to the final analytical steps of biomarker assessment involving nucleic acid–based and protein-based assays. Therefore, recognizing these preanalytical variables and optimizing specimen handling and processing techniques are critical for the overall success of molecular testing and instilling confidence in the test results from the specimen.

SPECIMEN ACQUISITION

One of the advantages in using cytology specimens for molecular testing in a minimally invasive aspiration setting is the ability to use rapid on-site evaluation (ROSE) to ensure specimen adequacy at the time of procurement and appropriately triage the sample for the necessary ancillary studies.[10–13] In the setting of ROSE, the cytopathologist/cytotechnologist can guide the proceduralist in procuring an adequate sample for diagnosis and directing additional passes to triage the remainder of the tissue collected for preparations amenable for downstream ancillary testing. For instance, if a hematolymphoid malignancy is suspected on ROSE, additional passes can be collected for flow

Department of Pathology, Division of Pathology and Laboratory Medicine, The University of Texas MD Anderson Cancer Center, 1515 Holcombe Boulevard Unit 85, Houston, TX 77030, USA
E-mail address: sroy2@mdanderson.org

Surgical Pathology 11 (2018) 669–677
https://doi.org/10.1016/j.path.2018.04.007

cytometric analysis and cell block for immunohisto-chemistry (IHC). Similarly, if ROSE shows evidence of infection, a sterile sample can be collected for microbiology and culture studies. In context of malignancies that may require molecular testing (eg, mutational assay or fluorescence in situ hybrid-ization [FISH]), once a diagnosis is made on the direct smears during ROSE, the protocol for col-lecting additional passes and the needle rinse depends on the individual laboratory/institutional practice and the molecular laboratory that often dictates the choice of substrate used for molecular testing.[14] For laboratories that perform molecular testing on FFPE cell blocks only, it is advisable to allocate most of the tissue into an appropriate collection medium with or without a fixative to be subsequently processed into a cell block. Although FFPE cell block material remains the most widely used substrate for molecular testing, several labo-ratories have moved away from using only FFPE substrates for molecular testing and have validated their assays on non-FFPE cytologic substrates, because they provide superior quality nucleic acid than their FFPE counterparts.[5,7,13,15–28] These include direct smears, touch preparations from core biopsies, and liquid-based cytology (LBC). Other preparations, such as fresh frozen samples and filter paper–based storage of unfixed cells (such as on Whatman FTA cards), also provide excellent quality DNA[29]; however, these have not gained popularity or widespread adaptation across laboratories due to the lack of direct morphologic evaluation, thus limiting its utility.

SPECIMEN PROCESSING

It is of paramount importance to recognize that multiple preanalytic factors associated with spec-imen processing can affect the quality and integ-rity of a sample, which in turn determine the confidence in the test results from the specimen. To obtain reliable, robust, and consistent molecu-lar test results, standardized protocols are imple-mented in individual molecular laboratories.[7] Some of the upstream variables associated with specimen processing, however, are outside the realm of the molecular laboratory. Although the availability of a variety of cytologic specimen sub-strates, including non-FFPE options, provides a range of molecular testing options, these speci-mens also suffer from a lack of standardization in terms of specimen collection, handling, process-ing, and storage.[7,9,14,30] Therefore, it is critical for individual cytology laboratories to work in close conjunction with their molecular laboratory, whether in house or a reference laboratory, to vali-date the various specimen preparations for the specific molecular assays to ensure confidence in the test results generated from these samples.

Although a range of media is used to collect tis-sue from aspiration procedures, which may be a nonfixative solution (eg, saline, Roswell Park Memorial Institute medium, or Dulbecco Minimal Eagle medium) or may include a fixative (eg, formalin, alcohol or CytoLyt), most cytopathology laboratories use 10% neutral buffered formalin as a fixative for cell block preparation. The ease of vali-dation of FFPE cell blocks, which is similar to that of histologic tissue blocks, makes FFPE the substrate of choice for molecular testing in most laboratories. Formalin fixation causes cross-linking of nucleic acids and proteins, however, and results in frag-mentation of nucleic acids and random polymerase errors in nucleotide incorporation.[31,32] In addition, a lack of adequacy assessment at the time of spec-imen acquisition often results in a paucicellular cell block that precludes ancillary studies, even when dedicated passes are allocated for the cell block preparation.[3,13,33] This in part has led to an increasing use of direct smeared cytologic material with air-dried, Diff-Quik–stained and alcohol-fixed Papanicolaou-stained smears, both providing excellent sources of cellular material for molecular testing. Not only do direct smears provide the abil-ity to assess for adequacy at the time of the proced-ure but also the lack of formalin fixation offers superior quality nucleic acid for mutation analysis. Tumor cells can be directly visualized on the stained smear preparations and scraped off or cell lifted from the slide by macrodissection or microdissection for nucleic acid extraction.[13,17,34] Molecular studies comparing results from stained direct smears versus FFPE material have shown higher-quality DNA as well as better sequencing metrics in the former.[15,16,35,36] FISH is also routinely performed on stained smears and frequently preferred over FFPE material, because whole cells present on smears are not subject to truncation artifacts as seen with the 4-μm to 5-μm sections from FFPE blocks.[37–41] Several institu-tions have also successfully used LBC slides for molecular testing[21,26,35,42–44] as well as the cell suspension directly from residual LBC.[22–24] Although RNA-based assays, such as reverse tran-scriptase (RT) polymerase chain reaction (PCR), prefer using fresh frozen samples as a substrate for analysis, because RNA tends to undergo rapid degeneration, several studies have also success-fully used archival stained smears, residual LBC preparations, and FFPE cell block preparations for RT-PCR analysis.[45–52] As with any other assay, preanalytical variables, such as type of fixative, length of fixation, processing, and length of stor-age, can affect the RNA quality, and optimizations steps may be necessary to stabilize and maintain RNA integrity prior to analysis.

Because each of these different cytologic substrates have to be individually validated in the molecular laboratory prior to clinical testing, this often results in an overall underutilization of non-FFPE cytologic material for molecular testing.[53,54] Nonetheless, the versatility of cytologic specimens provides an excellent source of nucleic acids that has received increasing recognition as evidenced by the revised lung molecular testing guidelines that endorsed the use of non–cell block cytopathology specimen preparations for molecular testing.[55]

SPECIMEN HANDLING

The cytopathologist plays a key role in the workflow of the molecular testing, from checking the appropriateness of the test request, to reviewing the archival cellular material to select the best tissue for the requested tests, to evaluating the specimen adequacy for cellularity and tumor fraction, to canceling the request if a specimen is insufficient for testing (eg, overall low cellularity or tumor cellularity falls below the analytical sensitivity of the assay), to determining which specimen preparation (eg, smears, cell block sections, or LBC) would be appropriate for specific tests (eg, mutational assay, FISH, and IHC), and to triaging the material to the different molecular testing platforms accordingly (Fig. 1).

Most molecular laboratories determine the lower limit of tumor content acceptable for testing and have individual specimen adequacy criteria for accepting or rejecting a sample. A critical parameter for the interpretation of mutational assays is the analytical sensitivity of the testing platform defined as the minimal tumor cell percentage necessary to reliably detect a specific mutation (ie, lowest limit of detection).[56] The reliability of detecting mutations, especially in samples of low tumor content that usually consists of a mixture of tumor cells (contributing both mutant and wild-type DNA) and non-neoplastic cells, such as background inflammatory cells, stromal elements, benign epithelial/mesothelial cells, and hematopoietic elements (contributing wild-type DNA), is a major concern. FNA samples have the distinct advantage of inherently enriched tumor cellularity due to low stromal content; nonetheless, an attempt to enrich tumor content by selecting tumor-rich areas for macrodissection or microdissection should be attempted, when feasible.[9,15,30,57] Cell blocks tend to be treated similarly to histologic tissue sections, where unstained sections from the block are lined up against a corresponding hematoxylin-eosin–stained section with circled tumor-rich areas to serve as a guide for tissue extraction. Direct smears frequently are more amenable to tumor enrichment due to the 3-D clumping of tumor cells that is easier to delineate from areas with high numbers of non-neoplastic cells.[9] The areas of interest are macro dissected or microdissected directly off the smears by either scraping using a scalpel blade or cell lifting or cell transfer techniques.[1]

MOLECULAR TESTING OF CYTOLOGIC SPECIMENS

The most commonly used molecular techniques using cytology specimens in a clinical setting involve PCR-based assays, sequencing, gene expression assays, and in situ hybridization. PCR is a widely used molecular technique that uses synthetically generated, strategically designed primers that bind to a target sequence followed by multiple cycles of amplification to generate numerous copies of the original target sequence. Although PCR is widely used as an amplification technique in DNA-based assays, it can also be used to amplify RNA sequence targets through RT-PCR by converting the RNA to complementary DNA.[58,59] Another popular variation of a PCR-based assay is the quantitative real-time PCR that uses fluorescent dyes and can detect and quantify the fluorescent signal after each amplification cycle. The technique can be used to detect and quantify the amount of target sequence present in a sample based on the time it takes for the signal amplification to achieve an exponential phase.[60] With regard to sequencing assays, Sanger sequencing has historically been considered the gold standard for DNA sequencing.[61] This widely popular method uses a chain termination technique based on random inhibition of an elongation process resulting in newly synthesized DNA fragments of various sizes that can be electrophoretically separated and visualized through automated readers. Pyrosequencing is an alternative to the conventional Sanger sequencing and uses DNA sequencing by synthesis with the generation of a pyrophosphate released during the DNA polymerase reaction resulting in production of visible light that can be detected as a signal.[62]

With increasing numbers of genes needed for mutation analysis to guide clinical decisions, the need for high-throughput sequencing technology is critical. The Sequenom MassARRAY (Sequenom, LabCorp, San Diego, California) genotyping platform uses matrix-assisted laser desorption/ionization time-of-flight mass spectrometry that provides a multigene testing approach to evaluate known somatic point mutations based on the mass

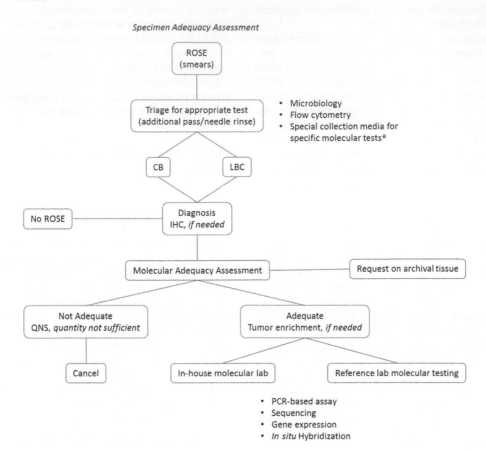

Fig. 1. Schematic illustrating the role of the cytopathologist in molecular testing. On samples requiring rapid on-site evaluation (ROSE), the cytopathologist can assess the sample for diagnostic adequacy and then triage the remainder of the specimen according to the downstream testing needs (eg, microbiology and flow cytometry). [a]Certain molecular tests require special collection, such as Afirma Gene Expression Classifier test (Veracyte, San Francisco, California), which requires dedicated passes collected in a special media (FNAprotect solution) for molecular testing of indeterminate thyroid fine needle aspirations (FNAs). The remainder of the specimen is then allocated to cell block (CB) and/or liquid-based cytology (LBC) preparation in anticipation of molecular tests that may be required after the cytologic diagnosis. If molecular testing is needed, the cytopathologist is responsible for evaluating molecular adequacy to ensure the specimen meets the analytical threshold of the assay and canceling a request if the specimen is insufficient (QNS, quantity not sufficient). For mutation testing on low tumor samples, the cytopathologist may need to enrich for tumor by delineating tumor-rich areas on the slide for macrodissection or microdissection prior to sending the tissue to the molecular laboratory for testing.

differences between the wild-type and the mutant products.[63,64] More recently, next-generation sequencing (NGS) has emerged as a novel disruptive technology that uses massively parallel sequencing and can simultaneously analyze multiple gene targets using minimal amounts of DNA.[65,66] The ability to analyze a panel of clinically relevant genes on a single platform simultaneously from nanograms of DNA is a game changer in the application of molecular testing in routine cytologic specimens[5,57,67,68] (**Fig. 2**). The NGS assay can be custom designed to detect single-nucleotide variants, insertions/deletions, copy number variations, and fusions on the same assay, thus providing a flexible and powerful tool to not only interrogate known therapeutic targets

but also identify potential targets with prognostic and predictive roles. Given the challenges of clinical validation of NGS panels, the interpretation of the data, and the bioinformatics challenges associated with the generation and storage of large amounts of genomic data, multiple professional societies are working in collaboration to establish consensus guidelines for NGS assay validation, interpretation, reporting and proficiency testing.[69,70]

Finally, in situ hybridization is another widely used technique that uses sequence specific probes often using fluorescent-labeled probes, as in FISH, to detect probe signal patterns in conjunction with morphology.[71] The number and location of the fluorescent signal(s) can identify

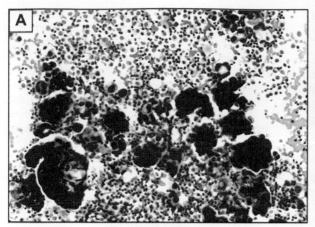
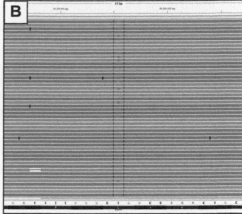

Fig. 2. NGS of a lung adenocarcinoma cytology sample. (*A*) Diff-Quik–stained smear (100×) showing 3-D clusters of malignant cells that were microdissected from tumor-rich areas by directly scraping the slide and used to extract DNA for NGS analysis; (*B*) NGS detects a missense mutation in exon 21 of the *EGFR* gene c.2573T>G p.L858R from the cytology sample, thus making the patient eligible for targeted therapy using a tyrosine kinase inhibitor.

chromosomal abnormalities, including gene amplification, gene deletion, or structural rearrangements, such as translocations.

The choice of selecting a molecular assay usually depends on the gene/genes of interest, the spectrum of mutations in a given gene of interest, the volume of patients to be screened, and the available infrastructure in the molecular laboratory for performing a variety of molecular assays. Although most academic medical centers have the capability of performing in-house molecular testing and may be able to cater to the specific needs and unique requirements associated with the use of cytologic specimens, a large fraction of molecular diagnostic assays are outsourced to reference laboratories. Therefore, the cytopathologist may often have to comply with the specific requirements of the molecular laboratory to meet the adequacy criteria for specimen selection. This underscores the critical need for clear communication between the cytopathology laboratory and the molecular laboratory in terms of minimum requirements for specimen adequacy, type of specimen preparations accepted for testing, molecular testing techniques used for different assays, analytical sensitivity of testing platform, ability to perform tumor enrichment by macrodissection or microdissection, and appropriate feedback for specimens that get rejected by the molecular laboratory.[1,14] In general, most current molecular diagnostic assays are either targeted to specific genes or generalized to analyze specific genes or groups of genes. Targeted mutation detection methods are popular in clinical diagnostic laboratories because of their ease of use. They can only be used, however, to detect known variants and, therefore, may need to be combined with other assays if a comprehensive mutational analysis is required.

Key Points
MOLECULAR TESTING OF CYTOLOGIC SPECIMENS

1. Advances in molecular techniques with adaptation of highly sensitive molecular testing using small amounts of tissue that provide clinically relevant information for patient care has been a paradigm shift in the practice of cytopathology.

2. The cytopathologist plays a key role not only in providing a timely and accurate diagnosis but also in processing the specimens appropriately and triaging the tissue judiciously for molecular testing.

3. There is a growing recognition of molecular-friendly cytologic substrates as an alternative to conventional FFPE tissue blocks.

4. Multiple preanalytic factors associated with specimen processing can affect the quality and integrity of a sample, which in turn determine the confidence in the test results from the specimen.

5. The most commonly used molecular techniques in a clinical setting involve PCR-based assays, sequencing, gene expression assays, and in situ hybridization.

6. The choice of selecting a molecular assay usually depends on the gene/genes of interest, the spectrum of mutations in a given gene of interest, the volume of patients to be screened, and the available infrastructure in the molecular laboratory for performing a variety of molecular assays.

APPLICATION OF MOLECULAR TESTING IN CYTOLOGIC SPECIMENS

Molecular testing in cytologic specimens is frequently used as an adjunct to diagnosis. Some key examples of ancillary molecular diagnostics include human papillomavirus testing in gynecologic cytology; human papillomavirus testing in determination of a possible oropharyngeal squamous cell carcinoma presenting with a neck mass; gene expression classifier testing, gene mutation/rearrangement assay, and micro-RNA analysis in the work-up of indeterminate thyroid nodules; identification of translocations, gene rearrangements, and amplifications in subclassification of salivary gland tumors, soft tissue neoplasms, and lymphomas by FISH and PCR-based assays; and the evaluation of urinary tract cytology and pancreaticobiliary brushings using FISH analysis.[2] In addition, the rapid evolution of high-throughput molecular platforms that can simultaneously test for a multitude of different genomic abnormalities using small amounts of DNA has resulted in a dramatic increase in the utilization of cytologic specimens to provide pertinent prognostic and predictive information and/or targeted therapeutic strategies. Some key examples of ancillary molecular testing for theranostic purposes include mutational analysis (such as epidermal growth factor receptor [*EGFR*] gene mutations) and anaplastic lymphoma kinase (*ALK*) and c-ros oncogene 1 (*ROS1*) gene rearrangements in non–small cell lung carcinoma; Kirsten Rat Sarcoma Viral Oncogene Homolog (*KRAS*) and v-raf murine sarcoma viral oncogene homolog B (*BRAF*) mutational analysis in colon adenocarcinoma, mutational analysis for *BRAF*, neuroblastoma v-ras oncogene homolog (*NRAS*), and v-kit Hardy-Zuckerman 4 feline sarcoma viral oncogene homolog (*KIT*) in melanoma; human epidermal growth factor receptor 2 (*ERBB2/HER2*) amplification in breast carcinoma and gastroesophageal adenocarcinoma by IHC and/or FISH analysis; and mutational analysis of *KIT* and Platelet Derived Growth Factor Receptor Alpha (*PDGFRA*) in gastrointestinal stromal tumors.[2]

SUMMARY

The ability to use highly sensitive molecular testing using small amounts of tissue and provide diagnostic, prognostic, and predictive information that can guide patient care has been a paradigm shift in the practice of cytopathology. The cytopathologist plays a key role in ensuring adequate tissue collection for diagnosis and molecular testing, appropriate processing and handling of the specimen, and finally judiciously using the limited tissue for the molecular tests that guide therapeutic decisions. As the era of precision medicine continues to evolve and expand, cytopathology remains a dynamic field with advances in the practice of molecular cytopathology providing new paradigms in clinical care.

REFERENCES

1. Bellevicine C, Malapelle U, Vigliar E, et al. How to prepare cytological samples for molecular testing. J Clin Pathol 2017;70:819–26.
2. VanderLaan PA. Molecular markers: implications for cytopathology and specimen collection. Cancer Cytopathol 2015;123:454–60.
3. Roh MH. The utilization of cytologic fine-needle aspirates of lung cancer for molecular diagnostic testing. J Pathol Transl Med 2015;49:300–9.
4. Rossi ED, Schmitt F. Pre-analytic steps for molecular testing on thyroid fine-needle aspirations: the goal of good results. Cytojournal 2013;10:24.
5. Roy-Chowdhuri S, Goswami RS, Chen H, et al. Factors affecting the success of next-generation sequencing in cytology specimens. Cancer Cytopathol 2015;123:659–68.
6. Schmitt FC. Molecular cytopathology and flow cytometry: pre-analytical procedures matter. Cytopathology 2011;22:355–7.
7. da Cunha Santos G. Standardizing preanalytical variables for molecular cytopathology. Cancer Cytopathol 2013;121:341–3.
8. da Cunha Santos G, Saieg MA. Preanalytic parameters in epidermal growth factor receptor mutation testing for non-small cell lung carcinoma: a review of cytologic series. Cancer Cytopathol 2015;123:633–43.
9. Roy-Chowdhuri S, Stewart J. Preanalytic variables in cytology: lessons learned from next-generation sequencing-The MD Anderson Experience. Arch Pathol Lab Med 2016. https://doi.org/10.5858/arpa.2016-0117-RA.
10. Collins BT, Murad FM, Wang JF, et al. Rapid on-site evaluation for endoscopic ultrasound-guided fine-needle biopsy of the pancreas decreases the incidence of repeat biopsy procedures. Cancer Cytopathol 2013;121:518–24.
11. da Cunha Santos G, Ko HM, Saieg MA, et al. "The petals and thorns" of ROSE (rapid on-site evaluation). Cancer Cytopathol 2013;121:4–8.
12. Fassina A, Corradin M, Zardo D, et al. Role and accuracy of rapid on-site evaluation of CT-guided fine needle aspiration cytology of lung nodules. Cytopathology 2011;22:306–12.

13. Knoepp SM, Roh MH. Ancillary techniques on direct-smear aspirate slides: a significant evolution for cytopathology techniques. Cancer Cytopathol 2013;121:120–8.

14. Roy-Chowdhuri S, Aisner DL, Allen TC, et al. Biomarker testing in lung carcinoma cytology specimens: a perspective from members of the pulmonary pathology society. Arch Pathol Lab Med 2016. https://doi.org/10.5858/arpa.2016-0091-SA.

15. Roy-Chowdhuri S, Chen H, Singh RR, et al. Concurrent fine needle aspirations and core needle biopsies: a comparative study of substrates for next-generation sequencing in solid organ malignancies. Mod Pathol 2017;30:499–508.

16. Gailey MP, Stence AA, Jensen CS, et al. Multiplatform comparison of molecular oncology tests performed on cytology specimens and formalin-fixed, paraffin-embedded tissue. Cancer Cytopathol 2015;123:30–9.

17. Betz BL, Roh MH, Weigelin HC, et al. The application of molecular diagnostic studies interrogating EGFR and KRAS mutations to stained cytologic smears of lung carcinoma. Am J Clin Pathol 2011; 136:564–71.

18. Khode R, Larsen DA, Culbreath BC, et al. Comparative study of epidermal growth factor receptor mutation analysis on cytology smears and surgical pathology specimens from primary and metastatic lung carcinomas. Cancer Cytopathol 2013;121: 361–9.

19. Treece AL, Montgomery ND, Patel NM, et al. FNA smears as a potential source of DNA for targeted next-generation sequencing of lung adenocarcinomas. Cancer Cytopathol 2016;124:406–14.

20. Velizheva NP, Rechsteiner MP, Wong CE, et al. Cytology smears as excellent starting material for next-generation sequencing-based molecular testing of patients with adenocarcinoma of the lung. Cancer 2017;125:30–40.

21. Reynolds JP, Zhou Y, Jakubowski MA, et al. Next-generation sequencing of liquid-based cytology non-small cell lung cancer samples. Cancer 2017; 125:178–87.

22. Tian SK, Killian JK, Rekhtman N, et al. Optimizing workflows and processing of cytologic samples for comprehensive analysis by next-generation sequencing: memorial sloan kettering cancer center experience. Arch Pathol Lab Med 2016. https://doi.org/10.5858/arpa.2016-0108-RA.

23. Fuller MY, Mody D, Hull A, et al. Next-generation sequencing identifies gene mutations that are predictive of malignancy in residual needle rinses collected from fine-needle aspirations of thyroid nodules. Arch Pathol Lab Med 2017. https://doi.org/10.5858/arpa.2017-0136-OA.

24. Wei S, Lieberman D, Morrissette JJ, et al. Using "residual" FNA rinse and body fluid specimens for next-generation sequencing: an institutional experience. Cancer Cytopathol 2016;124:324–9. https://doi.org/10.1002/cncy.21666.

25. Rosenblum F, Hutchinson LM, Garver J, et al. Cytology specimens offer an effective alternative to formalin-fixed tissue as demonstrated by novel automated detection for ALK break-apart FISH testing and immunohistochemistry in lung adenocarcinoma. Cancer Cytopathol 2014;122:810–21. https://doi.org/10.1002/cncy.21467.

26. Allegrini S, Antona J, Mezzapelle R, et al. Epidermal growth factor receptor gene analysis with a highly sensitive molecular assay in routine cytologic specimens of lung adenocarcinoma. Am J Clin Pathol 2012;138:377–81.

27. Hookim K, Roh MH, Willman J, et al. Application of immunocytochemistry and BRAF mutational analysis to direct smears of metastatic melanoma. Cancer Cytopathol 2012;120:52–61.

28. van Eijk R, Licht J, Schrumpf M, et al. Rapid KRAS, EGFR, BRAF and PIK3CA mutation analysis of fine needle aspirates from non-small-cell lung cancer using allele-specific qPCR. PLoS One 2011;6:e17791.

29. Saieg MA, Geddie WR, Boerner SL, et al. The use of FTA cards for preserving unfixed cytological material for high-throughput molecular analysis. Cancer Cytopathol 2012;120:206–14.

30. Bellevicine C, Vita GD, Malapelle U, et al. Applications and limitations of oncogene mutation testing in clinical cytopathology. Semin Diagn Pathol 2013; 30:284–97.

31. Srinivasan M, Sedmak D, Jewell S. Effect of fixatives and tissue processing on the content and integrity of nucleic acids. Am J Pathol 2002;161:1961–71.

32. Williams C, Pontén F, Moberg C, et al. A high frequency of sequence alterations is due to formalin fixation of archival specimens. Am J Pathol 1999; 155:1467–71.

33. Bellevicine C, Malapelle U, de Luca C, et al. EGFR analysis: current evidence and future directions. Diagn Cytopathol 2014;42:984–92.

34. Roy-Chowdhuri S, Chow CW, Kane MK, et al. Optimizing the DNA yield for molecular analysis from cytologic preparations. Cancer Cytopathol 2016;124:254–60.

35. Hwang DH, Garcia EP, Ducar MD, et al. Next-generation sequencing of cytologic preparations: an analysis of quality metrics. Cancer 2017. https://doi.org/10.1002/cncy.21897.

36. Karnes HE, Duncavage EJ, Bernadt CT. Targeted next-generation sequencing using fine-needle aspirates from adenocarcinomas of the lung. Cancer Cytopathol 2014;122:104–13.

37. Betz BL, Dixon CA, Weigelin HC, et al. The use of stained cytologic direct smears for ALK gene rearrangement analysis of lung adenocarcinoma. Cancer Cytopathol 2013;121:489–99.

38. Bravaccini S, Tumedei MM, Ulivi P, et al. ALK translocation detection in non-small cell lung cancer cytological samples obtained by TBNA or EBUS-TBNA. Cytopathology 2016;27:103–7.

39. Monaco SE, Teot LA, Felgar RE, et al. Fluorescence in situ hybridization studies on direct smears: an approach to enhance the fine-needle aspiration biopsy diagnosis of B-cell non-Hodgkin lymphomas. Cancer 2009;117:338–48.

40. Bozzetti C, Nizzoli R, Tiseo M, et al. ALK and ROS1 rearrangements tested by fluorescence in situ hybridization in cytological smears from advanced non-small cell lung cancer patients. Diagn Cytopathol 2015;43:941–6.

41. Bozzetti C, Personeni N, Nizzoli R, et al. HER-2/neu amplification by fluorescence in situ hybridization in cytologic samples from distant metastatic sites of breast carcinoma. Cancer 2003;99:310–5.

42. Rossi ED, Martini M, Capodimonti S, et al. BRAF (V600E) mutation analysis on liquid-based cytology-processed aspiration biopsies predicts bilaterality and lymph node involvement in papillary thyroid microcarcinoma. Cancer Cytopathol 2013; 121:291–7.

43. Minca EC, Lanigan CP, Reynolds JP, et al. ALK status testing in non-small-cell lung carcinoma by FISH on ThinPrep slides with cytology material. J Thorac Oncol 2014;9:464–8.

44. Minca EC, Portier BP, Wang Z, et al. ALK status testing in non-small cell lung carcinoma: correlation between ultrasensitive IHC and FISH. J Mol Diagn 2013;15:341–6.

45. Akoury DA, Seo JJ, James CD, et al. RT-PCR detection of mRNA recovered from archival glass slide smears. Mod Pathol 1993;6:195–200.

46. Chuaqui R, Cole K, Cuello M, et al. Analysis of mRNA quality in freshly prepared and archival Papanicolaou samples. Acta Cytol 1999;43:831–6.

47. Dimulescu II, Unger ER, Lee DR, et al. Characterization of RNA in cytologic samples preserved in a methanol-based collection solution. Mol Diagn 1998;3:67–71.

48. Dixon EP, King LM, Adams MD, et al. Isolation of RNA from residual BD SurePath liquid-based cytology specimens and detection of HPV E6/E7 mRNA using the PreTectt HPV-Proofer assay. J Virol Methods 2008;154:220–2.

49. Benchekroun M, DeGraw J, Gao J, et al. Impact of fixative on recovery of mRNA from paraffin-embedded tissue. Diagn Mol Pathol 2004;13: 116–25.

50. Chung JY, Braunschweig T, Hewitt SM. Optimization of recovery of RNA from formalin-fixed, paraffin-embedded tissue. Diagn Mol Pathol 2006;15: 229–36.

51. Krafft AE, Duncan BW, Bijwaard KE, et al. Optimization of the isolation and amplification of RNA from formalin-fixed, paraffin-embedded tissue: the armed forces institute of pathology experience and literature review. Mol Diagn 1997;2:217–30.

52. Annaratone L, Marchiò C, Renzulli T, et al. High-throughput molecular analysis from leftover of fine needle aspiration cytology of mammographically detected breast cancer. Transl Oncol 2012; 5:180–9.

53. Rekhtman N, Roy-Chowdhuri S. Cytology specimens: a goldmine for molecular testing. Arch Pathol Lab Med 2016;140:1189–90.

54. Clark DP. Seize the opportunity: underutilization of fine-needle aspiration biopsy to inform targeted cancer therapy decisions. Cancer 2009;117:289–97.

55. Lindeman NI, Cagle PT, Aisner DL, et al. Updated molecular testing guideline for the selection of lung cancer patients for treatment with targeted tyrosine kinase inhibitors: guideline from the College of American Pathologists, the International Association for the Study of Lung Cancer, and the Association for Molecular Pathology. Arch Pathol Lab Med 2018. https://doi.org/10.5858/arpa.2017-0388-CP.

56. Aisner DL, Sams SB. The role of cytology specimens in molecular testing of solid tumors: techniques, limitations, and opportunities. Diagn Cytopathol 2012; 40:511–24.

57. Vigliar E, Malapelle U, de Luca C, et al. Challenges and opportunities of next-generation sequencing: a cytopathologist's perspective. Cytopathology 2015; 26:271–83.

58. Mocharla H, Mocharla R, Hodes ME. Coupled reverse transcription-polymerase chain reaction (RT-PCR) as a sensitive and rapid method for isozyme genotyping. Gene 1990;93:271–5.

59. Miller WH Jr, Kakizuka A, Frankel SR, et al. Reverse transcription polymerase chain reaction for the rearranged retinoic acid receptor alpha clarifies diagnosis and detects minimal residual disease in acute promyelocytic leukemia. Proc Natl Acad Sci U S A 1992;89:2694–8.

60. Heid CA, Stevens J, Livak KJ, et al. Real time quantitative PCR. Genome Res 1996;6:986–94.

61. Sanger F, Nicklen S, Coulson AR. DNA sequencing with chain-terminating inhibitors. Proc Natl Acad Sci U S A 1977;74:5463–7.

62. Ahmadian A, Gharizadeh B, Gustafsson AC, et al. Single-nucleotide polymorphism analysis by pyrosequencing. Anal Biochem 2000;280:103–10.

63. Jurinke C, van den Boom D, Cantor CR, et al. The use of MassARRAY technology for high throughput genotyping. Adv Biochem Eng Biotechnol 2002;77: 57–74.

64. Jurinke C, van den Boom D, Cantor CR, et al. Automated genotyping using the DNA MassArray technology. Methods Mol Biol 2001;170:103–16.

65. Metzker ML. Sequencing technologies - the next generation. Nat Rev Genet 2010;11:31–46.

66. Liu L, Li Y, Li S, et al. Comparison of next-generation sequencing systems. J Biomed Biotechnol 2012; 2012:251364.

67. Kanagal-Shamanna R, Portier BP, Singh RR, et al. Next-generation sequencing-based multi-gene mutation profiling of solid tumors using fine needle aspiration samples: promises and challenges for routine clinical diagnostics. Mod Pathol 2014;27: 314–27.

68. Dumur CI, Kraft AO. Next-generation sequencing and the cytopathologist. Cancer Cytopathol 2015; 123:69–70.

69. Jennings LJ, Arcila ME, Corless C, et al. Guidelines for Validation of next-generation sequencing-based oncology panels: a joint consensus recommendation of the Association for Molecular Pathology and College of American Pathologists. J Mol Diagn 2017;19:341–65.

70. Li MM, Datto M, Duncavage EJ, et al. Standards and guidelines for the interpretation and reporting of sequence variants in cancer: a joint consensus recommendation of the Association for Molecular Pathology, American Society of Clinical Oncology, and College of American Pathologists. J Mol Diagn 2017;19:4–23.

71. Trask B, Pinkel D. Fluorescence in situ hybridization with DNA probes. Methods Cell Biol 1990;33: 383–400.

Circulating Tumor Cells
Applications in Cytopathology

Alarice C. Lowe, MD

KEYWORDS

- Circulating tumor cells • CTCs • Liquid biopsy • Cancer monitoring

Key points

- Circulating tumor cell (CTC) testing provides prognostic, predictive, and diagnostic information.
- CTC samples reflect tumor heterogeneity, are minimally invasive, and provide much of the information obtained by more invasive biopsies.
- CTC technology can be easily integrated into and enhance the practice of cytology.

ABSTRACT

Circulating tumor cells (CTCs) are rare tumor cells found in the blood of patients with cancer that can be reliably detected by CTC technologies to provide prognostic, predictive, and diagnostic information. CTC sampling reflects intratumoral and intertumoral heterogeneity better than targeted biopsy. CTC samples are minimally invasive and amenable to repeated sampling, allowing real-time evaluation of tumor in response to therapy-related pressures and possibly early detection. Cytology is the most natural arena for integration of CTC testing. CTC technology may also be deployed to enhance and facilitate the practice of cytology and surgical pathology.

OVERVIEW

The task of the oncologic pathologist/cytopathologist is to provide diagnostic, prognostic, and predictive tumor information to patients and their treating clinicians. This information is obtained through analysis of surgical pathology material, in the form of large resections, excisional biopsies, and more recently core biopsies. As the subspecialty of cytology began to develop, this same

information could be gleaned from single cells obtained by less invasive methods, such as fine-needle aspiration biopsies. The recent development of circulating tumor cell (CTC) technology suggests the possibility of being able to tackle some of these same questions, in a potentially more comprehensive manner, through the minimally invasive sampling of a blood draw.

This review covers the current demands on the field of pathology; the history of the CTC field; how CTCs may provide clinical prognostic, predictive, and diagnostic information; and how CTC technology may be incorporated into the practice of cytopathology.

THE CURRENT STATE OF PATHOLOGY

The task of the oncologic surgical pathologist is to provide clinically relevant information to patients and their treating clinicians. In the past century, this field has rapidly advanced and clinically relevant information has grown exponentially to encompass increasingly complex classification systems, including an increasing number of mutation specific defined tumors, tumor-specific prognostic factors, and a continuously growing list of therapeutic predictive factors. In addition, many of the diagnostic questions that clinicians are

---

Disclosures: None.
Cytology, Brigham and Women's Hospital, 75 Francis Street, MRB 308, Boston, MA 02115, USA
E-mail addresses: aclowe@partners.org; alowe@bwh.harvard.edu

Surgical Pathology 11 (2018) 679–686
https://doi.org/10.1016/j.path.2018.04.008
1875-9181/18/

asking to determine appropriate treatment are no longer static. As we gain experience treating with targeted inhibitors, we are learning which treatment-resistant genotypes or phenotypes may develop in the context of selective pressure; therefore, repeat sampling to assess for changes in these predictive factors, especially in the setting of recurrent and metastatic disease, is becoming the norm. Because patients with cancer are living longer through improved treatment of cancer, altered morphologic phenotypes of treated tumors are beginning to emerge, such as small cell transformation in lung and prostatic adenocarcinoma. Finally, there is a recognition that intratumoral and intertumoral heterogeneity exist and sampling from multiple sites has shown variable genotypic results. As the treatment armamentarium continues to advance, mechanisms for easy, repeated sampling of tumor are becoming more attractive. In the past 2 decades, the development of multiple different technologies has enabled recognizing that CTCs exist and may be able to fill this niche.

HISTORY AND OVERVIEW OF CIRCULATING TUMOR CELLS

CTCs are rare tumor cells found in the peripheral blood of patients with tumor. They were first described in 1869 by the Australian physician Dr Thomas Ashworth,[1] who at the time of autopsy noted the presence of tumor cells in a decedent's blood that were morphologically similar to the widely metastatic tumor that was the primary cause of death.

CTCs are intact cells containing a nucleus. Cytoplasmic fragments and circulating free nucleic acid are also components of the overarching term, "liquid biopsy", but are themselves insufficient to be CTCs.[2] The free nucleic acid represents dying tumor whereas CTCs represent intact tumor capable of seeding remote sites. CTCs are rare, comprising 1 in a million to 1 in a billion of the cells in the blood, even in patients with widely metastatic disease. The development of various highly sensitive technologies in the past few decades has allowed the reliable detection of these tumor cells by taking advantage of the biophysical and/or antigenic properties that distinguish them from the white blood cells and red blood cells that greatly outnumber them.[3] No single CTC system has been found to be universally superior. The CTCs captured (or missed) depend on the method used for enrichment. For example, filtration systems capture larger CTCs (but miss the smaller ones), and immunoaffinity systems that select for epithelial cell adhesion molecule (EpCAM)-positive cells capture EpCAM-positive carcinoma cells (but miss

melanoma or EpCAM-low or EpCAM-negative carcinoma cells).

The presence of CTCs is not limited to patients with metastatic disease and they have been found in patients with clinically localized (low-stage) disease, where their presence in increased numbers also portends poor prognosis.[4-8]

CTCs may not been found in all patients with metastatic disease; the reasons for this are likely multifactorial and interrelated.

- CTC systems vary with respect to sensitivity, specificity, and methods of capture and identification.[3] The Food and Drug Administration (FDA)-cleared CellSearch system (originally Immunicon/Veridex, currently Menarini Silicon Biosystems; Huntingdon Valley, Pennsylvania) is highly specific but does not show CTCs in all metastatic breast carcinoma patients when 7.5 mL of blood are evaluated.[9] Some highly sensitive methods, however, have found CTCs in almost all cancer patients, regardless of disease stage, when 2 mL of blood is evaluated, but also identify CTCs in healthy controls.[10]
- Cancer type may also affect the frequency of CTCs. Some cancers, such as small cell lung carcinoma, seem to yield high numbers of CTCs.[11,12]
- Most importantly, as discussed previously, the dynamic between tumor type and CTC technique used can have a significant effect on the number of CTCs identified. For example, CTCs from sarcoma patients are unlikely to be identified by CTC systems evaluating for surface EpCAM expression but can be readily identified by technology leveraging biophysical properties unique to CTCs.[13]
- Finally, differences in the underlying biology of patient cancers may be the most significant reason for variation in CTC count. This is exhibited in the prognostic significance of CTCs (discussed later). The mechanisms that underlie these differences are not yet understood but are of considerable interest.

Much of the focus has shifted from counting CTCs to isolating them. CTC isolation can provide a substrate for learning about the biology of metastasis and material to perform clinical predictive biomarker testing.

PROGNOSTIC SIGNIFICANCE OF CIRCULATING TUMOR CELLS—ENUMERATION

The CTC field began to blossom with the FDA clearance of CellSearch system. CellSearch is a highly specific antigen-based detection system that identifies EpCAM-positive and cytokeratin (CK) 8/18/19-positive CTCs. A study by Cristofanilli and colleagues[9] showed that patients with metastatic breast carcinoma and higher CTC counts had shorter overall survival and progression-free survival rates than metastatic breast cancer patients with lower CTC counts. This study set the threshold of a high CTC count as 5 or more CTCs per 7.5 mL of blood. Studies in patients with prostatic and colorectal adenocarcinoma showed similar results using the CellSearch system.[14,15] The CellSearch system continues to be the only FDA-cleared system.

Multiple other CTC systems using a variety of CTC detection methods have shown elevated CTC counts of prognostic significance in carcinoma from multiple different sites of origin (reviewed by Cabel and colleagues[16]). For example, the ISET system (Rarecells, Paris, France), which uses size-based filtration to capture CTCs that are greater than 8 μm in diameter, and the CTC-chip, which uses microfluidic enrichment coupled with antigenic capture, both show striking deceased overall survival in patients with high CTC counts. These CTC count thresholds are different and technology specific. The threshold for clinical significance in ISET in lung carcinoma was set at 50 CTCs/10 mL and the threshold for the CTC-chip in prostatic adenocarcinoma was set at 14 CTCs/mL.[17,18] CTC counts may vary with regard to different cancer types,[19] and therefore prognostic thresholds for clinical significance may be disease specific as well.

Data from the Southwestern Oncology Group S0500 trial further support that unfavorable CTC counts are prognostic in newly diagnosed metastatic breast cancer, across all breast cancer subtypes.[20] It also showed that switching cytotoxic chemotherapy regimens (clinician choice) in the context of a persistently elevated CTC count after 21 days of an initial therapy did not prolong overall survival.[20] This finding was disappointing to some investigators, but others thought it was not unexpected, because patients were switched from 1 pantoxic regimen to another without addressing the therapy-resistant clones that were evading the treatment regimens.[21] Although elevated CTC counts identify patient cohorts at risk for more aggressive disease, CTC profiling is needed to suggest effective treatment (discussed later).[21]

CTCs have prognostic significance even in clinically localized disease in breast cancer and lung cancer[4-8] and in the setting of neoadjuvant chemotherapy for clinically localized breast cancer where a decrease in CTC count post-treatment seems independent from pathologic complete response.[22]

The prognostic significance of CTC enumeration is clear but has not been incorporated into clinical practice guidelines.

PROGNOSTIC SIGNIFICANCE OF CIRCULATING TUMOR CELL CLUSTERS

Although the concentration of CTCs in the blood is of prognostic significance, the ability of CTCs to remain adherent to one another within the microcirculation appears to have greater significance. The presence of CTC clusters (groups of 2 or more cells) have a 50-fold or greater capacity to form metastases than single CTCs in cancer patients, and their presence, even in small numbers, is correlated with a significantly worse prognosis.[23,24] CTC clusters comprise a minority (<3%) of CTCs events.[23]

These clusters are capable of navigating through capillary-sized microfluidic chambers and zebrafish capillaries.[25] One study evaluating lung cancer patients undergoing surgery for clinically localized disease found an increased number of CTC clusters in pulmonary vein samplings compared with parallel samples drawn from the peripheral venous circulation (the standard site for obtaining CTC samples), suggesting many more are being shed than are identified in peripheral blood samples and that a majority of CTC clusters may be trapped in the microcirculation.[6] CTC clusters may be disrupted and dispersed into single cells over the course of CTC processing. The advent of CTC technology developed to specifically capture CTC clusters may allow them to be identified more reliably.[26] Studies to further evaluate the significance of CTC clusters are ongoing.[27]

PROGNOSTIC SIGNIFICANCE OF CIRCULATING TUMOR CELLS—CHARACTERIZATION

Prognostic significance in CTCs is not limited to enumeration of CTCs or CTC clusters. Many groups have characterized CTCs and found that the presence of certain CTCs phenotypes correlates with prognosis. So far, these findings have been limited to small cohorts, such as androgen receptor variant 7 (ARv7) in castrate resistant prostate cancer,[28] epithelial-to-mesenchymal transition–like CTCs in breast cancer,[29] and CTCs enriched for EGFR.[30] Although CTC characterization may be of prognostic significance, its greatest contribution likely will be with predictive testing.

EVALUATION OF PREDICTIVE BIOMARKERS VIA CIRCULATING TUMOR CELLS

CTC characterization also lends itself to real-time, minimally invasive, repeatable predictive biomarker testing, which may best represent the full diversity of a patient's metastatic tumor. Many of the markers that are evaluated daily in clinical practice on pathology or cytology specimens for clinical decision making have also been evaluated in CTCs. Characterization methods include surface antigen expression by antigenic capture or immunofluorescence; cytoplasmic, membranous, or nuclear expression by immunofluorescence (eg, ESR1[31] and ARv7[28]); immunocytochemistry (eg,Ki67[32]); and molecular methods to evaluate DNA somatic mutations (eg, EGFR T790M[33] and KRAS[34]) and RNA expression (eg, epithelial vs mesenchymal vs stem cell expression profiles monitored in patients undergoing therapy[35]). As research continues to explore CTC phenotypes, in mechanisms echoing those used currently to evaluate tissue biopsies/samples for predictive biomarkers, more such findings and correlation with clinical outcomes will be forthcoming. To be integrated into clinical testing, these protocols must be validated, and mechanisms to standardize and control for preanalytic[36] and analytic variables are needed.

TUMOR HETEROGENEITY MAY BE BETTER EVALUATED WITH CIRCULATING TUMOR CELLS

An increasing body of evidence supports the notion that cancer development is a heterogeneous process.[37] Most cancers are driven by genetic instability, which results in a constant evolution of tumor in response to the external pressures of treatment.[38] Tumor sampling by blood inherently allows more comprehensive sampling of the primary and metastatic sites that are shedding tumor cells.[39] Whole-exome sequencing performed on single CTCs and compared with known sequencing results from primary tumor and metastatic sites found CTCs to contain the expected driver and early trunk mutations seen in the primary tumor and metastases but also found additional mutations that were private to CTCs alone.[40] CTC testing may allow for more comprehensive characterization of tumors by testing that may be performed repeatedly over the course of treatment.

CIRCULATING TUMOR CELLS ISOLATION

Some techniques, such as CTC culture, require relative purity of CTCs. Such isolation may be achieved by single cell picking or bulk capture.

SINGLE CELL PICKING

Definitive sequencing of individual tumor cells is different from bulk processing of the nucleic acid present in a mixed sample.[41] Single cell sequencing allows evaluation of the co-occurrence of multiple DNA abnormalities within a cell. To achieve individual tumor cell sequencing, individual cells must be identified, isolated, and sequenced. Identification of tumor cells requires validated characterization, usually by exemplifying the target antigenic profile.[42] Specialized methods and bioinformatics approaches must be applied to achieve confident sequencing results.[43]

BULK CAPTURE

Bulk capture of CTCs can facilitate molecular interrogation of tumor cells because many molecular methods require a significant fraction of the sample to comprise target sequence to make a definitive call. CTC culture and drug sensitivity testing of tumor via CTCs currently require high purity of viable CTCs and large numbers of CTCs, which limit their widespread application.[31]

CIRCULATING TUMOR CELLS FOR EARLY SCREENING AND DIAGNOSIS

The presence of CTCs in early-stage cancer raises the possibility of early tumor diagnosis via blood sampling, ideally before a radiographically/clinically identifiable lesion is discovered. One small study prospectively evaluating COPD patients without cancer found that all the CTC-positive patients developed lung carcinoma within 4 years of their positive CTC screening test.[44] A larger study to confirm these findings is ongoing. Perhaps a combination of imaging and CTC testing will be the most fruitful in evaluating at-risk populations.[45,46] Another small study validated the use of a panel of immunofluorescent markers to determine the site of origin (lung vs prostate vs colorectal) of CTCs from patients with known carcinoma.[47] The suggestion of a site of origin of CTCs may assist in targeted screening of healthy or at-risk populations. Thorough evaluation of the accuracy of CTC screening must be achieved before clinical application can be considered.

INTEGRATION OF CIRCULATING TUMOR CELLS IN CYTOLOGY PRACTICE

PERFORMING CIRCULATING TUMOR CELLS TESTING IN CYTOLOGY LABORATORIES

CTC testing is broad and encompasses enumeration, characterization, and isolation. Enumeration and characterization are best deployed in the cytology environment due to the requirement of a morphologic assessment.

CTC identification for enumeration testing is the simplest form of CTC testing, but in my opinion is more nuanced than much of the high complexity testing that is performed in the clinical laboratories because of the element of morphologic interpretation. Although generally described as CK-positive, DAPI-positive, and CD45-negative, the definition of a CTC extends beyond those basic immunophenotypic requirements. In addition to this staining pattern, CTCs by the FDA-cleared CellSearch criteria must show cell-like morphology.[48] Guidance is also given for the allowable intensity of CK positivity, DAPI nuclear staining, and CD45 negativity, because none of these is binary.[48] Each of these criteria requires morphologic interpretation (**Fig. 1**). Although training and proficiency testing exist for CellSearch CTC enumeration, equivocal candidate CTC events exist. Much of the practice of enumeration mirrors performed the work daily by cytotechnologists and cytopathologists.

CTC characterization, which includes choosing which markers to evaluate in clinical context and which tumor cells should be scored as positive, adds additional layers of complexity. These tasks are part of the routine work performed in the cytopathology laboratory on cytology specimens and can easily be integrated into clinical practice.

CTC isolation in bulk form for CTC culture would not require a morphologic component, but single cell picking would require similar expertise to other CTC testing and would often be the next step in patient sample evaluation. Overall, establishment of the CTC clinical testing within cytology is most logical.

USING CIRCULATING TUMOR CELLS TECHNOLOGY TO FACILITATE CYTOLOGY DIAGNOSIS

Beyond performing CTC testing in the cytology environment, many common situations in cytology and general surgical pathology could benefit from integrating rare cell technology into daily practice. All CTC systems are designed to evaluate liquid samples. Although designed to evaluate blood, some protocols may be modified to evaluate nonblood liquid samples. Additionally, although most systems use unique chambers or microfluidic devices to visualize the specimen, some use routine glass slides for CTC evaluation. The glass slide–based systems may be able to analyze standard cytology or pathology slides for evaluation of rare cells.

Applications include

- Rare tumor cells in non-blood liquid cytology specimens (eg, cerebrospinal fluid, effusions, and fine-needle aspiration biopsies) processed by CTC technology
- Evaluation of rare tumor cells on cytology slides or histology slides (cell block or surgical pathology material)
- Multiparameter characterization of cells of interest on cytology or surgical pathology slides

Published reports for assessing nonblood liquid specimens by CTC testing methods have been limited to evaluating cerebrospinal fluid for metastatic tumor. In this setting, CTC technology has been shown a robust mechanism for identifying leptomeningeal metastasis.[49]

CTC technologies that process standard slides hold promise for being able to further evaluate rare atypical cells of uncertain etiology on specimens that have been stained and evaluated morphologically. Often these atypical cells are not present on other slides or deeper levels of the block. Modification of the multiparameter immunophenotyping performed by CTC systems could help confirm rare lesional cells (all CTC technologies evaluate at least 3 colors; 4 to 6 colors are becoming more common). This would be a significant advantage over the current practice of immunocytochemistry/immunohistochemistry performed routinely (usually 1 to 2 antigens).

In this era of precision medicine and personalized therapeutics, evaluating tumors for 1 or more relevant biomarkers is common. Turnaround time and conservation of tissue are paramount issues. Evaluating multiple markers concurrently, especially in the context of mutually exclusive biomarkers (eg, performing separate immunohistochemistry for ALK and ROS-1 while initiating EGFR molecular in lung cancer) saves time, but results in using more sample via multiparameter immunophenotyping, CTC technologies can perform multiple antigenic assessments on a single slide, providing rapid results using only limited sample. Tumor-specific panels could easily be established and used in all subspecialties of pathology.

CTC testing and CTC technologies have shown prognostic and predictive value and hold great promise for becoming a standard to evaluate blood and non-blood specimens. Although largely confined to the research space currently, incorporation of CTCs into clinical practice will be part of the future of cytology.

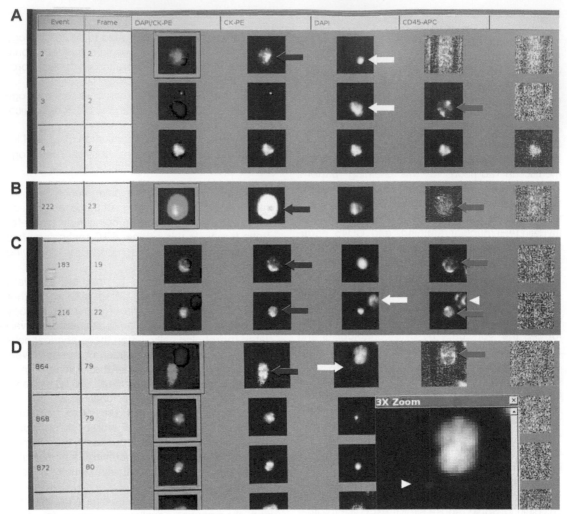

Fig. 1. Circulating tumor cell morphologic evaluation utilizing CellSearch criteria. (*A*) Typical CellSearch enumeration analysis screen. Each row represents a unique candidate CTC event evaluated by the CK, DAPI, and CD45 immunofluorescent filters, which are represented separately by the indicated column headers. The "DAPI/CK" column shows the CK (*colored green*) and DAPI (*colored pink*) windows superimposed upon each other. In this panel, the first row ("Event 2") shows a typical CTC with cytokeratin staining in the "CK" window (*red arrow*) with a superimposed smaller nucleus in the "DAPI" window (*white arrow*) and lack of CD45 staining in the "CD45" window. The second row ("Event 3") shows a white blood cell (WBC) which shows cytoplasmic CD45 staining (*blue arrow*) with a corresponding nucleus (*white arrow*). The third row ("Event 4") shows autofluorescent non-cellular material which shows a similar morphology in all columns, including the right most column, which represents the "open channel". This is not scored as a CTC. (*B*) Event 222 shows a typical CTC. Although signal is seen in the CD45 channel (*white arrow*), this is weak in comparison to the very strong corresponding CK signal (*red arrow*) and therefore is interpreted as representing spectral overlap. (*C*) Events 183 and 216 shows cells that should not be scored as CTCs. The CD45 signal (*blue arrows*) is too strong to represent spectral overlap from the relatively weak the CK (*red arrows*) and therefore is interpreted as true CD45 staining which excludes the cell from representing a CTC. A separate WBC is also present in Event 216 (*white arrow* and arrowhead highlight the nucleus and corresponding CD45-positive cytoplasm, respectively). (*D*) Event 864 shows a CTC (*red arrow*) with a very weak nucleus (*white arrow*), which is difficult to see on original magnification, but more conspicuous at higher magnification (*white arrowhead* of inset image). A WBC is also present (*blue arrow*).

REFERENCES

1. Ashworth T. A case of cancer in which cells similar to those in the tumours were seen in the blood after death. Aust Med J 1869;14:146–9.

2. Alix-Panabières C, Pantel K. Clinical applications of circulating tumor cells and circulating tumor DNA as liquid biopsy. Cancer Discov 2016;6(5):479–91.

3. Ferreira MM, Ramani VC, Jeffrey SS. Circulating tumor cell technologies. Mol Oncol 2016;10(3): 374–94.

4. Lucci A, Hall CS, Lodhi AK, et al. Circulating tumour cells in non-metastatic breast cancer: a prospective study. Lancet Oncol 2012;13(7):688–95.

5. Rack B, Schindlbeck C, Jückstock J, et al. Circulating tumor cells predict survival in early average-to-high risk breast cancer patients. J Natl Cancer Inst 2014;106(5), [pii:dju066].

6. Murlidhar V, Reddy RM, Fouladdel S, et al. Poor prognosis indicated by venous circulating tumor cell clusters in early-stage lung cancers. Cancer Res 2017;77(18):5194–206.

7. Dandachi N, Tiran V, Lindenmann J, et al. Frequency and clinical impact of preoperative circulating tumor cells in resectable non-metastatic lung adenocarcinomas. Lung Cancer 2017;113:152–7.

8. Janni WJ, Rack B, Terstappen LWMM, et al. Pooled analysis of the prognostic relevance of circulating tumor cells in primary breast cancer. Clin Cancer Res 2016;22(10):2583–93.

9. Cristofanilli M, Budd GT, Ellis MJ, et al. Circulating tumor cells, disease progression, and survival in metastatic breast cancer. N Engl J Med 2004; 351(8):781–91.

10. Chen JY, Tsai WS, Shao HJ, et al. Sensitive and specific biomimetic lipid coated microfluidics to isolate viable circulating tumor cells and microemboli for cancer detection. PLoS One 2016;11(3): 1–21.

11. Allard WJ, Matera J, Miller MC, et al. Tumor cells circulate in the peripheral blood of all major carcinomas but not in healthy subjects or patients with nonmalignant diseases tumor cells circulate in the peripheral blood of all major carcinomas but not in healthy subjects or patients with non. Clin Cancer Res 2005;10:6897–904.

12. Foy V, Fernandez-Gutierrez F, Faivre-Finn C, et al. The clinical utility of circulating tumour cells in patients with small cell lung cancer. Transl Lung Cancer Res 2017;6(4):409–17.

13. Balasubramanian P, Kinders RJ, Kummar S, et al. Antibody-independent capture of circulating tumor cells of non-epithelial origin with the ApoStream® system. PLoS One 2017;12(4):e0175414.

14. De Bono JS, Scher HI, Montgomery RB, et al. Circulating tumor cells predict survival benefit from treatment in metastatic castration-resistant prostate cancer. Clin Cancer Res 2008;14(19):6302–9.

15. Cohen SJ, Punt CJA, Iannotti N, et al. Relationship of circulating tumor cells to tumor response, progression-free survival, and overall survival in patients with metastatic colorectal cancer. J Clin Oncol 2008;26(19):3213–21.

16. Cabel L, Proudhon C, Mariani P, et al. Circulating tumor cells and circulating tumor DNA: what surgical oncologists need to know? Eur J Surg Oncol 2017; 43(5):949–62.

17. Hofman V, Bonnetaud C, Ilie MI, et al. Preoperative circulating tumor cell detection using the isolation by size of epithelial tumor cell method for patients with lung cancer is a new prognostic biomarker. Clin Cancer Res 2011;17(4):827–35.

18. Stott SL, Hsu C-H, Tsukrov DI, et al. Isolation of circulating tumor cells using a microvortex-generating herringbone-chip. Proc Natl Acad Sci U S A 2010;107(43):18392–7. Available at: www. pnas.org/cgi/doi/10.1073/pnas.1012539107.

19. Krebs MG, Hou J-M, Ward TH, et al. Circulating tumour cells: their utility in cancer management and predicting outcomes. Ther Adv Med Oncol 2010;2(6):351–65.

20. Smerage JB, Barlow WE, Hortobagyi GN, et al. Circulating tumor cells and response to chemotherapy in metastatic breast cancer: SWOG S0500. J Clin Oncol 2014;32(31):3483–9.

21. Cruz MR, Costa R, Cristofanilli M. The truth is in the blood: the evolution of liquid biopsies in breast cancer management. 2017. Available at: https://am. asco.org/truth-blood-evolution-liquid-biopsies-breast-cancer-management. Accessed January 19, 2018.

22. Fei F, Du Y, Di G, et al. Are changes in circulating tumor cell (CTC) count associated with the response to neoadjuvant chemotherapy in local advanced breast cancer? A meta-analysis. Oncol Res Treat 2014;37(5):250–4.

23. Aceto N, Bardia A, Miyamoto DT, et al. Circulating tumor cell clusters are oligoclonal precursors of breast cancer metastasis. Cell 2014;158(5): 1110–22.

24. Cheung KJ, Padmanaban V, Silvestri V, et al. Polyclonal breast cancer metastases arise from collective dissemination of keratin 14-expressing tumor cell clusters. Proc Natl Acad Sci 2016;113(7):E854–63.

25. Au SH, Storey BD, Moore JC, et al. Clusters of circulating tumor cells traverse capillary-sized vessels. Proc Natl Acad Sci 2016;113(18):4947–52.

26. Au SH, Edd J, Haber DA, et al. Clusters of circulating tumor cells: a biophysical and technological perspective. Curr Opin Biomed Eng 2017;3:13–9.

27. Hong Y, Fang F, Zhang Q. Circulating tumor cell clusters: what we know and what we expect (Review). Int J Oncol 2016;49(6):2206–16.

28. Scher HI, Lu D, Schreiber NA, et al. Association of AR-V7 on circulating tumor cells as a treatment-specific biomarker with outcomes and survival in castration-resistant prostate cancer. JAMA Oncol 2016;2(11):1441–9.

29. Bulfoni M, Gerratana L, Del Ben F, et al. In patients with metastatic breast cancer the identification of circulating tumor cells in epithelial-to-mesenchymal transition is associated with a poor prognosis. Breast Cancer Res 2016;18(1):1–15.

30. Vila A, Abal M, Muinelo-Romay L, et al. EGFR-based immunoisolation as a recovery target for low-EpCAM CTC subpopulation. PLoS One 2016; 11(10):1–20.

31. Yu M, Bardia A, Aceto N, et al. Ex vivo culture of circulating breast tumor cells for individualized testing of drug susceptibility. Science 2014; 345(6193):216–20.

32. Lowe AC, Pignon JC, Carvo I, et al. Young investigator challenge: application of cytologic techniques to circulating tumor cell specimens: Detecting activation of the oncogenic transcription factor STAT3. Cancer Cytopathol 2015;123(12): 696–706.

33. Sundaresan TK, Sequist LV, Heymach JV, et al. Detection of T790M, the acquired resistance EGFR mutation, by tumor biopsy versus noninvasive blood-based analyses. Clin Cancer Res 2016;22(5): 1103–10.

34. Kondo Y, Hayashi K, Kawakami K, et al. KRAS mutation analysis of single circulating tumor cells from patients with metastatic colorectal cancer. BMC Cancer 2017;17(1):1–10.

35. Markou A, Lazaridou M, Paraskevopoulos P, et al. Multiplex gene expression profiling of in vivo isolated circulating tumor cells in high-risk prostate cancer patients. Clin Chem 2017; 64(2):297–306.

36. Rodríguez-Lee M, Kolatkar A, McCormick M, et al. Effect of blood collection tube type and time to processing on the enumeration and high-content characterization of circulating tumor cells using the high-definition single-cell assay. Arch Pathol Lab Med 2017;137(9):1255–61.

37. McGranahan N, Favero F, De Bruin EC, et al. Clonal status of actionable driver events and the timing of mutational processes in cancer evolution. Sci Transl Med 2015;7(283):1–12.

38. Merlo LMF, Pepper JW, Reid BJ, et al. Cancer as an evolutionary and ecological process. Nat Rev Cancer 2006;6(12):924–35.

39. Zhang C, Guan Y, Sun Y, et al. Tumor heterogeneity and circulating tumor cells. Cancer Lett 2016; 374(2):216–23.

40. Lohr JG, Adalsteinsson VA, Cibulskis K, et al. Whole exome sequencing of circulating tumor cells provides a window into metastatic prostate cancer. Nat Biotechnol 2014;32(5):479–84.

41. Zong C, Lu S, Chapman AR, et al. Genome-wide detection of single-nucleotide and copy-number variations of a single human cell. Science 2012; 338(6114):1622–6.

42. Stilwell JL, et al. RareCyte® CTC analysis step 3: using the CytePicker® module for individual cell retrieval and subsequent whole genome amplification of circulating tumor cells for genomic analysis. In: Magbanua M, Park JW, Varshavskaya P, editors. Circulating tumor cells. Methods in molecular biology, vol. 1634. New York: Humana Press; 2017. p. 181–92.

43. De Bourcy CFA, De Vlaminck I, Kanbar JN, et al. A quantitative comparison of single-cell whole genome amplification methods. PLoS One 2014; 9(8):e105585.

44. Ilie M, Hofman V, Long-Mira E, et al. "Sentinel" circulating tumor cells allow early diagnosis of lung cancer in patients with Chronic obstructive pulmonary disease. PLoS One 2014;9(10):4–10.

45. He Y, Shi J, Shi G, et al. Using the new CellCollector to capture circulating tumor cells from blood in different groups of pulmonary disease: a cohort study. Sci Rep 2017;7(1):9542.

46. Murray NP, Miranda R, Ruiz A, et al. Diagnostic yield of primary circulating tumor cells in women suspected of breast cancer: the BEST (Breast Early Screening Test) study. Asian Pac J Cancer Prev 2015;16(5):1929–34.

47. Lu SH, Tsai WS, Chang YH, et al. Identifying cancer origin using circulating tumor cells. Cancer Biol Ther 2016;17(4):430–8.

48. Veridex, LLC. CellTracks analyzer II: user guide. Cell interpretation guidelines. Raritan (NJ): Veridex, LLC; 2013. p. 47–52.

49. Lin X, Fleisher M, Rosenblum M, et al. Cerebrospinal fluid circulating tumor cells: a novel tool to diagnose leptomeningeal metastases from epithelial tumors. Neuro Oncol 2017;19(9):1248–54.